Causes, Prevention and Management of Liver Disorders

Causes, Prevention and Management of Liver Disorders

Editor: Daisy Truman

FOSTER ACADEMICS
www.fosteracademics.com

www.fosteracademics.com

FOSTER ACADEMICS

Cataloging-in-Publication Data

Causes, prevention and management of liver disorders / edited by Daisy Truman.
p. cm.
Includes bibliographical references and index.
ISBN 978-1-63242-684-0
1. Liver--Diseases. 2. Liver--Diseases--Etiology. 3. Liver--Diseases--Prevention.
4. Liver--Diseases--Treatment. I. Truman, Daisy.
RC845 .C38 2019
616.362--dc23

Foster Academics,
118-35 Queens Blvd., Suite 400,
Forest Hills, NY 11375, USA

ISBN 978-1-63242-684-0 (Hardback)

Printed and bound in China.

Contents

Preface

Liver disorders are the conditions of the liver that cause damage to the liver or inhibit normal functioning. Such disorders can be inherited (genetic) or caused due to viral infections, alcohol use and even obesity. Infections with hepatitis virus A, B, C, D and E cause hepatitis which is a severe condition. Some of these may be transmitted sexually. Immune system abnormalities often lead to autoimmune liver diseases such as primary sclerosing cholangitis, primary biliary cirrhosis, autoimmune hepatitis, etc. Some genetic liver diseases are alpha-1 antitrypsin deficiency, hemochromatosis and Wilson's disease, besides many others. Primary liver cancer often manifests as cholangiocarcinoma or hepatocellular carcinoma. Sometimes, primary cancers of the gastrointestinal tract can metastasize and cause secondary lesions or liver malignancies. Liver diseases can be prevented by drinking alcohol in moderation, getting vaccinations, maintaining a healthy weight, avoiding risky behavior pertaining to drug use, sex, etc. Medical and surgical procedures may be used for the management and treatment of the conditions of the liver. Much research on the possibility of using stem cells for the generation of an artificial liver is also being done. This book unravels the recent studies in liver disorders. Also included in this book is a detailed explanation of the various causes of liver disorders and their prevention and management strategies. It is a resource guide for experts as well as students.

After months of intensive research and writing, this book is the end result of all who devoted their time and efforts in the initiation and progress of this book. It will surely be a source of reference in enhancing the required knowledge of the new developments in the area. During the course of developing this book, certain measures such as accuracy, authenticity and research focused analytical studies were given preference in order to produce a comprehensive book in the area of study.

This book would not have been possible without the efforts of the authors and the publisher. I extend my sincere thanks to them. Secondly, I express my gratitude to my family and well-wishers. And most importantly, I thank my students for constantly expressing their willingness and curiosity in enhancing their knowledge in the field, which encourages me to take up further research projects for the advancement of the area.

Editor

1

A new paradigm evaluating cost per cure of HCV infection

Stephen T. Barclay[1], Graham S. Cooke[2], Elizabeth Holtham[3], Aline Gauthier[4], Jeremie Schwarzbard[4], Petar Atanasov[4], William L. Irving[3,5*] and On behalf of HCV Research UK

Abstract

Background: New interferon (IFN)-free treatments for hepatitis C are more effective, safer but more expensive than current IFN-based therapies. Comparative data of these, versus current first generation protease inhibitors (PI) with regard to costs and treatment outcomes are needed. We investigated the real-world effectiveness, safety and cost per cure of 1st generation PI-based therapies in the UK.

Methods: Medical records review of patients within the HCV Research UK database. Patients had received treatment with telaprevir or boceprevir and pegylated interferon and ribavirin (PR). Data on treatment outcome, healthcare utilisation and adverse events (AEs) requiring intervention were collected and analysed overall and by subgroups. Costs of visits, tests, therapies, adverse events and hospitalisations were estimated at the patient level. Total cost per cure was calculated as total median cost divided by SVR rate.

Results: 154 patients from 35 centres were analysed. Overall median total cost per cure was £44,852 (subgroup range,: £35,492 to £107,288). Total treatment costs were accounted for by PI: 68.3 %, PR: 26.3 %, AE management: 5.4 %. Overall SVR was 62.3 % (range 25 % to 86.2 %). 36 % of patients experienced treatment-related AEs requiring intervention, 10 % required treatment-related hospitalisation.

Conclusions: This is the first UK multicentre study of outcomes and costs of PI-based HCV treatments in clinical practice. There was substantial variation in total cost per cure among patient subgroups and high rates of treatment-related discontinuations, AEs and hospitalisations. Real world safety, effectiveness and total cost per cure for the new IFN free combinations should be compared against this baseline.

Keywords: Hepatitis C, Protease inhibitors, Cost, SVR

Background

Hepatitis C virus (HCV) infection remains a global public health issue with most recent estimates suggesting that more than 180 million people have been infected worldwide [1]. The combination of peginterferon alfa (IFN), ribavirin (RBV) and one of the first generation protease inhibitors (PI), boceprevir (BOC) or telaprevir (TVR) was the standard care for genotype 1 HCV up to 2014 [2, 3].

IFN based HCV treatment is able to cure HCV (as defined by sustained virological response, SVR) [2] which is associated with improved clinical outcomes [4–6]. However, common adverse events (AEs) associated with traditional 1st generation PI-based therapies include skin rashes, pruritus, anaemia, neutropaenia, nausea and dysgeusia [7]. In addition, treatment with IFN may cause psychiatric adverse events such as depression [8]. Evidence suggests that treatment-related AEs have a negative impact on health-related quality of life (HRQoL) leading to higher rates of premature discontinuation and lower SVR rates than reported from clinical trials [9, 10]. Evidence from clinical trials suggests that in treatment naïve genotype 1 patients, triple therapy of PR + 1st generation PIs results in SVR rates of between 65–75 % [11–14] however, lower effectiveness has been reported in real-world studies (44–55 %) [15–18].

* Correspondence: will.irving@nottingham.ac.uk
[3]NIHR Nottingham Digestive Diseases Biomedical Research Unit, University of Nottingham, Nottingham, UK
[5]Microbiology, Queen's Medical Centre, Nottingham NG7 2UH, UK
Full list of author information is available at the end of the article

The treatment landscape of HCV is changing rapidly with the emergence of novel highly effective all oral combination therapies active against genotype 1 [2]. With better efficacy, improved safety and substantially shortened treatment durations, these IFN – and RBV-free treatments are expected to become the cornerstone of HCV therapy, [19–23]; these advances represent a major treatment improvement for patients. However, current pricing, combined with the likely increased patient demand, means these regimens pose a significant budgetary impact in developed healthcare systems [24]. Recently, the concept of "cost per SVR" has evolved to take account of opportunity costs (i.e. the loss of potential gain from other alternatives when one alternative is chosen) in HCV management. More data is required to understand the total cost per SVR of existing IFN-based therapies to allow meaningful comparison with newer interferon free regimens.

To date there have been no published real-world studies assessing the cost per cure, safety and effectiveness of PR + 1st generation PI triple therapy in the UK. This study aimed to estimate the total cost per HCV patient cured associated with first generation PI-based therapy in a real world setting, across a large number of centres. As secondary objectives, this study also aimed at estimating the effectiveness, safety and tolerability of these regimens.

Methods

Study design and patients

This was a retrospective observational multi-centre study of patients enrolled in the HCV Research UK biobank, who received a first generation PI-based regimen between July 2012 and July 2014 through National Health Service (NHS) hospitals following recommendation by the National Institute for Health and Care Excellence (NICE) [25, 26] and the Scottish Medicines Consortium. HCV Research UK is a cohort of 10,000 patients, plus database and biorepository, enrolled with informed consent from 59 centres across England, Scotland and Wales [27]. Patients within HCV Research UK were considered eligible for this analysis if they were 18 years of age or older, had HCV genotype 1 infection and had received either TVR or BOC in association with PEG + RBV with a known treatment outcome. Patients were randomly selected for this study from all eligible patients using a number generator. A TVR: BOC sample ratio of 2:1 was chosen to reflect use in clinical practice among the HCV Research UK cohort.

Data collection

Baseline data available from within the HCV Research UK database were supplemented by a detailed clinic case note review. Data collected included patient characteristics at initiation of the PI-based treatment (age, gender, ethnicity, liver disease status, genotype, blood test results, comorbidities recorded in the HCV Research UK database relating to renal failure, diabetes, HIV co-infection, depression, haemophilia and cancer (other than HCC)), previous HCV therapy (type of treatment and associated response), details regarding the PI-based therapy, treatment outcome, safety and healthcare resource use (nurse and physician visits, tests and investigations, medications used to treat AEs, and hospitalisations). Details on comorbidities at baseline were gathered through a review of the patient's clinical notes as well as patient questionnaire. IL28B genotyping at locus rs12979860 was performed (by Micropathology Ltd, Coventry, UK) post-hoc using a Roche Hybprobe kit and meltcurve analysis.

Assessment of outcomes

The outcomes of interest included SVR, which was assessed at 12 or 24 weeks. The incidence and type of adverse events (AEs) requiring therapeutic intervention, healthcare resource use, treatment discontinuation and/or hospitalisation was collected by the study centre through a standardised questionnaire and quality controlled by a study coordinator. The relationship of HCV therapy to each AE was assessed independently by two physicians (STB, GSC), and categorised as "likely", "unlikely" or "can't tell". Any discrepancy between assessments was resolved by discussion. In total, there were 12 discrepancies after the initial individual assessments, all of which were agreed on after discussion with no further action needed.

Costs were estimated from the NHS perspective. The unit costs to be applied were derived from the British National Formulary for drugs [28]. The cost of managing HCV was estimated by applying the national unit costs to the number of physician and nurse visits, medications and tests [29]. The cost of hospitalisations was estimated based on Health Resource Group (HRG) codes classifying the reasons for hospitalisation and procedures undertaken during the stay [30]. Corresponding unit costs were obtained from the NHS reference costs [31]. Total costs were estimated and cost per cure was calculated as total median cost divided by SVR rate. For the conversion of UK pound (£) to US dollar ($), the Bank of England exchange rate was applied (£1 = $1.4905) [32].

Statistical analysis

Sample size was not formally assessed and the number of patients enrolled was based on time and resource constraints. Descriptive statistics were analysed according to treatment status (naïve vs experienced) and liver disease status (cirrhosis vs no cirrhosis) at baseline. The proportion of patients achieving SVR was determined overall, by treatment (BOC vs TVR) and by liver disease status. The calculation of SVR took into account all patients, including those who discontinued therapy prematurely. The statistical significance was tested for each comparison using a Chi-square test.

Logistic regression was conducted to assess the impact of patient characteristics on the probability of reaching SVR. The list of covariates was specified a priori and included age, liver disease status, gender, treatment naïve vs experienced, HIV co-infection, IL28B subtypes, history of depression, diabetes, genotype and race. A stepwise procedure was run to identify the most significant covariates.

The incidence of AEs and of AEs assessed as "likely" to be related to HCV treatment was estimated overall and by type of AE. The incidence of AEs leading to treatment discontinuation and/or to hospitalisation was also estimated.

To identify factors which have an impact on the probability of experiencing an AE, a logistic regression was conducted. The list of covariates included age, gender, treatment regimen, past treatment history, liver disease status, HIV status, history of depression and diabetes.

Sensitivity analyses were performed to assess the impact of PI drug price discounts of 30 %, 40 % and 50 % and the impact of including management costs of 'can't tell' AEs on the total cost per cure.

Results

Baseline characteristics

From the initial 160 patients selected for this study from the HCV Research UK database, 8 patients did not in fact start TVR/BOC therapy, 3 patients were switched from one PI to the other, 1 patient had a genotype 3 infection, and for 5 patients, the clinics concerned notified us that they would not be able to retrieve and return the data within our specified timeframe, resulting in a total of 17 patients being excluded. An additional 11 patients were randomly selected, resulting in a total of 154 patients entered into this study derived from 35 centres.

Table 1 shows the baseline characteristics of all patients enrolled in this study. Of all patients, 63/154 (40.9 %) had at least one comorbidity and 8/154 (5.2 %) had at least two. The most common comorbidities at baseline were reported history of depression (40/154, 26 %), HIV co-infection (10/154, 6.5 %), diabetes (8/154, 5.2 %), haemophilia (8/154, 5.2 %), cancer (6/154, 3.9 %) and renal failure (1/154, 0.7 %). Over half the patients were treatment experienced (80/154, 52 %), the majority having been treated with PEG + RBV (62/80, 77.5 %). The nature of the previous treatment regimen was not available for the other 18 patients. Among treatment-experienced patients, 35/80 (43.7 %) were relapsers and 36/80 (45.0 %) were non-responders. This information was not available for 9 patients.

Table 1 Baseline characteristics for total cohort

	All patients ($n = 154$)
Age [Mean, (SD)]	49.6 (9.01)
Gender	
Male [%]	73.4 %
Female [%]	26.6 %
Ethnicity	
White [%]	94.2 %
Liver disease (Metavir stage)	
Non-cirrhotic (F0-F3) [%]	78.6 %
Cirrhotic (F4 including 1 HCC) [%]	21.4 %
Treatment history	
Experienced [%]	52.0 %
Naïve [%]	48.0 %
Response to previous therapy	
Relapse [%]	43.7 %
No response [%]	45.0 %
Missing [%]	11.3 %
HCV genotype	
Genotype 1a [%]	51.3 %
Genotype 1b [%]	18.8 %
G1 subtype Missing [%]	29.9 %
HCV therapy	
Telaprevir treatment [%]	69.1 %
Boceprevir treatment [%]	33.1 %
IL28B status (SNP rs12979860)	
Heterozygous CT [%]	56.9 %
Homozygous CC [%]	29.4 %
Homozygous TT [%]	13.7 %
Missing [%]	0.7 %
Comorbidities	
Depression [%]	26.0 %
HIV co-infection [%]	6.5 %
Diabetes [%]	5.2 %
Haemophilia [%]	5.2 %
Cancer [%]	3.9 %
Renal failure [%]	0.7 %

More treatment-experienced patients had cirrhosis compared to treatment-naïve (24/80 (30.0 %) vs 9/74 (12.2 %); $p = 0.007$). Patients with cirrhosis were significantly older than those with milder liver disease (stages F0 – F3) (55.6 years (SD: 7.16) vs 48.1 years (SD: 8.9); $p < 0.0001$).

Effectiveness results

Overall 96/154 (62.3 %) patients achieved SVR. SVR rate in patients treated with BOC was 63.1 % (65/103) and

60.8 % (31/51) in patients treated with TVR ($p = 0.89$). The SVR rate among patients who were treatment-naïve was 51/74 (68.9 %) compared to 12/36 prior non- responders (33.3 %; $p = 0.004$, Table 2). Patients with cirrhosis showed consistently lower SVR compared to those with milder liver disease regardless of previous treatment status. The logistic regression found age, cirrhotic status and IL28b genotype to be significant predictors of SVR (Table 3). Patients with cirrhosis were almost 3 times less likely to achieve SVR compared to those with milder liver disease (F0 – F3) (OR = 0.35; 95 %CI: 0.13, 0.94). Patients with a CC genotype of IL28b were around 9 times more likely to achieve SVR than those with non-CC genotype (OR = 0.116; 95 %CI: 0.037, 0.365).

Safety analysis

Over the study period 70/154 (45 %) of the study population experienced at least one AE requiring intervention. The total number of AEs requiring intervention was 178 (see Additional file 1 for details). 141/178 (79.2 %) of these were assessed as "likely" to be related to treatment. Twenty-two of the 178 (12.4 %) AEs requiring intervention were due to anaemia. This was managed by ribavirin dose reduction (16/22, 72.7 %), treatment with erythropoietin analogues (6/22, 27.3 %) and/or blood transfusion (15/22, 68.2 %). All the patients who required intervention for neutropaenia, ($n = 6$) were treated with GCSF, and the single case of thrombocytopenia ($n = 1$) was managed with a dose reduction.

Fifty-five out of 154 (33 %) patients stopped therapy prematurely – of those 17/55 (30.9 %) because of adverse events, 24/55 (43.6 %) patients failed stopping rules, 12/55 (21.8) patients withdrew themselves from therapy, and for 2/55 (3.6 %) patients the physician withdrew therapy. There were 36 hospitalisations amongst 29 patients and, of those, 16 (44.4 %) hospitalisations were classified as "likely" to be treatment related, comprising of 15 hospitalisations due to anaemia (all were associated with blood transfusion) and 1 due to severe headache (see Supplementary material).

Using logistic regression, liver disease status, treatment regimen, gender and past treatment experience were statistically significant predictors of the incidence of any AE (see Supporting material). Cirrhotic patients had a 3-fold increased risk of experiencing an AE compared with patients with no cirrhosis ($p = 0.0206$). Patients on TVR were twice as likely to experience an AE compared to patients on BOC ($p = 0.0445$). Females had approximately a 2-fold increased risk of AEs compared to males ($p = 0.0384$) as did treatment-naïve patients compared to experienced patients ($p = 0.0476$).

Economic assessment

The overall median total cost per HCV cure was £44,852 ($66,852). Median cost per HCV cure varied according to prior treatment status: £83,948 ($125,125) for previous non-responders, £39,150 ($58,353) for prior relapsers and £37,958 ($56,576) for treatment naïve patients (Table 4).

Patients with cirrhosis consistently showed higher costs per cure compared to those with milder liver disease across subgroups - £61,496 ($91,660) vs £35,492 ($52,900) in treatment naïve patients; £49,016 ($73,058) vs £37,455 ($55,827) in prior relapsers; £107,288 ($159,913) vs £73,098 ($108,953) in non-responders.

Using NHS list prices for the base case analysis total direct cost associated with the management of the 154 HCV patients was estimated to be £4,289,909 ($6,394,109). The total drug costs for the 154 patients associated with PI therapies accounted for 68.3 % of total cost (£2,930,769; $4,368,311), PEG accounted for 19.5 % (£834,485; $1,243,800) and RBV, 6.8 % (£290,975; $433,698) (Table 5). In the base case analysis, 'other' costs accounted for 5.4 % of total costs (£233,780; $348,449), comprising of consultant/nurses visits (59.9 %; £139,992); tests (22.5 %; £52,616); medications for adverse events (including blood transfusions) (7.4 %; £17,233); other investigations (6.3 %; £14,576) and hospitalisations (3.9 %; £9,209) (Table 5). Management of depression accounted for a small fraction of these costs.

All but 1 (13/14) patient experiencing a 'likely' treatment-related hospitalisation had a single hospital

Table 2 SVR rate by regimen, cirrhosis status and prior treatment history

Total ($n = 145$[a])	Treatment-naïve patients ($n = 74$)	Prior relapsers ($n = 35$)	Prior non-responders ($n = 36$)
SVR rate	68.9 % [57.1;79.2]	82.9 % [66.4;93.4]	33.3 % [18.6;51.0]
By regimen			
BOC triple therapy ($n = 48$)	66.7 % [47.2;82.7] ($n = 30$)	75.0 % [34.9;96.8] ($n = 8$)	30.0 % [6.7;65.2] ($n = 10$)
TVR triple therapy ($n = 97$)	70.4 % [54.8;83.2] ($n = 44$)	85.2 % [66.3;95.8] ($n = 27$)	34.6 % [17.2;55.7] ($n = 26$)
By liver disease stage			
No-cirrhosis (n = 114)	73.8 % [61.5;84.0] ($n = 65$)	86.2 % [68.3;96.1] ($n = 29$)	40.0 % [19.1;64.0] ($n = 20$)
Cirrhosis or HCC ($n = 31$)	33.3 % [7.5;70.1] ($n = 9$)	66.7 % [22.3;95.7] ($n = 6$)	25.0 % [7.3;52.4] ($n = 16$)

[a] Previous treatment outcome status was not available for 9 patients

Table 3 Logistic regression: Probability of achieving SVR

Parameter	OR	95 % Wald Confidence Limits		Standard Error	*P* value
Age	0.94	0.90	0.99	0.03	0.02
Gender	1.20	0.49	2.93	0.23	0.69
Female (vs male)					
Liver disease	0.35	0.13	0.94	0.25	0.04
Cirrhosis (vs no cirrhosis)					
Treatment status	0.84	0.35	1.99	0.22	0.69
Experienced (vs naïve)					
HIV co-infection ($n = 10$)	2.56	0.44	14.77	0.45	0.29
Absence (vs presence)					
Depression ($n = 40$)	0.88	0.35	2.22	0.24	0.79
Absence (vs presence)					
Diabetes ($n = 8$)	4.94	0.62	39.56	0.53	0.13
Absence (vs presence)					
IL28b	0.12	0.04	0.37	0.29	0.0002
Non-CC (vs CC)					
Genotype	1.09	0.37	3.22	0.29	0.28
G1a (vs G1b)					
Race	0.31	0.04	2.42	0.52	0.27
Other (vs white)					

episode with 1 patient being admitted twice. The mean number of hospital days spent per hospitalisation was 3.5.

In the UK, treatment is generally supervised by a clinical nurse specialist, however 78/154 (51 %) of patients had at least one consultant (hepatology or infectious diseases) visit and 17/154 (11 %) patients required at least one dermatologist visit during treatment. The mean number of consultant visits per patient during the follow-up was 1.2, with a mean number of nurse visits of 14.5. During the follow-up period, patients had, on average, 13 liver function tests, 10 electrolyte tests and 5 HCV viral load tests. In total 'other healthcare costs' accounted for approximately £1,500 per patient; £232,573 per 154 patients.

The PI price sensitivity analysis (30 %, 40 %, 50 % discount) indicated that a 10 % drop in PI drug price was associated with a decrease of 7 % in the cost per cure (Table 5). Discount rates sensitivity analyses stratified according to outcome of previous therapy as well as liver disease status showed clearly that no response to previous therapy as well as the presence of cirrhosis is associated with increases in total costs per cure (see Supporting material).

In the base case analysis, only 'likely' hospitalisations and AEs were included. 141 AEs were deemed 'likely' and 24 'can't tell' (the remaining 13 being deemed "unlikely"). The impact of inclusion of cost for 'can't tell' classified AEs in the sensitivity analysis had only a negligible impact on total median cost per SVR - £38,027 vs £37,958 with and without respectively.

Discussion

The fact that HCV infection will incur a significant future healthcare burden is now commonly accepted. Use of highly effective therapies has been proven to improve

Table 4 Cost per HCV cure – by prior treatment and cirrhotic status

Total ($n = 154$)	Treatment naïve patients ($n = 74$)	Prior relapsers ($n = 35$)	Prior non-responders ($n = 36$)	Prior treatment status unknown ($n = 9$)
Overall	£ 37,958	£ 39,150	£ 83,948	£ 61, 804
By liver disease stage				
Non cirrhotic ($n = 114$)	£ 35,492	£ 37,455	£ 73,098	£ 49,070
Cirrhotic ($n = 31$)	£ 61,496	£ 49,016	£ 107,288	NA

Table 5 Total costs

Costs	Base case Total cost (in £)	%	30 % discount on PI	%	40 % discount on PI	%	50 % discount on PI	%
PIs	2,930,769	68.3	2,051,538	60.2	1,758,461	56.4	1,465,385	51.9
PegINF	834,485	19.5	834,485	24.5	834,485	26.8	834,485	29.6
Ribavirin	290,975	6.8	290,975	8.5	290,975	9.3	290,975	10.3
Physician visits	139,992	5.4	232,573	6.8	232,573	7.5	232,573	8.2
Tests	52,616							
Other investigation	14,576							
Hospitalisation	9,209							
Adverse events	17,233							
Depression & hypnotics	54							
Total	4,289,909	100.0	3,409,571	100.0	3,116,494	100.0	2,823,418	100.0
Total median cost per cure (£)	44,852	-	34,416	-	30,968	-	27,233	-

SVR rates and therefore reduce HCV related morbidity and mortality [33]. The first IFN-free combinations of directly acting antivirals (DAAs) against hepatitis C (HCV) have been licensed and more are likely to follow in the coming years. These treatments are significantly shorter in duration, yield higher SVR and have fewer AEs [34] than traditional IFN-based therapies. With expected high costs of therapy, it is important to evaluate the cost per SVR in order to maximise efficient use of scarce healthcare resources.

We set out to describe the effectiveness, safety and costs per cure for first generation protease inhibitor based treatment of genotype 1 hepatitis C (the most common genotype), in a real-world UK setting.

Differences between SVR results achieved in trials (efficacy) and those in clinical practice (effectiveness) with PR + 1st generation PIs have been previously documented [11–18]. Such differences have been attributed to the restrictive inclusion criteria of clinical trials with respect to certain groups of patients including those with advanced disease, cirrhosis and high co-morbidity burden.

While we found an overall SVR of 63 % in our sample, comparable with registration trials, there was (as expected) significant variation, with cirrhotic patients and prior non-responders having worse SVR outcomes.

Just over a third (35.7 %) of patients did not complete treatment. The discontinuation rate due to treatment related AE amongst our sample was 11 %. Nearly half of patients in our sample experienced an AE requiring an intervention with 79 % of those AE considered 'likely' to be treatment-related. Almost 10 % of all patients required hospitalisation 'likely'- related to treatment.

Overall median total cost per cure for our sample in the base case analysis was £44,852; however, there was substantial variation among subgroups ranging from £35,492 in treatment naive non-cirrhotics to £107,288 in cirrhotic prior non-responders. In the base case analysis for 154 patients, HCV triple therapy costs accounted for 94.6 % of the total cost (£4,056,229).

The characteristics of our UK cohort and the overall SVR rates are very similar to a study carried out in Germany, although the costs per cure estimated here were significantly lower, a difference driven to a large extent by the higher costs attributed to antivirals in Germany (see Table 6). A recent US study of similar size found a lower overall SVR rate, reflecting in part a slightly older population and a higher proportion of African-Americans, a group where a higher prevalence of IL28b T allele has been associated with poorer treatment outcomes. Despite these differences, cost per cure in the US was substantially higher, likely due to sample differences (e.g. proportion of high cost prior non-responders 46 % US: 22 % UK) as well as differences in clinical AE management (e.g. anaemia) and drug costs).

The strength of this study is that it represents a large randomly drawn sample, representing 35 UK centres treating hepatitis C, taken from a large UK database (HCV Research UK) and is thus likely to be representative of overall UK practice. The overall case-mix of patients considered for treatment in coming years is likely to change and the breakdown of outcomes presented according to sub-groups allows comparative analysis for different patient groups.

There are a number of factors which may underestimate the 'true' total cost per cure in our analysis. Firstly, we conducted our analysis from the direct health service perspective only, we did not consider additional indirect (such as loss in economic productivity due to treatment related side effects) or intangible costs (e.g. loss in HRQoL). Secondly, perhaps of greater impact on the definitive cost-per-cure per patient, we have not taken into

Table 6 Comparison with recent US and German studies

Patients characteristics	Current study (*n* = 154)	Stahmeyer et al. (GER) [35] (*n* = 858)*	Bichoupan et al. (US) [17] (*n* = 147)
Age, years [Mean, (SD)]	49.6 (9.0)	49.2 (11.2)	56 (IQR = 51–61)
Gender, Male [%]	73.4	58	68
Ethnicity, %			
Caucasian [%]	94.20 %	97.30 %	Not reported
Asian [%]	2.70 %	0.90 %	Not reported
African [%]	1.30 %	0.80 %	19 %
Hispanic [%]	Not reported	0.50 %	Not reported
Other [%]	1.80 %	Not reported	Not reported
SVR rate by therapy			
BOC [%]	60.8	58.1	Not reported
TVR [%]	63.1	68.4	44
Cirrhosis [%]	21.40 %	Not reported	36 %
Prior non-responders [%]	22.10 %	Not reported	46 %
Cost drivers			
Drug costs	94.60 %	94.6–97.7 %	89 %
PIs	68.30 %	Not reported	Not reported
TVR	Not reported	Not reported	61
PegIFN	19.50 %	Not reported	24 %
RBV	6.80 %	Not reported	4 %
Outpatient and inpatient care (incl AEs & follow-up)	5.40 %	5.4-3.3 %	8 %
Cost per SVR ($)			
Treatment naïve	56,576	73,473–82,756	Not reported
Relapsers	58,353	78,529–93,758	Not reported
Non-responders	125,125	127,1049–132,204	Not reported
Overall	Not reported	Not reported	189,000

*Costs from Stahmeyer et al. were converted from euros to US dollars (conversion rate: €1 = $1.0985 based on European Central Bank exchange rates, March 2015)

account the additional costs of retreating the 37.7 % of patients who failed PI treatment.

Analysis of cost-effectiveness is inevitably something that will change as prices of drugs, which make up the bulk of treatment costs, change. It is reasonable to expect that as there is more competition, prices will fall. Table 5 shows the effect of discount on cost-per-cure and given the high proportion of overall costs due to PI, discounts have a significant impact on cost-per-cure. However the results also show the proportional increase of non-discountable 'other' (largely AE management related) healthcare costs. This study provides valuable data to allow clinicians and healthcare decision makers to evaluate the real world total cost-per-cure amongst patients treated with current and future therapies. In particular, we provide a baseline dataset against which with the total cost per cure of emerging, all oral therapies can be compared and contrasted.

Conclusion

The future healthcare burden of HCV in the UK, as in many countries, is significant. Further prospective real world safety, effectiveness and total cost data is needed for the new IFN free treatment combinations from different healthcare settings. Comparison with this data can provide evidence to inform future treatment decisions to ensure scarce healthcare resources are able to maximize patient outcomes.

Abbreviations

AE: adverse event; BOC: boceprevir; HCC: hepatocellular carcinoma; HCV: hepatitis C virus; HRG: Health Resource Group; HRQoL: health-related quality of life; IFN: interferon; NHS: National Health Service; NICE: National Institute of Health and Care Excellence; PEG: pegylated interferon;

PI: protease inhibitor; PR: pegylated interferon and ribavirin; RBV: ribavirin; SVR: sustained viral response; TVR: telaprevir.

Competing interests

Dr Stephen Barclay: Consultant: Abbvie, BMS, Gilead, Janssen, MSD; Grants: Gilead, Janssen, MSD; Sponsored lectures: Gilead, Janssen, MSD, Roche. Dr Graham Cooke: Consultant: Janssen, BI, Gilead and Merck; Grants: Janssen, BMS and Gilead. Miss Elizabeth Holtham: N/A. Ms Aline Gauthier: analysis funded by Gilead. Mr Jeremie Schwarzbard: analysis funded by Gilead. Mr Petar Atanasov: analysis funded by Gilead. Prof William Irving: Consultant: Merck, Novartis, BMS; Grants: Pfizer, GSK, Gilead; Educational grants: Boehringer Ingelheim, Gilead, Merck; Sponsored lectures: Janssen.
None of the authors have hold any stocks or shares in an organization that may in any way gain or lose financially from the publication of this manuscript, either now or in the future.

Authors' contributions

WI contributed to study concept, design and methodology. EH developed the data collection tool and led on data collection. AG, JS, PA undertook the statistical and health-economic analysis. STB, GSC and WI lead on interpretation and appraisal of results. All authors contributed to development and critical revisions of the manuscript for important intellectual content. All authors read and approved the final manuscript.

Acknowledgements

HCV Research UK is funded by grant number C0365 from the Medical Research Foundation. GC is supported by the BRC of Imperial College NHS Trust. WI and GC are members of the STOP-HCV consortium, which is funded by the Medical Research Council.

HCV Research UK contributors

Abouda G (Hull Royal Infirmary), Agarwal K (Kings College Hospital, London), Aldersley M (St James's University Hospital, Leeds), Alexander G (Addenbrookes Hospital, Cambridge), Aspinall R (Queen Alexandra Hospital, Portsmouth), Barclay S (Glasgow Royal Infirmary), Barnes E (John Radcliffe Hospital, Oxford), Brown A (St Mary's Hospital, London), Butterworth J (Royal Shrewsbury Hospital), Ch'ng C (Singleton Hospital, Swansea), Chadwick D (James Cook University Hospital, Middlesbrough), Cramp M (Derriford Hospital, Plymouth), Datta S (Southern General Hospital & Glasgow Victoria Hospital), Dillon J (Ninewells Hospital, Dundee), Forton D (St George's Hospital, London), Foster G (The London Hospital), Fraser A (Aberdeen Royal Infirmary), Gelson W (Addenbrookes Hospital, Cambridge), Goldberg D (Health Protection Scotland), Gorard D (Wycombe General Hospital), Gore C (Hepatitis C Trust), Hayes P (Royal Infirmary of Edinburgh), Heydtmann M (Royal Alexandra Hospital, Glasgow), Higham A (Royal Lancaster Infirmary), Holtham E (Queen's Medical Centre, Nottingham), Hubscher S (Queen Elizabeth Hospital, Birmingham), Hutchinson S (Glasgow Caledonian University), Irving W (University of Nottingham), Jenkins N (Birmingham Heartlands Hospital), Kelly D (Birmingham Children's Hospital), Khakoo S (Southampton General Hospital), Langford A (British Liver Trust), Lawson A, (Royal Derby Hospital), Leen C (Western General Hospital, Edinburgh), McDonald S (University of Glasgow), McLauchlan J (University of Glasgow), McPherson S (Freeman Hospital, Newcastle), Mills P (Gartnavel General Hospital, Glasgow), Moreea S (Bradford Royal Infirmary), Mutimer D (Queen Elizabeth Hospital, Birmingham), Neal K (Public Health England), Patel A (University of Glasgow), Prince M (Manchester Royal Infirmary), Quinlan P (University of Nottingham), Ramsay M (Public Health England), Reddy Y (Royal Blackburn Hospital), Richardson P (Royal Liverpool University Hospital), Rosenberg W (Royal Free Hospital & University College Hospital), Ryder S (Queen's Medical Centre, Nottingham), Shields P (Royal Preston Hospital), Shorrock C (Blackpool Victoria Hospital), Singhal S (Sandwell & City Hospitals, Birmingham), Sreedharan A (Lincoln County Hospital), Srirajaskanthan R (University Hospital Lewisham), Stone B (Royal Hallamshire Hospital, Sheffield), Thursz M (St Mary's Hospital, London), Ustianowski, A (North Manchester General Hospital), Wilkes B (University of Nottingham), Wiselka M (Leicester Royal Infirmary).

Author details

[1]Walton Liver Clinic, Glasgow Royal Infirmary, Glasgow, UK. [2]Division of Infectious diseases, Imperial College London, London, UK. [3]NIHR Nottingham Digestive Diseases Biomedical Research Unit, University of Nottingham, Nottingham, UK. [4]Amaris Ltd, London, UK. [5]Microbiology, Queen's Medical Centre, Nottingham NG7 2UH, UK.

References

1. Messina JP, Humphreys I, Flaxman A, Brown A, Cooke GS, Pybus OG, et al. Global distribution and prevalence of hepatitis C virus genotypes. Hepatology. 2015;61(1):77–87. doi:10.1002/hep.27259.
2. Eurpean Association for the Srudy of the Liver (EASL). EASL recommendations on treatment of hepatitis C 2014. J Hepatol. 2014;61(2): 373–95. doi:10.1016/j.jhep.2014.05.001.
3. EASL Recommendations on Treatment of Hepatitis C 2015. J Hepatol. 63(1): 199–236. doi:10.1016/j.jhep.2015.03.025
4. Morgan RL, Baack B, Smith BD, Yartel A, Pitasi M, Falck-Ytter Y. Eradication of hepatitis C virus infection and the development of hepatocellular carcinoma: a meta-analysis of observational studies. Ann Intern Med. 2013; 158(5 Pt 1):329–37. doi:10.7326/0003-4819-158-5-201303050-00005.
5. Veldt BJ, Heathcote EJ, Wedemeyer H, Reichen J, Hofmann WP, Zeuzem S, et al. Sustained virologic response and clinical outcomes in patients with chronic hepatitis C and advanced fibrosis. Ann Intern Med. 2007;147(10): 677–84.
6. Smith-Palmer J, Cerri K, Valentine W. Achieving sustained virologic response in hepatitis C: a systematic review of the clinical, economic and quality of life benefits. BMC Infect Dis. 2015;15(1):19. doi:10.1186/s12879-015-0748-8.
7. Park C, Jiang S, Lawson KA. Efficacy and safety of telaprevir and boceprevir in patients with hepatitis C genotype 1: a meta-analysis. J Clin Pharm Ther. 2014;39(1):14–24. doi:10.1111/jcpt.12106.
8. Udina M, Castellvi P, Moreno-Espana J, Navines R, Valdes M, Forns X, et al. Interferon-induced depression in chronic hepatitis C: a systematic review and meta-analysis. J Clin Psychiatry. 2012;73(8):1128–38. doi:10.4088/JCP. 12r07694.
9. Gao X, Stephens JM, Carter JA, Haider S, Rustgi VK. Impact of adverse events on costs and quality of life in protease inhibitor-based combination therapy for hepatitis C. Expert Rev Pharmacoecon Outcomes Res. 2012;12(3):335–43. doi:10.1586/erp.12.10.
10. Cotler SJ, Patil R, McNutt RA, Speroff T, Banaad-Omiotek G, Ganger DR, et al. Patients' values for health states associated with hepatitis C and physicians' estimates of those values. Am J Gastroenterol. 2001;96(9):2730–6. doi:10. 1111/j.1572-0241.2001.04132.x.
11. Bacon BR, Gordon SC, Lawitz E, Marcellin P, Vierling JM, Zeuzem S, et al. Boceprevir for Previously Treated Chronic HCV Genotype 1 Infection. N Engl J Med. 2011;364(13):1207–17. doi:10.1056/NEJMoa1009482.
12. Jacobson IM, McHutchison JG, Dusheiko G, Di Bisceglie AM, Reddy KR, Bzowej NH, et al. Telaprevir for Previously Untreated Chronic Hepatitis C Virus Infection. N Engl J Med. 2011;364(25):2405–16. doi:10.1056/ NEJMoa1012912.
13. Poordad F, McCone J, Bacon BR, Bruno S, Manns MP, Sulkowski MS, et al. Boceprevir for Untreated Chronic HCV Genotype 1 Infection. N Engl J Med. 2011;364(13):1195–206. doi:10.1056/NEJMoa1010494.
14. Zeuzem S, Andreone P, Pol S, Lawitz E, Diago M, Roberts S, et al. Telaprevir for Retreatment of HCV Infection. N Engl J Med. 2011;364(25):2417–28. doi: 10.1056/NEJMoa1013086.
15. Ioannou GN, Beste LA, Green PK. Similar effectiveness of boceprevir and telaprevir treatment regimens for hepatitis C virus infection on the basis of a nationwide study of veterans. Clin Gastroenterol Hepatol. 2014;12(8):1371–80. doi:10.1016/j.cgh.2013.12.011.
16. Price JC, Murphy RC, Shvachko VA, Pauly MP, Manos MM. Effectiveness of telaprevir and boceprevir triple therapy for patients with hepatitis C virus infection in a large integrated care setting. Dig Dis Sci. 2014;59(12):3043–52. doi:10.1007/s10620-014-3294-0.
17. Bichoupan K, Martel-Laferriere V, Sachs D, Ng M, Schonfeld EA, Pappas A, et al. Costs of telaprevir-based triple therapy for hepatitis C: $189,000 per sustained virological response. Hepatology. 2014;60(4):1187–95. doi:10.1002/ hep.27340.

18. Gordon SC, Muir AJ, Lim JK, Pearlman B, Argo CK, Ramani A, et al. Safety profile of boceprevir and telaprevir in chronic hepatitis C: Real world experience from HCV-TARGET. J Hepatol. 2015;62(2):286–93. doi:10.1016/j.jhep.2014.08.052.
19. Lawitz E, Mangia A, Wyles D, Rodriguez-Torres M, Hassanein T, Gordon SC, et al. Sofosbuvir for Previously Untreated Chronic Hepatitis C Infection. N Engl J Med. 2013;368(20):1878–87. doi:10.1056/NEJMoa1214853.
20. Jacobson IM, Dore GJ, Foster GR, Fried MW, Radu M, Rafalsky W, et al. Simeprevir with pegylated interferon alfa 2a plus ribavirin in treatment-naive patients with chronic hepatitis C virus genotype 1 infection (QUEST-1): a phase 3, randomised, double-blind, placebo-controlled trial. Lancet. 2014;384(9941):403–13. doi:10.1016/s0140-6736(14)60494-3.
21. Manns M, Marcellin P, Poordad F, de Araujo ES, Buti M, Horsmans Y, et al. Simeprevir with pegylated interferon alfa 2a or 2b plus ribavirin in treatment-naive patients with chronic hepatitis C virus genotype 1 infection (QUEST-2): a randomised, double-blind, placebo-controlled phase 3 trial. Lancet. 2014;384(9941):414–26. doi:10.1016/s0140-6736(14)60538-9.
22. Forns X, Lawitz E, Zeuzem S, Gane E, Bronowicki JP, Andreone P, et al. Simeprevir with peginterferon and ribavirin leads to high rates of SVR in patients with HCV genotype 1 who relapsed after previous therapy: a phase 3 trial. Gastroenterology. 2014;146(7):1669–79. doi:10.1053/j.gastro.2014.02.051. e3.
23. Pol S, Ghalib RH, Rustgi VK, Martorell C, Everson GT, Tatum HA, et al. Daclatasvir for previously untreated chronic hepatitis C genotype-1 infection: a randomised, parallel-group, double-blind, placebo-controlled, dose-finding, phase 2a trial. Lancet Infect Dis. 2012;12(9):671–7. doi:10.1016/s1473-3099(12)70138-x.
24. The price of good health. Nat Med. 2014;20(4):319-. doi:10.1038/nm.3538.
25. National Institute for Health and Care Excellence. NICE technology appraisal guidance [TA252]: Telaprevir for the treatment of genotype 1 chronic hepatitis C. 2012. https://www.nice.org.uk/guidance/ta252. Accessed 06 March 2015.
26. National Institute for Health and Care Excellence. NICE technology appraisal guidance [TA253]: Boceprevir for the treatment of genotype 1 chronic hepatitis C. 2012. https://www.nice.org.uk/guidance/ta253. Accessed 06 March 2015.
27. UK HR. HCV Biobank. 2015. https://www.hcvresearchuk.org/hcv/databases. Accessed 15 April 2015.
28. British National Formulary. BNF March 2014. 2015. http://www.bnf.org/bnf/index.htm. Accessed 28 Aug 2014.
29. Department of Health. NHS Reference Costs. 2014. https://www.gov.uk/government/collections/nhs-reference-costs. Accessed 28 Aug 2014.
30. Health & Social Care Information Centre. Payment groupers. 2014. http://www.hscic.gov.uk/article/3938/HRG4-201415-Payment-Grouper. Accessed 28 Aug 2014.
31. Department of Health. NHS reference costs. 2014. https://www.gov.uk/government/collections/nhs-reference-costs. Accessed 06 March 2016.
32. Bank of England. Statistical Interactive Database - daily spot exchange rates against Sterling. 2015. http://www.bankofengland.co.uk/boeapps/iadb/Rates.asp. Accessed 16 March 2015.
33. van der Meer AJ, Veldt BJ, Feld JJ, Wedemeyer H, Dufour JF, Lammert F, et al. Association between sustained virological response and all-cause mortality among patients with chronic hepatitis C and advanced hepatic fibrosis. JAMA. 2012;308(24):2584–93. doi:10.1001/jama.2012.144878.
34. Kohli A, Shaffer A, Sherman A, Kottilil S. Treatment of hepatitis C: a systematic review. JAMA. 2014;312(6):631–40. doi:10.1001/jama.2014.7085.
35. Stahmeyer JT, Rossol S, Bert F, Abdelfattah AM, Mauss S, Heyne R et al. P1147 Outcomes and costs of treating hepatitis C with protein inhibitors: results from a multi-centre study. J Hepatol. 60(1):S464-S5. doi:10.1016/s0168-8278(14)61307-6.

2

Concordance between self-reported and measured HIV and hepatitis C virus infection status among people who inject drugs

Stine Nielsen[1,2*], Martyna Gassowski[1], Benjamin Wenz[1], Norbert Bannert[3], Claus-Thomas Bock[4], Claudia Kücherer[3], R. Stefan Ross[5], Viviane Bremer[1], Ulrich Marcus[1], Ruth Zimmermann[1] and the DRUCK study group

Abstract

Background: People who inject drugs (PWID) are disproportionately affected by both HIV and hepatitis C infection (HCV). Awareness of infection status is essential to ensure linkage to appropriate healthcare for those infected, who need treatment and regular follow-up, as well as for uninfected individuals, who need access to targeted testing and counselling services. In this paper we compare self-reported HIV and HCV status with serological markers of infection among PWID recruited through respondent driven sampling.

Methods: From 2011 through 2014, biological and behavioural data was collected from 2,077 PWID in Germany. Dried blood spots from capillary blood samples were collected and screened for HCV antibodies, HCV RNA and HIV-1/-2 antibodies. HIV reactive samples were confirmed by Western blot.

Results: Laboratory testing revealed that 5 % were infected with HIV and 81 % were aware of being infected. Chronic HCV infection was detected in 41 % of the participants, 2 % had an acute HCV infection, 22 % had a cleared infection, and 34 % were unexposed to HCV. The concordance between self-reported and measured HCV status was lower than for HIV, with 73 % of those with chronic HCV infection being aware of their infection.

Conclusions: We found a relatively high awareness of HIV and HCV infection status among PWID. Nevertheless, access to appropriate testing, counselling and care services targeted to the needs of PWID should be further improved, particularly concerning HCV.

Keywords: People who inject drugs, Germany, Hepatitis C, HIV, Testing, Knowledge, Self-report, Validity, Undiagnosed, Respondent driven sampling

* Correspondence: stine.nielsen12@gmail.com
[1]Department for Infectious Disease Epidemiology, Division for HIV/AIDS, STI and Blood-borne Infections, Robert Koch Institute, Berlin, Germany
[2]Charité University Medicine, Berlin, Germany
Full list of author information is available at the end of the article

Background

Accurate knowledge of infection status is important as it gives infected individuals the opportunity to seek appropriate healthcare and may encourage people to engage in preventive behaviours, which can protect themselves and others from infections. People who inject drugs (PWID) have a high risk and burden of both HIV and Hepatitis C infection (HCV) [1–4]. Determining HIV infection status is relatively straightforward since there is no clearance or cure. In contrast, screening for HCV antibodies (anti-HCV) will identify if a person has ever been in contact with the virus, but this person may have cleared the infection either with treatment or spontaneously, or the person may have a chronic HCV infection, characterised by being both anti-HCV and HCV RNA positive. A person who has cleared the infection can later be re-infected with HCV. Since the acquisition of both HIV and HCV is often asymptomatic or the occurrence of non-specific symptoms may be attributed to other problems, and since serious sequelae may take several decades to develop, people infected with these two viruses may remain unaware of being infected for a long period of time. Annual routine unlinked anonymous monitoring (UAM) of HIV and hepatitis among PWID in England, Wales and Northern Ireland has shown that the proportion of infected PWID unaware of their infection varied between 4 %-15 % for HIV and 45 %-53 % for HCV in the period 2010–2014 [5]. In a recent systematic review including 11 studies from five EU countries the proportion of undiagnosed HCV infections among PWID varied between 24 %-76 % (IQR: 38 %-64 % and median: 49 %) [4]. Several previous studies only looked at anti-HCV status and did not include HCV RNA status, which is needed to assess current infection status [4–6].

With new, highly effective and well tolerable HCV therapy options being available as well as the potential of HIV-treatment as prevention also among PWID [7], it is of growing importance to increase awareness of infection status.

In order to assess the level of awareness of infection status among PWID in Germany, we used data from a recent, cross-sectional bio-behavioural survey of this population to compare self-reported HIV and HCV status with serological markers of infection.

Methods

The DRUCK-study collected biological and behavioural data from 2,077 PWID in eight large German cities in the years 2011–2014 [8]. The respondents were recruited using respondent driven sampling. Inclusion criteria were a minimum age of 16 years, having injected drugs in the given study city in the last 12 months, and providing informed consent for study participation. All participants went through a questionnaire-assisted interview and provided a capillary blood sample, collected as dried blood spots (DBS). Samples and questionnaires were marked with the same unique identifier. The study was piloted in two cities and then implemented in the remaining six. Before starting the data collection we trained interviewers to increase their understanding of HIV and HCV, and laboratory staff for collection of DBS and handling and shipping of the samples in each of the study cities to ensure the comparability of results. All samples were screened for anti-HIV-1/-2 by EIA, and reactive samples were confirmed by Western blot. In six of the eight study cities, all samples were screened for both anti-HCV by EIA and analysed for the presence of HCV-RNA using nested RT-PCR. Anti-HCV positive samples were confirmed by immunoblot. In the two pilot cities all samples were screened for anti-HCV by EIA and RT-PCR was performed on all anti-HCV positive samples and on anti-HCV negative samples if test results did not correspond to self-reported results. The test specificity was 100 % for all three markers: anti-HIV, anti-HCV and HCV RNA. The same was true for the sensitivity for HIV and HCV RNA, whereas the sensitivity for anti-HCV was 97.8 % [9]. Further information about study design, data collection and laboratory methods etc. has been published elsewhere [8, 9].

Defining self-reported HIV status

The self-reported HIV status was determined using two questions: if the participant had ever been tested for HIV and if yes, what the result of their latest test was. Based on the answers participants were categorised as HIV negative, HIV positive or never tested. Participant's self-reported HIV status were categorised as unclear when they were not sure if they had ever been tested or if they did not know their last test result. Participants who reported having been diagnosed with HIV were asked about month and year of their first positive HIV test in order to calculate how long they had been aware of being infected.

Defining measured HIV status

We defined samples as HIV positive if testing positive for anti-HIV with EIA and being confirmed by Western blot. EIA-reactive samples with indeterminate immunoblot pattern were excluded from this analysis. Anti-HIV negative samples were determined as HIV negative.

Defining self-reported HCV status

To determine the self-reported HCV status several questions were used. Participants were asked if they had ever been tested for anti-HCV. Those who had not were categorised as never tested. The participants who reported testing for HCV were further asked if they had ever received a positive anti-HCV test result. Those who had not were categorised as uninfected. Participants reporting having ever received a positive anti-HCV test result were further asked if they had ever been successfully treated or had cleared the infection spontaneously. Those who responded no to both questions were categorised as infected, while those who responded yes to either of the questions were defined as previously infected. As for HIV, participants who were either not sure if they had ever been tested or did not know their last test result, were categorised as unclear.

Defining measured HCV status

We defined chronic HCV infection as testing anti-HCV and RNA positive, acute infection (HCV infection acquired within the last 4–6 weeks) as anti-HCV negative, but RNA positive, cleared infection as anti-HCV positive and HCV RNA negative, and unexposed as testing anti-HCV and RNA negative.

An example of the questionnaire used to guide the interviews can be found online [10].

Results

In total, 2,077 PWID from eight German cities were included in the study, with the proportion of female participants ranging between 19 %-35 % in the respective cities, and a median age ranging between 29–41 years.

HIV status

The laboratory testing revealed 100 participants (4.8 %) to be positive for HIV, and 1976 (95.2 %) to be negative. One sample had a reactive EIA result but an indeterminate immunoblot, and was thus excluded from the analysis. Of the 100 HIV positive cases, 81 % were aware of their infection while 16 % reported their last HIV test to be negative. One HIV positive participant reported no previous testing.

Among the participants testing negative for HIV, 90 % reported a negative test result at last test, while 7 % reported never having had an HIV test. Of the HIV negative participants, six individuals (0.3 %) reported having received a positive HIV-test result. Two HIV positive and one HIV negative participant declined to answer the question on HIV-status. The concordance of the self-reported HIV status and laboratory test results is displayed in Table 1.

Among the 81 self-reported HIV infected, 5 % reported receiving their diagnosis in the last year, 17 % 1–5 years ago, 22 % 6–10 years ago and 47 % more than 10 years ago. Seven cases (9 %) did not provide information on time of their HIV diagnosis.

Table 1 Concordance of self-reported and measured HIV status, *n*=2076 (excluding one sample with indeterminate HIV status)

	HIV laboratory test results	
Self-reported status	HIV negative (AB-)	HIV positive (AB+)
Concordant	1784 (90 %)	81 (81 %)
Discordant	6 (0,3 %)	16 (16 %)
Never tested	133 (7 %)	1 (1 %)
Unclear	52 (3 %)	0 (0 %)
Answer declined	1 (0,1 %)	2 (2 %)
Total	1976	100

Unclear means not sure if tested or did not get last test result.
AB antibodies

HCV status

The laboratory tests found 716 (34 %) participants to be unexposed to HCV, 857 (41 %) participants to have a chronic HCV infection and 457 (22 %) participants with a cleared HCV infection. In 47 (2 %) participants HCV-RNA but no anti-HCV was detected, indicating an acute infection. As the participants were only asked about anti-HCV test results, this group was excluded from the analysis.

The concordance between the self-reported HCV status and the laboratory test results was 47 % among those unexposed, while 27 % reported an HCV status discordant to the laboratory findings (Table 2). Of these, 56 % reported a current HCV infection and 44 % a previous one (Table 3). Of all unexposed individuals, 16 % reported never to have had a test for HCV. In the group with confirmed, chronic HCV infections, 73 % reported a status concordant to the laboratory test results, whereas 19 % reported a differing HCV status. In 37 % of these discordant cases, participants reported to be uninfected and in 63 % a cleared infection. Among participants positive only for anti-HCV but not HCV-RNA, i.e., with a cleared infection, 38 % correctly reported to have cleared the infection. Of those reporting a discordant status, 89 % reported to be currently infected and 11 % reported an uninfected status.

Discussion

In our study population of PWID, the concordance of self-reported and measured HIV status was relatively high. The proportion of HIV positive participants aware of their infection was 81 %. These data compare well with the data from both the UAM in England, Wales and northern Ireland from 2010–2014 where 85-96 % of HIV positive PWID were aware of their HIV infection [5] and the latest HIV modelling data from Germany, where it was estimated that 89 % (81-93 %) of all HIV infected PWID living in Germany in 2014 had received an HIV diagnosis [11]. According to the same HIV modelling data for Germany, the proportion of HIV infected individuals who are aware of their HIV status is higher

Table 2 Concordance of self-reported and measured HCV status, *n*=2030 (excluding cases with acute infection)

	HCV laboratory test results		
Self-reported status	Unexposed (AB-, RNA-)	Chronic infection (AB+, RNA+)	Cleared infection (AB+, RNA-)
Concordant	339 (47 %)	622 (73 %)	174 (38 %)
Discordant	194 (27 %)	163 (19 %)	254 (56 %)
Never tested	113 (16 %)	37 (4 %)	15 (3 %)
Unclear	69 (10 %)	35 (4 %)	14 (3 %)
Answer declined	1 (0,1 %)	0 (0 %)	0 (0 %)
Total	716	857	457

Unclear means not sure if tested or did not get last test result
AB antibodies

among PWID compared to other groups such as men who have sex with men (MSM) (82 % (79-85 %)) and non-injecting heterosexuals (74 % (66-80 %)). This might partly be explained by the fact that the majority of HIV infections among PWID in Germany were acquired in the 1980ies and 90ies, which is also seen by the high proportion of known HIV infections being diagnosed more than 10 years ago. This means that the majority of HIV infected PWID have had many years to get a diagnosis and begin therapy. Increasing treatment rates among PWID may have a relatively large impact on reducing potential sources of HIV transmission within this population [7]. A low rate of newly acquired HIV infections is also indicated by the fact that <1 % of PWID not yet tested for HIV were found to be anti-HIV positive in our study. The one sample with a reactive AB test and indeterminate immunoblot could be a recent infection in the stage of seroconversion. We tried to receive a second blood sample from this participant to repeat the testing, but the person did not show up in the drug service again.

The finding that 17 % of those positive for HIV reported a negative HIV status or to never have been tested, underlines the undiminished importance of ensuring access to targeted HIV testing and counselling services for PWID in Germany, e.g., in low threshold settings.

For the disconcerting finding of six self-reported infections in participants without measurable anti-HIV several possible explanations exist. One possibility is the failure to detect antibodies in excessively diluted samples if the original amount of capillary blood was inadequately small, resulting in a higher dilution of the antibodies as compared to the standardized and validated protocol. Further we cannot rule out the communication of false positive test results to study participants, in particular if reactive screening test results were not confirmed, which can happen if respondents were not linked into care. Processing mistakes during sample collection or during testing of DBS, or the disappearance of HIV antibodies if treatment has been started early and viral load has remained suppressed continuously are further, though in our view less likely possibilities.

The results of the HCV testing revealed that 34 % were unexposed to HCV, 2 % had an acute HCV infection, 41 % of participants had a chronic infection and 22 % had a cleared infection. It is possible that a few acute HCV infections might have been missed in the two first pilot cities where PCR was only done for anti-HCV negative respondents with a self-reported HCV diagnosis. The concordance between self-reported and actual HCV status was much lower than for HIV. Concordance was highest (73 %) among those with a chronic infection, 47 % among those unexposed to HCV and just 38 % among those with a cleared infection.

The somewhat surprising finding of 27 % of those with no markers of HCV infection reporting to be infected (chronic or cleared HCV), might partly be explained by confusion about the different types of hepatitis, e.g., participants may previously have received a positive test result for hepatitis B. Another explanation could be the failure to detect antibodies e.g., due to excessive dilution, as described above for HIV or a false negative anti-HCV

Table 3 Discordance of self-reported and measured HCV status, *n*=611

	HCV laboratory test results		
Self-reported status	Unexposed (AB-, RNA-)	Chronic infection (AB+, RNA+)	Cleared infection (AB+, RNA-)
Uninfected		61 (37 %)	29 (11 %)
Infected	109 (56 %)		225 (89 %)
Previously infected (cleared infection)	85 (44 %)	102 (63 %)	
Total	194	163	254

AB antibodies

test result which is not unlikely given the estimated sensitivity of 97.8 %.

Of the participants with a chronic HCV infection, 27 % falsely believed to be uninfected, to have cleared the infection or had never been tested or were not sure of their test result. This rate is much lower than what is reported from the UAM in England, Wales and northern Ireland where 45-53 % of anti-HCV positive were unaware of their HCV infection in the years 2010–2014 [5]. Also the recent systematic review on HCV in PWID in Europe found higher rates of undiagnosed HCV: 24-76 % (IQR: 38-64 % and median: 49 %) [4]. An Australian study of 352 active injectors under the age of 30, found rates of concordance similar to our study: 68 % among those with a chronic infection and 46 % among those with a cleared HCV infection [12]. Also data from a French study of HCV among PWID found that only 22 % of PWID were unaware of their HCV infection [13, 14]. A recently published study from Spain presents data on the proportion of undiagnosed HCV infection among PWID stratified by migration status and duration of injecting. This study reports rates of undiagnosed HCV from 15 % among Spanish long-term injectors up to 57 % among migrant new injectors [6]. All these data suggest that awareness of HCV infection status among PWID in Germany is relatively high. This is also true when comparing with data for the general population in Europe, where between 40 % and 80 % of people with chronic hepatitis are believed to be unaware of their infection [15]. However, the persons indicating a true positive anti-HCV test result often do not necessarily also know their PCR test result. In times of effective treatment options for HCV this will become increasingly important.

In our study, the majority (63 %) of those with a chronic HCV infection with a discordant self-reported status were aware of having been exposed to the virus but believed to have cleared the infection. These participants might have simply assumed to be healed (we did not collect data on whether the reported clearance had been laboratory confirmed) or they might indeed have cleared the virus but later become re-infected. These results show the need of special screening efforts of PWID who have once cleared their HCV infection, as re-infections can only be diagnosed by detecting the viral RNA.

From a public health point of view, the most undesirable discordant status is being infected and either not being aware of being infected or believing to be uninfected. This discrepancy between perception and reality limits the access to appropriate health care and may increase the risk of unknowingly transmitting infections. However, the evidence about the association between knowledge of HCV status and risk behaviours in PWID is conflicting. Some longitudinal studies have observed a reduction in risky injecting drug use following notification of HCV-positive status [16, 17], while other studies found either no reduction or even increased risky injection behaviours among PWID receiving a diagnosis of HCV infection [18, 19]. This means that believing to be infected, while actually being uninfected may turn out to become a self-fulfilling prophecy. As mentioned in the results, it was common among both unexposed participants, as well as participants with a cleared infection, to wrongly believe they were currently infected. It might be that those who have been at risk assume they are infected and/or do not believe their test results.

Studying HCV infection status and HCV test status is complicated and not only our study participants, but in our experience also both non-medical and medical staff often had difficulties in distinguishing between the two HCV tests (AB and RNA) and in interpreting the combination of the two test results. Our findings, as are those from other, similar studies, are limited by the lack of clarity regarding HCV test and infection status among both interviewers and respondents. Several qualitative studies among PWID have shown that confusion and uncertainty regarding the meaning of a positive HCV test and HCV risk exist in this group and that HCV is often perceived as an almost inevitable consequence of drug injecting [20–22].

Our data is collected from eight large cities in Germany, but is not likely to be representative for all PWID living in Germany. E.g. our study sample might be more knowledgeable about their infection status than PWID living in smaller cities due to better access to drug user services, testing and treatment in larger cities.

Conclusion

In our study, 17 % of HIV positive PWID and 27 % of those with chronic HCV infection were unaware of their infections. These results indicate that the majority of the study population is aware of their infection status, however still more than a quarter of those with infectious HCV and nearly one in five of HIV infected PWID in our study sample did not know their status, although they were often attached to opioid substitution therapy or other harm reduction services. Not being aware of the infection status implies that they cannot access appropriate health care and they risk unknowingly transmitting the disease to others.

In line with several other studies, we also believe that the quality of post-test counselling is crucial for increasing awareness of infection status as well as for ensuring a positive impact on risk behaviours and ensuring linkage to care and appropriate medical services for both infected and uninfected PWID. In the era of highly effective antiviral HCV-treatment options, the opportunity is there to clear infection in almost all HCV-infected PWID, if infected persons become aware of their status and are linked to care.

Abbreviations

AB, antibodies; DBS, dried blood spots; HCV, Hepatitis C infection; MSM, men who have sex with men; PWID, people who inject drugs; RKI, Robert Koch Institute; UAM, unlinked anonymous monitoring

Acknowledgements

The authors would like to thank all study participants and all staff members of the low-threshold-drug services for the cooperation. During the pilot, Jessica Ackermann, Ewa Bayrambasi, Ulrike Büttner, Sylvia Dziubek, Irina Jakobsche, Britta Krellenberg, Jadwiga Piejek, Anna Metcalf, Silke Saar, and Melanie Schröter gave technical assistance in the laboratory. We are grateful for the excellent technical assistance of Claudia Zymelka, Ute Obst, Sabrina Neumann, Katrin Arndt, Hanno von Spreckelsen, Joana Tziolis, Estelle Kenfack Guepi and Guido Vogt who assisted with the laboratory work for the data collected in the last six study cities. Thanks also to the sequencing service of the RKI (ZBS1) for support of the study: Andreas Nitsche, Julia Tesch and Sylvia Muschter.

We also acknowledge Rieke Barbek, Serdar Danis, Maria Friedrich, Sami Marzougi, Doreen Nitschke, Eva Pedersen, Andrea Teti and Weidong Zhang for their contributions in questionnaire design, logistic assistance, data entry and validation during the study, and Matthias an der Heiden and Ramona Scheufele for giving statistical advice.

*"The DRUCK Study group" includes the following people (all in Germany): Vikas Bapat (Fixpunkt Step Hannover gGmbH; vikas.bapat@step-hannover.de); Johannes Bombeck (Suchthilfe direkt Essen gGmbH; bombeck@suchthilfe-direkt.de); Kerstin Dettmer (Fixpunkt Berlin e.V.; K.Dettmer@fixpunkt.org); Andreas Hecht (Sozialdienst Katholischer Männer e.V.; andreas.hecht@skm-koeln.de); Werner Heinz (Jugendberatung und Jugendhilfe e.V.; werner.heinz@jj-ev.de); Christiane Kerres (Step -Paritätische Gesellschaft für Sozialtherapie und Pädagogik mbH; christiane.kerres@step-hannover.de); Jürgen Klee (Aids-Hilfe Frankfurt e.V.; Juergen.Klee@frankfurt.aidshilfe.de); Astrid Leicht (Fixpunkt Berlin e.V.; A.Leicht@fixpunkt.org); Sylke Léin (Stadt Leipzig, Gesundheitsamt – Suchtbeauftragte; sylke.lein@leipzig.de); Bärbel Marrziniak (Suchthilfe direkt Essen gGmbH; marrziniak@suchthilfe-direkt.de); Olaf Ostermann (Condrobs e.V.; olaf.ostermann@condrobs.de); Prof. Dr. Norbert Scherbaum (Klinik für abhängiges Verhalten und Suchtmedizin, LVR-Klinikum Essen, Kliniken/Institut der Universität Duisburg-Essen; norbert.scherbaum@uni-due.de); Dirk Schäffer (Deutsche Aids-Hilfe e.V.; dirk.schaeffer@dah.aidshilfe.de); Ina Stein (Stadt Leipzig, Gesundheitsamt; ina.stein@leipzig.de); Lutz Wiederanders (Stadt Leipzig, Amt für Jugend, Familie und Bildung – Straßensozialarbeit; lutz.wiederanders@leipzig.de).

Authors' contributions

SN did the analyses and drafted the manuscript together with MG, UM and RZ. RZ and UM designed the study. SN and BW were scientific coordinators of the study during the data collection period. RSR validated laboratory procedures for DBS testing and analysed the samples during the pilot phase of the study in 2011. CK, CTB and NB validated and performed laboratory testing since 2012. The manuscript was critically revised by MG NB, CTB, CK, RSR, NB, BW, VB, UM and RZ. All authors participated in the critical discussion of the results, and contributed to and have approved the final manuscript.

Authors' information

SN is currently a PhD-student at the Charité University Medicine, Berlin, Germany.

Competing interests

All authors declare that they have no competing interest.

Author details

[1]Department for Infectious Disease Epidemiology, Division for HIV/AIDS, STI and Blood-borne Infections, Robert Koch Institute, Berlin, Germany. [2]Charité University Medicine, Berlin, Germany. [3]Department for Infectious Diseases, Division for HIV and other Retroviruses, Robert Koch Institute, Berlin, Germany. [4]Department for Infectious Diseases, Division for Viral Gastroenteritis and Hepatitis Pathogens and Enteroviruses, Robert Koch Institute, Berlin, Germany. [5]Institute of Virology, National Reference Centre for Hepatitis C, University Hospital Essen, University of Duisburg-Essen, Essen, Germany.

References

1. European Monitoring Centre for Drugs and Drug Addiction (EMCDDA). Drug-related infectious diseases in Europe: update from the EMCDDA expert network. Luxembourg: Publications Office of the European Union; 2015.
2. Platt L, Jolley E, Hope V, Latypov A, Vickerman P, Hickson F, Reynolds L, Rhodes T. HIV Epidemics in the European Region: Vulnerability and Response. Washington: Directions in Development–Human Development; 2015.
3. Hope VD, Eramova I, Capurro D, Donoghoe MC. Prevalence and estimation of hepatitis B and C infections in the WHO European Region: a review of data focusing on the countries outside the European Union and the European Free Trade Association. Epidemiol Infect. 2014;142:270–86.
4. Wiessing L, Ferri M, Grady B, Kantzanou M, Sperle I, Cullen KJ, group ED, Hatzakis A, Prins M, Vickerman P, et al. Hepatitis C virus infection epidemiology among people who inject drugs in Europe: a systematic review of data for scaling up treatment and prevention. PLoS One. 2014;9:e103345.
5. Public Health England (PHE). Data tables of the Unlinked Anonymous Monitoring Survey of HIV and Hepatitis in People Who Inject Drugs. London: Public Health England; 2015.
6. Folch C, Casabona J, Espelt A, Majo X, Merono M, Gonzalez V, Wiessing L, Colom J, Brugal MT. High prevalence and incidence of HIV and HCV among new injecting drug users with a large proportion of migrants-is prevention failing? Subst Use Misuse. 2016;51:250–60.
7. Wood E, Milloy MJ, Montaner JSG. HIV treatment as prevention among injection drug users. Current Opinion in HIV and AIDS. 2012;7:151–6.
8. Zimmermann R, Marcus U, Schaffer D, Leicht A, Wenz B, Nielsen S, Santos-Hovener C, Ross RS, Stambouli O, Ratsch BA, et al. A multicentre sero-behavioural survey for hepatitis B and C, HIV and HTLV among people who inject drugs in Germany using respondent driven sampling. BMC Public Health. 2014;14:845.
9. Ross RS, Stambouli O, Gruner N, Marcus U, Cai W, Zhang W, Zimmermann R, Roggendorf M. Detection of infections with hepatitis B virus, hepatitis C virus, and human immunodeficiency virus by analyses of dried blood spots-performance characteristics of the ARCHITECT system and two commercial assays for nucleic acid amplification. Virol J. 2013;10:72.
10. Sample Questionnaire used for the DRUCK Studie [in German] [http://www.rki.de/DE/Content/InfAZ/H/HIVAIDS/Studien/DRUCK-Studie/Fragebogen_Muster.pdf?__blob=publicationFile].
11. Robert Koch Institut (RKI). Schätzung der Prävalenz und Inzidenz von HIV-Infektionen in Deutschland, Stande Ende 2014. EpiBull. 2015;45:475–90.
12. O'Keefe D, Aitken C, Higgs P, Dietze P. Concordance between self-reported and actual hepatitis C virus infection status in a cohort of people who inject drugs. Drug and alcohol review. 2013;32:208–10.
13. Brouard C, Le Strat Y, Larsen C, Jauffret-Roustide M, Lot F, Pillonel J. he undiagnosed chronically-infected HCV population in France. Implications for expanded testing recommendations in 2014. PLoS One. 2015;10:e0126920.
14. Weill-Barilet L, Pillonel J, Semaille C, Léon L, Le Strat Y, Pascal X, Barin F, Jauffret.Roustide M: Hepatitis C virus and HIV seroprevalences, sociodemographic characteristics, behaviors and access to syringes among drug users, a comparison of geographical areas in France, ANRS-Coquelicot 2011 survey. Rev Epidemiol Sante Publique 2016. http://dx.doi.org/10.1016/j.respe.2015.10.003.
15. Hahne SJ, Veldhuijzen IK, Wiessing L, Lim TA, Salminen M, Laar M. Infection with hepatitis B and C virus in Europe: a systematic review of prevalence and cost-effectiveness of screening. BMC Infect Dis. 2013;13:181.

16. Bruneau J, Zang G, Abrahamowicz M, Jutras-Aswad D, Daniel M, Roy E. Sustained drug use changes after hepatitis C screening and counseling among recently infected persons who inject drugs: a longitudinal study. Clin Infect Dis. 2014;58:755–61.
17. Aspinall EJ, Weir A, Sacks-Davis R, Spelman T, Grebely J, Higgs P, Hutchinson SJ, Hellard ME. Does informing people who inject drugs of their hepatitis C status influence their injecting behaviour? Analysis of the Networks II study. Int J Drug Policy. 2014;25:179–82.
18. Spelman T, Morris MD, Zang G, Rice T, Page K, Maher L, Lloyd A, Grebely J, Dore GJ, Kim AY, et al. A longitudinal study of hepatitis C virus testing and infection status notification on behaviour change in people who inject drugs. J Epidemiol Community Health. 2015;69:745–52.
19. Korthuis PT, Feaster DJ, Gomez ZL, Das M, Tross S, Wiest K, Douaihy A, Mandler RN, Sorensen JL, Colfax G, et al. Injection behaviors among injection drug users in treatment: the role of hepatitis C awareness. Addict Behav. 2012;37:552–5.
20. Jones L, Atkinson A, Bates G, McCoy E, Porcellato L, Beynon C, McVeigh J, Bellis MA. Views and experiences of hepatitis C testing and diagnosis among people who inject drugs: systematic review of qualitative research. Int J Drug Policy. 2014;25:204–11.
21. Rhodes T, Davis M, Judd A. Hepatitis C and its risk management among drug injectors in London: Renewing harm reduction in the context of uncertainty. Addiction. 2004;99:621–33.
22. Jordan AE, Masson CL, Mateu-Gelabert P, McKnight C, Pepper N, Bouche K, Guzman L, Kletter E, Seewald RM, Des-Jarlais DC, et al. Perceptions of drug users regarding hepatitis C screening and care: a qualitative study. Harm Reduct J. 2013;10:10.

3

Coverage of different health insurance programs and medical costs associated with chronic hepatitis C infection

Hai-yang Zhou[1], Shuang Liu[2], Su-jun Zheng[2], Xiao-xia Peng[3], Yu Chen[2], Carol Duan[1], Qing-fen Zheng[2,4], Zhao Wang[1] and Zhong-ping Duan[2*]

Abstract

Background: Hepatitis C virus (HCV) imposes a considerable disease burden in China, with at least 10 million people chronically infected. Little is known about the financial impact of the HCV epidemic, nor about the extent to which various forms of insurance are providing HCV patients with financial protection. A cross-sectional multi-site study was conducted to acquire data that will aid policy-makers and other stakeholders in developing effective strategies to address this situation.

Methods: At 29 hospitals across China, inpatients and outpatients with chronic HCV were surveyed about their insurance coverage and medical costs. Percentages, means and medians were calculated, and differences in continuous variables among multiple groups were analyzed using the Kruskal-Wallis test or Wilcoxon two-sample test.

Results: Many inpatients ($N = 593$) and outpatients ($N = 523$) reported being covered by one of three major types of government health insurance, but 13 % of inpatients and 43 % of outpatients reported having no insurance. Among inpatients, the total median cost per hospitalization per patient was 8212 Renminbi (RMB). The category of expenditure with the highest median cost per hospitalization was Western medicine, followed by lab tests and Chinese medicine. The median cost per hospitalization was far higher for patients who had hepatocellular carcinoma than for those with less severe forms of liver disease. Outpatient antiviral therapy costs ranged from a median of 377 RMB for ribavirin to a median of 37,400 RMB for pegylated interferon-alpha for up to one year of treatment.

Conclusions: For uninsured chronic HCV patients in China, inpatient and outpatient costs may be financially devastating. Research is needed on how different approaches to financing HCV treatment and care might improve health outcomes as well as achieve cost savings by enabling more people to be cured of HCV.

Keywords: Medical costs, Chronic HCV infection, Coverage of health insurance, Mainland China

* Correspondence: duan2517@163.com
[2]Beijing Youan Hospital, Capital Medical University, Beijing, China
Full list of author information is available at the end of the article

Background

In China, chronic hepatitis C virus (HCV) infection is increasingly recognized as a public health problem that has major consequences for individuals, families and society in general. At least 10 million people in mainland China are chronically infected with HCV [1–3], and annual HCV incidence has increased considerably in recent years [4]. Chronic hepatitis C infection is one of the leading causes of cirrhosis and hepatocellular carcinoma (HCC). Usually, 10 to 15 % of HCV-infected patients are expected to develop cirrhosis, and the risk of HCC in persons with cirrhosis is approximately 2–4 % per year [5, 6]. Therefore China is thought to have a considerable burden of HCV-associated cirrhosis and HCC.

Hepatitis C is a curable disease [6, 7], and advances in HCV therapy have resulted in steadily higher cure rates. New direct-acting antivirals (DAAs) represent a major breakthrough in the treatment of HCV infection, but these drugs are not generally available in mainland China. Currently either interferon or peg-interferon (PEG-IFN) combined with ribavirin (RBV) is still the first-line HCV treatment in China [4, 5]. The use of PEG-IFN/RBV has resulted in sustained viral response rates ranging from 44 to 83 % in a number of Chinese studies [4], representing somewhat better outcomes than those observed worldwide for PEG-IFN/RBV. While PEG-IFN/RBV is much cheaper than the DAA regimens, the cost of PEG-IFN/RBV still imposes a heavy financial burden on many HCV patients in China.

The Chinese health system incorporates multiple types of insurance that offset medical costs for covered individuals, although a lack of comprehensive national data makes it difficult to determine the extent to which people are utilizing different types of insurance to meet their health needs. Major categories of insurance include the government employee program; government public program for urban areas; government public program for rural areas; commercial health insurance; and government-provided catastrophic health insurance. The government employee program, which is provided by the national government, is only for civil servants who are national or local government employees. The government public program for urban areas is provided by the national government for urban residents, and the insured individual must submit an annual co-pay. The government public program for rural areas is offered to farmers by national and local governments, and farmers also have a co-pay. Commercial health insurance, provided by private insurance companies, is available to anyone who meets the specified requirements. Catastrophic health insurance provided by the national government is a kind of supplementary insurance for basic national health insurance plans including the government employee program, government public program for urban areas, and government public program for rural areas. If the patient suffers from a life-threatening or highly debilitating disease, or if medical expenses exceed the limitation of the basic national health insurance coverage, the additional amount will be paid through catastrophic medical insurance. There are other types of insurance for populations such as military personnel and college students. Some people do not purchase any government or private health insurance, and thus are responsible for meeting all of their health care costs.

The financial impact of the HCV epidemic in China is not well known. This evidence gap threatens to undermine efforts to develop strategies that will improve outcomes for HCV patients. In this study, we conducted cross-sectional multisite surveys of outpatients and inpatients with chronic HCV infection. Our purpose was to acquire data that will guide policy-makers and other relevant stakeholders in making decisions that will contribute to reducing the burden of HCV disease in China.

Methods

Study population

China is a very large country with many different regions and with different levels of development across regions. In an effort to reflect the overall national situation, we conducted a cross-sectional survey at 29 hospitals in 20 provinces in all regions of China (North, Northeast, East, Middle, South and Northwest) (Fig. 1). Sixteen of the 29 participating hospitals were tertiary hospitals and 13 were secondary hospitals. The 29 hospitals included 11 infectious disease specialty hospitals.

Inpatients and outpatients with a diagnosis of chronic hepatitis C were eligible to participate in the study if they were at least 18 years old and if they had tested serum-positive for anti-HCV Ab or HCV-RNA (confirmed by either HCV-RNA quantitative real-time PCR test or qualitative test) at least six months before study enrollment. Inpatients had undergone at least one hospital admission. Outpatients were only eligible to participate in the study if they had been seen for at least one year at the hospital where study enrollment was taking place. Patients were excluded from study participation if they had HIV, other forms of viral hepatitis, cancer, cardiovascular disease or other serious health conditions; if they had underlying liver disease due to other factors such as autoimmune factors, alcohol consumption or drug use; or if they were pregnant or breastfeeding. Hepatocellular carcinoma was regarded differently since it was a condition of interest for investigators, and having HCC did not disqualify patients from study participation.

Data collection

To ensure consistency in how data were collected, the principal investigators from all study sites underwent training at Beijing Youan Hospital before study enrollment

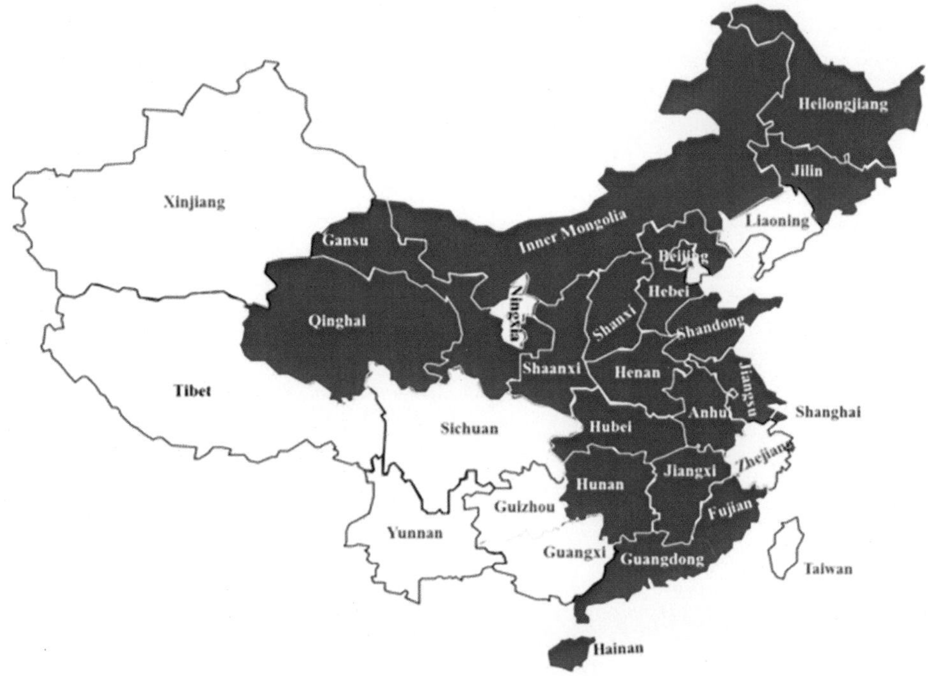

Fig. 1 Geographic distribution of participating hospitals. Legend: Provinces with hospitals that participated in the study appear in blue

began. The training curriculum explained the inclusion and exclusion criterion, as well as introducing standard procedures for how to communicate with patients and how to instruct them to complete the study questionnaires. Each site was asked to enroll 40 to 45 individuals, including at least 20 inpatients and 20 outpatients. Sites stopped enrolling new study participants when they reached this target. Outpatients completed questionnaires in the waiting room of the outpatient department. Inpatients completed questionnaires in a quiet room in the inpatient department. Physicians provided in-person instruction to patients regarding how to complete the questionnaires. Data collection took place from 1 May to 31 December 2011. During this time, a designated clinical associate from Beijing Youan Hospital was charged with responding immediately to questions from the study sites.

Different questionnaires were used for outpatients and inpatients. Both questionnaires included the same four sections. The first section asked for the patient's name and for demographic information such as age, sex and place of residence. The second section addressed the patient's general condition, including the following information: the age when he or she was diagnosed with hepatitis C; insurance status; disease stage; disease complications; and time of hospitalization. The third section asked about the patient's treatment history, including whether the patient received antiviral therapy; the names of antiviral medications; whether therapy to protect liver function was received; and whether traditional Chinese medicines were utilized. The fourth section collected information about various medical costs. Inpatients were asked about costs per hospitalization, including the cost of Western medication, traditional Chinese medicine, laboratory tests, bed charges and nursing. For HCC patients, additional questions were asked about the costs of HCC-specific treatment and HCC-related surgery. For outpatients, antiviral treatment costs were requested.

The questionnaire was designed in the Chinese language. All questions were expressed in short simple sentences such as "Where do you come from?" and "How old are you?". Study investigators explained questions to patients who could not read. After each patient completed his or her questionnaire, the answers were checked against the patient's medical records for accuracy. If differences were identified, the information in the medical record was used. Data management was performed by a professional statistician to ensure the soundness of the data.

Study participants were categorized according to disease severity using the following criteria. People who had chronic HCV but did not have a diagnosis of either cirrhosis or HCC were designated as "chronic HCV, no cirrhosis or HCC". The diagnosis of chronic hepatitis C was based on the criteria used by the Chinese Society of Hepatology and the American Association for the Study of Liver Diseases (AASLD) [5, 8]. People who had been diagnosed with cirrhosis via liver biopsy or imaging but did not have a diagnosis of HCC were "chronic HCV plus cirrhosis". People who had been diagnosed with

HCC, including those with and without a diagnosis of cirrhosis, were "chronic HCV plus HCC". The diagnosis of HCC was based on AASLD guidance and utilized radiology, AFP serology, and/or biopsy [9].

Data analysis

Statistical analysis was performed using IBM SPSS Statistics for Windows, version 19.0 (IBM Corp, Armonk, NY, USA). Data were expressed as the mean (standard deviation), median or number (percentage). If the data had non-normal distributions, differences in continuous variables among multiple groups were analyzed using the Kruskal-Wallis Test or Wilcoxon Two-Sample Test between two groups. A two-sided p-value of <0.05 was considered statistically significant. For the comparison of inpatient costs by type of insurance, four categories were used: one for no insurance and the other three for the three types of insurance that cover nearly 85 % of Chinese citizens: government employee program, government urban public program and government rural public program [10].

Research ethics

The study protocol was approved by the Institutional Review Board of Beijing Youan Hospital, Capital Medical University and the study was performed in accordance with the provisions of the Declaration of Helsinki 1975 and its revision. Written informed consent was obtained from all study participants. Personal information collected by investigators was only used for study purposes. Data were managed using identification numbers that were assigned to protect the privacy of study participants.

Results

Among 1149 questionnaires submitted, 1116 (97.1 %) fulfilled data collection requirements (593 from inpatients and 523 from outpatients). Fifty-three percent of these 1116 respondents were male and 47 % were female. More than 90 % of respondents were aged 30 or older. A higher number of outpatients than inpatients were younger than 30 years, while more inpatients than outpatients were older than 60 years. An average of 18 months had elapsed from the first confirmed diagnosis of HCV infection to the time of study enrollment (Table 1).

Health insurance coverage

Compared with outpatients, more inpatients were covered by the government public programs for urban and rural health (46.4 % versus 30.0 % and 25.6 % versus 12.4 %, respectively). Up to 43.0 % of all outpatients reported paying for medical expenses on their own, while

Table 1 Sociodemographic characteristics of study participants

		Total patients ($n = 1116$)	Inpatients ($n = 593$)	Outpatients ($n = 523$)
Gender (%)	Female	529 (47.4)	276 (46.5)	253 (48.4)
	Male	587 (52.6)	317 (53.5)	270 (51.6)
Age, mean (standard deviation)		47.5 (13.1)	49.1 (12.8)	45.5 (13.3)
Age, median (P25, P75)		48.00 (39,57)	48.0 (40,58)	46.00 (37, 55)
Age, range (minimum, maximum)		68 (18,86)	68 (18,86)	65 (18, 83)
Age, n/%	<30	109 (9.8)	39 (6.9)	70 (13.4)
	30–39	196 (17.6)	97 (16.4)	99 (18.9)
	40–49	334 (29.9)	178 (30.0)	156 (29.8)
	50–59	278 (24.9)	153 (25.8)	125 (23.9)
	60–69	148 (13.3)	96 (16.2)	52 (9.9)
	≥70	51 (4.5)	30 (5.1)	21 (4.0)
Months elapsed since diagnosis, mean (standard deviation)		35.5 (47.9)	34.0 (47. 6)	37.4 (48.4)
Months elapsed since diagnosis, median (P25, P75)		18.0 (11.0, 38.0)	18.0 (8.0, 37.3)	22.0 (12.0,39.0)
Months elapsed since diagnosis, range (minimum, maximum)		333.0 (0.0, 333.0)	325.0 (0.0, 325.0)	333.0 (0.0, 333.0)
Region, n/%	North	201 (18.0)	109 (18.4)	92 (17.6)
	Northeast	96 (8.6)	54 (9.1)	42 (8.0)
	East	304 (27.2)	158 (26.6)	146 (27.9)
	Middle	283 (25.4)	141 (23.8)	142 (27.1)
	South	81 (7.3)	40 (6.7)	41 (7.8)
	Northwest	151 (13.5)	91 (15.3)	60 (11.5)

only 13.3 % of all inpatients reported paying on their own. (Table 2).

Inpatient cost per hospitalization and major categories of expenditure

The total median cost for hospitalization per time per patient was 8212 RMB. While Western medicine was the category of expenditure with the highest median cost (4701 RMB), mean costs for lab tests and Chinese medicine both exceeded 1000 RMB (Table 3). Since traditional Chinese medicine has been in existence for thousands of years, it is worth noting that the mean cost of Chinese medicine was about 8 % of the total cost of hospitalization.

Inpatient costs by type of insurance

We further analyzed inpatient medical costs per time per person by comparing inpatients with insurance coverage through the government employee program to those covered through the government urban public program and government rural public program, as well as those who were uninsured. The median total cost per hospitalization before insurance payout was 12,117 RMB for patients in the government employee program, 9535 RMB for patients in the government urban public program and 6340 RMB for patients in the government rural public program. Patients without insurance reported a median total cost per hospitalization of 6937 RMB. The differences were statistically significant ($X^2 = 41.27, p < 0.0001$) (Table 4).

Relationship between cost of hospitalization and level of hospital

Two hundred and sixty-four inpatients (44.5 %) were treated in secondary hospitals and 329 (55.5 %) were treated in tertiary hospitals. The median total cost of one hospitalization per time per patient in RMB was significantly higher in tertiary hospitals than in secondary hospitals (9778 vs 6780) ($p < 0.0001$) (Table 5).

Table 2 Health insurance coverage

	Inpatients ($n = 593$)		Outpatients ($n = 523$)	
	N	(%)	N	(%)
Government employee program (total)	75	12.7	73	14.0
With catastrophic health insurance	(2)			
Government public program, urban (total)	275	46.4	157	30.0
With catastrophic health insurance	(1)		(5)	
With commercial health insurance	(1)		(2)	
Government public program, rural (total)	152	25.6	65	12.4
With commercial health insurance	(2)			
With catastrophic health insurance	(1)			
Other types of health insurance	12	2.0	3	0.6
Uninsured	79	13.3	225	43.0

Table 3 Inpatient costs, total and by category of expenditure (in Renminbi)

	N	Mean cost	Standard deviation	Median cost	P25	P75
Total	593	12,720	14,595	8212	5098	15,358
Western medicine	577	8255	11,192	4701	2539	9610
Lab tests	569	1574	1386	1302	709	1977
Chinese medicine	245	1038	2861	314	120	812

Hospitalization expenses in relation to disease stage

Inpatient costs were assessed by disease stage, with patients classified as "chronic HCV, no cirrhosis or HCC", "chronic HCV plus cirrhosis" or "chronic HCV plus HCC". The median total cost increased significantly with the severity of the disease stage, from 8112 RMB to 8399 RMB to 14,425 RMB (p = 0.0353) (Table 6).

Outpatient expenses for antiviral therapy

Among the 404 outpatients who had received antiviral therapy, the following median costs were reported for a treatment duration of up to one year: 37,400 RMB for pegylated interferon-alpha ($N = 197$), 6798 RMB for interferon-alpha (N =185) and 377 RMB for ribavirin ($N = 341$) (Table 7).

Discussion

To our knowledge, this is the first study to examine medical costs associated with management of chronic HCV infection in mainland China. Although fairly high proportions of both inpatients and outpatients reported being covered by one of China's three major types of government health insurance, 13 % of inpatients and 43 % of outpatients reported having no insurance. Among inpatients, the total median cost per hospitalization per patient was 8212 RMB. The category of expenditure with the highest median cost per hospitalization was Western medicine, followed by lab tests

Table 4 Inpatient costs by type of insurance (in Renminbi)

	N	Median cost	P25	P75	X^2	P value*
Government employee program	67[a]	12,117	7531	17,989	41.27	<0.0001
Government urban public program	274[b]	9535	5623	16,667		
Government rural public program	152	6340	4262	9056		
Uninsured population	83[c]	6937	5061	18,273		

*The Kruskal-Wallis test was used for comparisons
[a]8 responses were excluded from analysis because the information was incomplete or implausible
[b]1 response was excluded from analysis because the information was incomplete or implausible
[c]25 responses were excluded from analysis because the information was incomplete or implausible

Table 5 Hospitalization expenses and level of hospital (in Renminbi)

	N	Mean cost	Standard deviation	Median cost	P25	P75	Z*	*P* value*
Secondary Hospitals	264	10,268	11,181	6780	4016	12,196	−5.7639	<0.0001
Tertiary Hospitals	329	14,687	16,599	9778	6075	17,633		

*The Wilcoxon Two-Sample Test was used for comparisons

and Chinese medicine. The median cost per hospitalization was much higher for patients who had hepatocellular carcinoma than for those with less severe forms of liver disease. Additionally, outpatients reported high costs for antiviral drugs.

Beginning in the late 1990s, the Chinese government implemented a series of reforms for the purpose of making health care more affordable, but it is not clear whether the intended benifits are being realized [11, 12]. Our study of chronic HCV patients found that even while study participants reported utilizing all three major types of government health insurance, a high proportion of patients had no insurance of any kind. The impact of this situation on individual and household financial well-being may be devastating in light of the high costs associated with HCV disease.

The median cost per hospitalization for uninsured inpatients in our study was reported to be almost 7000 RMB. Although this study did not disaggregate outpatient antiviral therapy costs by insurance status, the fact that more than two in five outpatients were uninsured suggests that a considerable number of people paid out-of-pocket for pegylated interferon-alpha, interferon alpha and ribavirin. The median costs reported for these medicines were 37,400 RMB, 6798 RMB and 377 RMB respectively. To put these inpatient and outpatient costs in context, China had an annual per-capita income of 23,979 RMB in cities and towns in 2011, while the annual per-capita income for rural residents was 6977 RMB [13]. Thus it would be unsurprising for a single hospitalization to consume one-third of an uninsured urban HCV patient's annual income or the entirety of an uninsured rural HCV patient's annual income. The costs of the PEG-IFN/RBV and IFN/RBV regimens for outpatients are also far out of proportion to what the average Chinese person earns.

Insurance coverage gaps for HCV patients may also have grave implications for patient outcomes. In our study, the median inpatient cost per hospitalization for uninsured patients was 6937 RMB – slightly more than the median for patients covered by the government rural public insurance program. In contrast, median costs per hospitalization were more than 9500 RMB and more than 12,000 RMB for inpatients covered by the government employee insurance program and government urban public insurance program respectively. While this difference might be attributable to multiple reasons, one troubling possibility is that uninsured inpatients are receiving less of the health care services that they need because of perceived or actual inability to pay. The finding thus points to an important issue that warrants further attention from Chinese researchers and policy-makers. Research elsewhere has directly assessed the health consequences of a lack of insurance for HCV patients. A recent study by Younossi et al. reported that during the years 2005 to 2009, uninsured HCV patients in the United States had a 49 to 72 % greater chance of dying during a hospitalization than HCV patients who had insurance [14] .

Our analysis of the cost of hospitalization in relation to HCV disease stage indicated that a hospitalization for an HCV patient with hepatocellular carcinoma was typically far more costly than a hospitalization for an HCV patient who did not have HCC. Research from Canada and the United States also has found higher costs to be associated with more advanced HCV disease stage. A Canadian study that utilized modeling data for the estimated national population of HCV-infected people projected increasingly higher lifetime HCV costs for patients at more advanced disease stages [15]. In a large US cohort, chronic HCV patients with end-stage liver disease had far higher all-cause health care costs than chronic HCV patients with noncirrhotic liver disease or those with compensated cirrhosis. Approximately half of costs were HCV-related, with a higher proportion of HCV-related costs concentrated among patients with end-stage liver disease [16].

While this relationship between cost and disease stage is not unexpected, it bears emphasizing in light of the

Table 6 Inpatient costs by disease stage (in Renminbi)

	N	Median	P25	P75	X^2	P*
Chronic HCV, no cirrhosis or HCC	485	8112	5144	15,344	6.685	0.0353
Chronic HCV plus cirrhosis	95	8399	4746	15,004.0		
Chronic HCV plus HCC	13	14,425	14,114	25,995		

*The Kruskal-Wallis test was used for comparisons

Table 7 Outpatient antiviral therapy costs (in Renminbi)[a]

	N	Mean	Standard deviation	Median	P25	P75
Pegylated interferon-alpha	197	37,968	22,182	37,400	17,550	59,424
Interferon-alpha	185	7256	6397	6798	2790	9877
Ribavirin	341	643	1055	377	172	660

[a]The amount attributed to each antiviral drug was for up to one year of treatment

fact that HCV is a curable disease. The cost of providing treatment to chronic HCV patients in China may be well less than the cost of managing patients with untreated chronic HCV, and research is urgently needed to explore cost-benefit dynamics in the Chinese context. A US study quantified the direct economic burden of HCV infection and PEG-IFN/RBV treatment for HCV from 2002 to 2007, and found that PEG/IFN-RBV-treated patients had higher total direct medical costs than untreated HCV patients (US $28,547 vs. US $21,752; $P < 0.001$) [17]. Other research has found that despite the high cost of antiviral treatment, compared to discontinued therapy patients, chronic hepatitis C patients who completed interferon therapy and presumably had a higher rate of achieving sustained viral response were found to have lower levels of healthcare resource utilization and costs post-therapy [18]. Also, Federico et al. [19] showed that Canadian patients who had cleared the virus had the lowest time and out-of-pocket costs. Thus it seems feasible that increasing the use of antiviral therapy for HCV in China can reduce the overall economic burden in addition to improving health outcomes, and it is important for policy-makers to explore the potential for expansions in insurance coverage to contribute to overall financial gains in this regard.

This study has some limitations. First it is a cross-sectional investigation which does not reflect the dynamic changes in medical costs for all HCV patients. Second, the sample size is not large enough. A larger investigation needs to be conducted to acquire a more comprehensive dataset that can reliably guide health policy decision-making. Finally, there might be some recall bias in this study, such as the exact time of HCV diagnosis. Since we investigated outpatient medical cost within one year and per hospitalization cost, we consider it played a minor impact on the analysis of medical costs.

Conclusions

For uninsured chronic HCV patients in China, inpatient and outpatient costs may be financially devastating. Chinese policy-makers need a better knowledge base in order to develop informed strategies for expanding insurance coverage. Research is needed on how different approaches to financing HCV treatment and care might improve health outcomes as well as achieve cost savings by enabling more people to be cured of HCV.

Abbreviations

AASLD: American association for the study of liver diseases; DAAs: direct-acting antivirals; HCC: hepatocellular carcinoma; HCV: hepatitis C virus; PEG-IFN: peg-interferon; RBV: Ribavirin; RMB: Renminbi.

Competing interests

The authors declare that they have no competing interests.

Authors' contributions

HYZ, SJZ and SL participated in the design of the study and drafted the manuscript. QFZ, YC, and CD collected the data. XXP performed the statistical analysis. ZPD and ZW conceived the study and participated in its design and coordination. All authors read and approved the final manuscript.

Acknowledgements

We thank all health workers from the 29 study sites for donating much time to this investigation.

Funding

This work was supported by the Bristol-Myers Squibb Foundation.

Author details

[1]Wu Jieping Medical Foundation, Beijing, China. [2]Beijing Youan Hospital, Capital Medical University, Beijing, China. [3]Department of Epidemiology and Biostatistics, School of Public Health and Family Medicine, Capital Medical University, Beijing, China. [4]Department of Gastroenterology, The First Affiliated Hospital of Zhengzhou University, Zhengzhou, China.

References

1. Sievert W, Altraif I, Razavi HA, Abdo A, Ahmed EA, Alomair A, et al. A systematic review of hepatitis C virus epidemiology in Asia, Australia and Egypt. Liver Int. 2011;31 Suppl 2:61–80. doi:10.1111/j.1478-3231.2011.02540.x.
2. Wang FS, Fan JG, Zhang Z, Gao B, Wang HY. The global burden of liver disease: the major impact of China. Hepatology. 2014;60(6):2099–108. doi:10.1002/hep.27406.
3. Gower E, Estes C, Blach S, Razavi-Shearer K, Razavi H. Global epidemiology and genotype distribution of the hepatitis C virus infection. J Hepatol. 2014;61(1 Suppl):S45–57. doi:10.1016/j.jhep.2014.07.027.
4. Duan Z, Jia JD, Hou J, Lou L, Tobias H, Xu XY, et al. Current challenges and the management of chronic hepatitis C in mainland China. J Clin Gastroenterol. 2014;48(8):679–86. doi:10.1097/mcg.0000000000000109.
5. The Chinese medical association of liver branch idapeboCma. Guidelines on the management of hepatitis C. Chin J Hepatol. 2004;12(1674–7380):194–8.
6. World Health Organization. Guidelines for the screening, care and treatment of persons with hepatitis C infection. 2014.
7. Hepatitis C guidance. AASLD-IDSA recommendations for testing, managing, and treating adults infected with hepatitis C virus. Hepatology. 2015;62(3):932–54. doi:10.1002/hep.27950.
8. Ghany MG, Strader DB, Thomas DL, Seeff LB. Diagnosis, management, and treatment of hepatitis C: an update. Hepatology. 2009;49(4):1335–74. doi:10.1002/hep.22759.
9. Bruix J, Sherman M. Management of hepatocellular carcinoma: an update. Hepatology. 2011;53(3):1020–2. doi:10.1002/hep.24199.
10. Wang Z, Zhang Y, Xiong F, Li H, Ding Y, Gao Y, et al. Association between medical insurance type and survival in patients undergoing peritoneal dialysis. BMC Nephrol. 2015;16:33. doi:10.1186/s12882-015-0023-7.
11. Zhang L, Liu N. Health reform and out-of-pocket payments: lessons from China. Health Policy Plan. 2014;29(2):217–26. doi:10.1093/heapol/czt006.
12. Long Q, Xu L, Bekedam H, Tang S. Changes in health expenditures in China in 2000s: has the health system reform improved affordability. Int J Equity Health. 2013;12:40. doi:10.1186/1475-9276-12-40.
13. China NBoSotPsPo. Chinese economy continues to maintain steady and rapid development in 2011. 2011. http://www.stats.gov.cn/tjsj/zxfb/201201/t20120117_12777.html. Accessed January 17, 2012.
14. Younossi ZM, Otgonsuren M, Henry L, Arsalla Z, Stepnaova M, Mishra A, et al. Inpatient resource utilization, disease severity, mortality and insurance coverage for patients hospitalized for hepatitis C virus in the United States. J Viral Hepat. 2015;22(2):137–45. doi:10.1111/jvh.12262.
15. Myers RP, Krajden M, Bilodeau M, Kaita K, Marotta P, Peltekian K, et al. Burden of disease and cost of chronic hepatitis C infection in Canada. Can J Gastroenterol Hepatol. 2014;28(5):243–50.
16. Gordon SC, Pockros PJ, Terrault NA, Hoop RS, Buikema A, Nerenz D, et al. Impact of disease severity on healthcare costs in patients with chronic hepatitis C (CHC) virus infection. Hepatology. 2012;56(5):1651–60. doi:10.1002/hep.25842.
17. Solomon M, Bonafede M, Pan K, Wilson K, Beam C, Chakravarti P, et al. Direct medical care costs among pegylated interferon plus ribavirin-treated and untreated chronic hepatitis C patients. Dig Dis Sci. 2011;56(10):3024–31. doi:10.1007/s10620-011-1802-z.

4

Urgent action to fight hepatitis C in people who inject drugs

John F. Dillon[1*], Jeffrey V. Lazarus[2] and Homie A. Razavi[3]

Abstract

Hepatitis C virus (HCV) infection is a leading cause of liver cirrhosis and liver cancer, is curable in most people. Injecting drug use currently accounts for 80 % of new HCV infections with a known transmission route in the European Union (EU). HCV has generally received little attention from the public or policymakers in the EU, with major gaps in national-level strategies, action plans, guidelines and the evidence base. Specifically, people who inject drugs (PWID) are often excluded from treatment owing to various patient, healthcare provider and health system factors.

All policymakers responsible for health services in EU countries should ensure that prevention, treatment, care and support interventions addressing HCV in PWID are developed and implemented. According to current best practice, PWID should have access to comprehensive, evidence-based multiprofessional harm reduction (especially opioid substitution therapy and clean needles and syringes) and support/care services based in the community and modified with community involvement to accommodate this hard-to-reach population. Other recommended components of care include vaccination against hepatitis B and other infections; peer support interventions; HIV testing, prevention and treatment; drug and alcohol services; psychological care as needed; and social support services. HCV testing should be performed regularly in PWID to identify infected persons and engage them in care. HCV-infected PWID should be considered for antiviral treatment (based on an individualised assessment and delivered within multidisciplinary care/support programmes) both to cure infected individuals and prevent onward transmission. Modelling data suggest that the HCV disease burden can only be cut substantially if antiviral treatment is scaled up together with prevention programmes. Measures should be taken to reduce stigma and discrimination against PWID at the provider and institutional levels.

In conclusion, strategic action at the policy level is urgently needed to increase access to HCV prevention, testing and treatment among PWID, the group at highest risk of HCV infection. Such action has the potential to substantially reduce the number of infected persons, along with the disease burden and related care costs.

Keywords: Antiviral therapy, Harm reduction, Hepatitis C, People who inject drugs, Risk reduction behaviour

Background

According to the World Health Organization (WHO), 14 million people in the European Region are chronically infected with hepatitis C virus (HCV), a blood-borne infection of the liver [1]. Another recent study has estimated that there are 3.6 million people with viraemic HCV infections in the EU [2]. HCV is a leading cause of liver cirrhosis and liver cancer and around 70,500 infected people die each year in the European Union as a result of these complications [3]. Without action, the burden of HCV disease is expected to rise in the coming years owing to the ageing of the infected population, ongoing new infections and low levels of treatment uptake [4–6]. For example, the number of HCV-related cirrhosis cases in England is expected to increase by 50 % by 2030, while HCV-related deaths will almost double [4].

Injecting drug use currently accounts for 80 % of new HCV infections in the European Union with a known transmission route [7]. Globally, two out of three people who inject drugs (PWID) have HCV infection [8], with rates in European Union countries varying between 14 % and 84 % [9]. However, HCV remains a hidden epidemic. A pooled analysis of data from studies in Denmark, France, Poland, Spain and the United Kingdom estimated

* Correspondence: j.f.dillon@dundee.ac.uk
[1]Division of Molecular and Clinical Medicine, School of Medicine, University of Dundee, Ninewells Hospital, Dundee, UK
Full list of author information is available at the end of the article

that a median of 49 % of HCV-infected PWID were undiagnosed (range: 24–76 %) [10]. HCV is transmitted more easily than HIV and globally there are more than three times as many PWID infected with HCV than with HIV [8]. When formulating strategies to address the problem of HCV infection, especially if considering treatment as prevention strategies, it is important to differentiate between individuals who are currently active drug injectors and those who are former injectors. In addition, among active injecting drug users, it is important to distinguish between those who share injecting equipment and those who do not. HCV is spread between PWID primarily by the sharing of injection equipment and thus the vast majority of new infections occurs in active injectors who share.

The window of opportunity for HCV prevention is narrow, as infection is likely to occur soon after initiation of injection drug use. The time to infection is shortest among individuals with many contacts within their network of drug users and among those who inject most frequently [11]. Furthermore, the incidence of infection is highest among individuals who do not utilise existing harm reduction services such as opioid substitution therapy (OST) and sterile needle and syringe programmes (NSP). HCV in PWID is preventable and curable, and therefore efforts to reduce the incidence and transmission of HCV infection must aim to increase access to testing, risk reduction and treatment in this population, with a strong focus on active injectors. Treatment with antiviral medicines is as effective in PWID as in non-drug users [12], and guidelines published by international and European organisations identify the prevention and treatment of HCV among PWID as major components of protecting the public from blood-borne viruses [13–16].

The European Commission recognises PWID as a key target group in its ongoing activities to address blood-borne viruses, and in October 2015 it launched a three-year Joint Action that engaged representatives of 18 Member States in efforts to intensify the response to HIV and viral hepatitis among PWID [17] and followed this up with a second Joint Action on these issues in 2016. However, considering the extent of the public health threat, HCV has generally received little attention from the public or policymakers in the European Union, with major gaps in international and national-level strategies, action plans, guidelines and in the evidence base more generally [10, 18–20]. This paper discusses barriers to improving HCV care for PWID and current best practices in HCV prevention, diagnosis and treatment in PWID in the context of recent data and relevant policy initiatives. It concludes by making policy recommendations to address unmet needs in PWID and thereby strengthen the response to HCV in the European Union.

Barriers to improving HCV care for PWID

A recent study of the EU countries found an overall diagnosis rate for HCV infection of 33 % and a treatment rate of 3.7 % [2]. Median treatment rates specifically among diagnosed PWID have been estimated at around 10–30 % [10, 21], but this masks wide variation within and between countries and of course many PWID are not even diagnosed. A study of seven sites in the UK found that treatment rates among PWID varied from <5 to >25 per 1000 PWID [22]. Of course, many more PWID are not even diagnosed. Access to prevention, testing and treatment is even more limited in prisons than in the community, despite high rates of HCV in the prison population internationally [23, 24] as well as legal and human rights obligations for governments to provide health care to prison inmates.

A fundamental dilemma is that PWID, in whom HCV infection is most common and in whom treatment to prevent onward transmission is particularly important, are generally difficult to engage in formal healthcare services. PWID are often wrongly excluded from treatment, and uptake rates are low even where treatment is offered. The main barriers to PWID accessing care for HCV include [21, 25–28]:

- *Patient-related factors*, such as lack of awareness of diagnosis or HCV status; limited knowledge or negative perceptions of HCV and how it is treated; low levels of health literacy; negative relations with the healthcare system, including fear of or experience of stigmatization; social, medical and psychiatric co-morbidities; lack of insurance; low socioeconomic status; homelessness or unstable housing; and factors relating to migrant status or ethnic/cultural minority status;
- *Healthcare provider-related factors*, such as limited expertise in HCV care for PWID; misperceptions that treatment is less effective or is associated with high re-infection rates in PWID versus non-PWID groups; and discrimination or stigmatization toward PWID;
- *System-related and institutional factors*, such as lack of infrastructure or treatment settings adapted or conveniently located for PWID; lack of coordination or collaboration among providers of different services; lack of suitable training programmes; high treatment fees; criminalisation of PWID; and a lack of validated, shared, systematic national data on the health and economic impact of HCV to inform service investment and planning.

Programmes for HCV treatment as prevention will only work if high levels of coverage and adherence are achieved and maintained. In light of the known barriers, HCV services need to be modified to effectively deliver harm reduction interventions and antiviral treatment to hard-to-reach populations. Survey data suggest that the majority of PWID may be willing to receive treatment for HCV if it is available to them [29]. However, whether individuals undertake and adhere to treatment in practice will depend on how they prioritise this option in relation to various competing priorities and challenges [26]. Some individuals may need particular encouragement, making advocacy and peer support important features of efforts to scale up treatment.

The question of whether further measures to incentivise PWID into care should be employed, and what form these should take, has received little attention to date. In conventional health services, patients with symptoms are motivated to seek health care as a means of obtaining relief from the symptoms. Similarly, patients are motivated to participate in HCV testing programmes because of their recognition that a diagnosis can lead to the timely initiation of treatment, reducing the risk of complications from the disease. In both cases, health-seeking behaviour is rewarded. In the PWID population, these mechanisms may be much less powerful. PWID often have quite nihilistic views of the future [30, 31], and as HCV is frequently asymptomatic, there are few drivers for treatment-seeking behaviour. This is compounded further if early treatment is perceived to principally benefit society (in terms of prevention of transmission, as discussed below) rather than infected individuals. Such perceptions may result from the asymptomatic nature of early infection or a lack of knowledge or concern about the long-term consequences of chronic HCV infection among some PWID. Additionally, for treatment as prevention strategies to work, the uptake of treatment needs to be high, as a small number of individuals at key points in networks could reinfect many people who have been cured. Therefore, incentives or contingency management programs should be considered. Assessed in a variety of diseases and populations by the National Institute for Health and Care Excellence in England and Wales and found to be cost-effective and acceptable [32], these should be considered a key component of motivating active PWID populations into treatment.

Crucially, many countries lack national evidence-based best practice programmes such as the one implemented and evaluated in Scotland [33]. In 2006, the Scottish Government launched its Hepatitis C Action Plan for the purposes of improving services to prevent transmission of HCV infection (particularly among PWID), identifying those infected, and ensuring that those infected receive optimal treatment, care and support [33]. The comprehensive plan was based on evidence from national monitoring systems and models showing the potential benefit of scaling up therapy and the mounting cost of inaction, and was informed by stakeholder consultations. It was implemented by national and local multidisciplinary, multi-agency networks, coordinated by Health Protection Scotland and supported by substantial government investment. Achievements include an increase of approximately 50 % in the proportion of the infected population diagnosed (38 % to 55 %); a nearly three-fold increase in the annual number of PWID initiating therapy, and a reversal of the upward trend in the overall number of people living with chronic HCV infection [33].

Prevention, harm reduction and testing

There is currently no vaccine against HCV. However, HCV infection among PWID can be greatly reduced using a combination of prevention strategies [13, 34]. PWID should have access to comprehensive harm reduction and support/care services. These services should also be based in the community, to facilitate access by PWID and to aid service expansion. Guidelines by WHO [13], the Joint United Nations Programme on HIV/AIDS [35], the European Centre for Disease Prevention and Control (ECDC)/European Monitoring Centre for Drugs and Drug Addiction [14] and other experts [15, 16, 36] all recommend packages of services that include the following elements (Fig. 1).

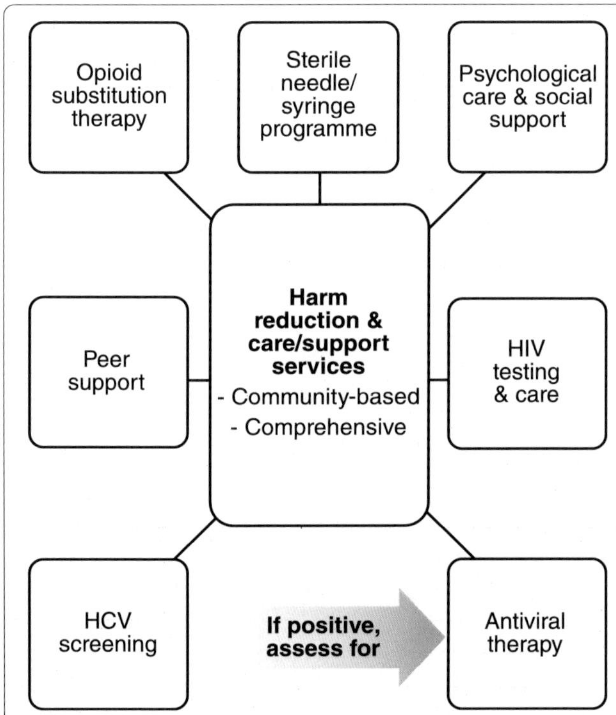

Fig. 1 Components of comprehensive hepatitis C virus (HCV) care services to which people who inject drugs should have access

Prevention and harm reduction

PWID should have easy access to harm reduction services, two key components of which are OST and NSP [13, 14, 35]. As well as reducing HCV risk behaviour and transmission through injecting drug use, these interventions can serve as a platform to promote HCV care. While harm reduction services are often grouped together, it is important to differentiate them and their potential utility in efforts to combat HCV. NSP programmes by definition are focussed on those still injecting and aim to make the act of injecting safer. Such services greatly reduce the rate of transmission. Therefore, it is logical to make this group the focus of treatment-as-prevention strategies. OST services take many forms across countries and regions depending on local legal requirements and regulations; some are very open to unstable and active injectors while others require PWID to modify their drug use to varying degrees as a condition for initiating or continuing OST. The design of the OST service model has considerable implications for the efficacy of OST as a prevention tool for HCV, with the only likely prevention benefit being seen in the context of low-threshold early access leading to reduced injecting frequency. The use of peer support interventions within these services is recommended [13, 14, 35]. Various models of peer support exist [37], including those that promote education, engagement in services, and treatment uptake and assessment [37–40]. HIV testing, prevention and care should be provided in concert. Available data suggest that the prevalence of HIV/HCV co-infection ranges widely across Europe, depending on the prevalence of HIV [10]. Other recommended components of care for PWID include: vaccination against other infections (e.g. hepatitis A and B, tetanus), psychological care for selected cases, and social support services [13–16, 35, 41].

The 2013–2016 European Commission Action Plan on Drugs charges Member States with ensuring that treatment and outreach services incorporate greater access to risk and harm reduction options to reduce the consequences of drug use including transmission of blood-borne viruses [42]. There are examples of good practice underway in Europe [33, 43], but the unmet need is still high [44, 45].

Testing

Many individuals with chronic HCV infection are diagnosed after being infected for many years and enter care only when they develop clinical symptoms, despite having been engaged by the healthcare system earlier [46]. Late diagnosis of HCV is associated with worse outcomes [46] and with the risk of onward transmission. Many opportunities for timely diagnosis of HCV infection are missed, especially in PWID populations. Active testing of PWID who are current injectors is rarely undertaken. It is argued that treatment of such patients is too difficult, too expensive and the risk of re-infection too high, although the developing evidence base clearly shows that this is not the case. Additionally, the diagnosis of HCV may change behaviour in the short term or identify patients who could be followed up for treatment in the future before presenting with liver failure. Recently, the European Association for the Study of the Liver and the HIV in Europe initiative developed a new consensus definition of late presentation for viral hepatitis [47]. This is an important performance indicator of success for programmes aiming to improve the identification and management of viral hepatitis.

HCV testing should be performed regularly in PWID to identify infected persons and engage them in care and treatment [13–16]. HCV antibody testing is recommended, and if the result is positive, a more sensitive HCV RNA test should be performed to determine whether or not there is current infection [13, 16]. Targeted HCV testing linked to treatment increases diagnosis rates and treatment uptake [48] and is a cost-effective way to reduce the disease burden [49]. New types of rapid and point-of-care HCV tests (e.g. dried blood spot tests) can help to increase the number of tested individuals, especially in hard-to-reach groups [13, 50]. However, according to a 2013 survey, only six of 44 countries in the European Region provided hepatitis B and C virus testing to PWID at no charge [20].

Antiviral treatment: individual benefit and transmission prevention

HCV antiviral treatment aims to cure, or eradicate, HCV infection in individuals, thereby preventing its complications and death [15]. HCV treatments are assessed according to the sustained virological response rate (SVR), defined as the proportion of patients with undetectable HCV RNA measured after 12 or 24 weeks according to defined methods. Patients who achieve an SVR remain free of the virus in 99 % of cases and hence are considered cured [15, 51]. An SVR has been associated with significantly reduced risks of 10-year all-cause mortality, and liver-related mortality or transplantation, among HCV-infected individuals with advanced hepatic fibrosis [52].

The introduction of direct-acting antiviral (DAA) therapies in recent years has revolutionised the treatment of HCV. Previously, pegylated interferon/ribavirin (peg-IFN/RBV) regimens were only moderately effective (depending on the HCV genotype), required IFN injections and variable treatment durations up to 48 or even 72 weeks, and were associated with significant toxicities. New all-oral IFN-free DAA regimens, given for 8–24 weeks, are much more effective (achieving SVR rates of ≥90 % in clinical trials), and are generally well tolerated [13, 15, 53]. It can be extrapolated that the much higher SVRs achieved will still be associated with the reduced liver and all-cause mortality seen with interferon-based regimens.

Currently, treatment priority is based on fibrosis stage, risk of progression to more advanced disease, presence of extrahepatic manifestations of infection and cirrhosis. It should also take into account the risk of transmission [15]. European and international guidelines recommend that all patients with chronic HCV — including PWID — should be considered for antiviral treatment based on an individualised assessment [13–16, 35]. According to a systematic review of studies, the effectiveness of peg-IFN/RBV treatment among PWID who are eligible and committed to starting HCV treatment (including active injectors) is similar to that in non-drug users, with high levels of adherence, low rates of treatment discontinuation, and a low rate of reinfection among PWID [12]. These findings support current treatment recommendations and refute misperceptions about poor effectiveness and high rates of re-infection in PWID that can lead to their exclusion from treatment. Indeed, PWID are among the groups that should be prioritised for treatment, regardless of fibrosis stage or extra-hepatic manifestations, in view of their risk of transmitting HCV [15]. Patients who are co-infected with HCV and HIV should also be prioritised for HCV treatment [15]. Importantly, HCV treatment for PWID should be delivered within multidisciplinary care/support programmes that include harm reduction and support services [13–16, 35], including measures to limit alcohol intake and to address obesity, smoking and drug usage.

Curing HCV infection not only benefits infected individuals, but also has the potential to prevent onward viral transmission and hence to reduce the disease burden at the population level [13]. The impact of treatment on HCV prevalence depends on its effectiveness and on the levels of treatment uptake. Modelling studies in various countries consistently suggest that current levels of treatment using conventional peg-IFN/RBV regimens are unlikely to significantly reduce or even stabilise the disease burden over the next 10 to 15 years [4–6, 54]. According to models, the HCV disease burden can only be cut substantially if antiviral treatment is scaled up together with prevention programmes [22, 54–60]. For example, using dynamic modelling, researchers in the United Kingdom projected that a 50 % reduction in the prevalence of chronic HCV in PWID (from a baseline of 20 %, 40 % or 60 %) could be achieved within 10 years by combining OST, NSP and antiviral treatment. A halving of the prevalence was made more achievable (i.e. fewer treatments were needed) if DAAs were used instead of peg-IFN/RBV, and also if harm reduction were scaled up [55]. Further modelling, based on real-world data on treatment rates and outcomes from 538 PWID in seven centres in the United Kingdom, suggested that the introduction of DAA therapies combined with the scaling up of treatment to rates already achieved in some centres – to 26 per 1000 PWID – could allow all seven sites to achieve at least a 15 % absolute reduction in HCV prevalence after 10 years, with prevalence more than halved in three sites [22]. In Scotland, doubling treatment uptake and prioritising PWID was projected to reduce incident infection to negligible levels (<50 cases per year) by 2025 and to stabilise rates of severe liver morbidity by 2028 [61]. Targeting those with moderate/advanced fibrosis would stabilise severe liver morbidity five years earlier, but would be significantly less effective in reducing new infections. In Sweden, modelling suggests that doubling the number of DAA treatments overall would bring about 65–70 % reductions in both the incidence of hepatocellular cancer and liver-related deaths by 2030 [59]. Targeting only patients with advanced fibrosis would only stabilise the incidence of serious complications with minimal impact on the total number of HCV infections. Internationally, other analyses suggest that a 90 % reduction in total HCV infections and/or disease burden within 15 years is feasible in most countries studied, provided there is upscaling of testing, harm reduction and efficacious treatment [5, 57].

Antiviral treatment among PWID, in combination with harm reduction services, is therefore a critical component of primary prevention of HCV. Despite implementation challenges, treatment uptake rates of 20–22 % have already been reported in dedicated services linking OST and community hepatitis care [22, 62–64]. Furthermore, experience from Scotland shows that a scale-up of antiviral therapy can be achieved without compromising SVR rates, including among PWIDs [65].

The cost of DAA treatments is a barrier to their wide usage in HCV management strategies in most European Union countries. However, PWID were not widely treated even during the previous era of lower cost therapies, underlining the point that particular barriers such as discrimination exist for this group. Economic models indicate that HCV treatment using DAAs is cost-effective owing to a reduction in the costs of HCV-related complications [66–69]. Few studies have assessed the cost-effectiveness of antiviral treatment specifically for PWID (Table 1). Modelling data from Australia and the United Kingdom suggest that treating active or former PWID with peg-IFN/RBV at mild stages of HCV is cost-effective compared with no antiviral treatment, resulting in incremental cost-effectiveness ratios (ICER, measured as cost per quality adjusted life-years [QALY]) below standard local thresholds for cost-effectiveness [70, 71]. The Australian study and the UK study both took into account the costs of disease progression, together with deleterious aspects such as reinfection, but only one also took into account the prevention effects of treatment on transmission [70].

Table 1 Studies modelling the cost-effectiveness of antiviral therapy for hepatitis C virus infection in people who inject drugs (PWID)

Reference	Country/setting	Design	Intervention and population	Cost impact
PegIFN/RBV therapy				
Martin et al. 2012 [70]	United Kingdom	Dynamic disease progression and transmission model	pegIFN/RBV at mild stage vs no treatment (best supportive care) in:	ICER for treating current PWID vs no treatment, according to baseline chronic HCV prevalence:
		Probablistic cost-utility analysis	Current PWID	20 % prevalence: ICER treat PWID vs no treatment = £521/QALY
		Direct medical costs (2010 prices)	Non/ex PWID	40 % prevalence: ICER vs no treatment = £2539/QALY
			N = 1000 individuals	60 % prevalence: ICER = £7675[a]/QALY
				Treatment of non/ex-PWID dominant at 60 % prevalence; ICER £6803/QALY vs no treatment
Visconti et al. 2013 [71]	Australia	Markov decision-analytic model	pegIFN/RBV at mild (F0/1) stage vs no treatment (best supportive care) in:	Current PWID: $AUS 7941/QALY
		Direct medical costs (2011 prices)	Current PWID	Former PWID: $AUS 5808/QALY
			Former PWID	Non-injectors: $AUS 3985/QALY
			Non-injectors	Treatment at mild stage dominated treatment at later stages for all cohorts
			N = 1000 individuals	
DAA therapy				
Bennett et al. 2015 [58]	United Kingdom	Dynamic model of disease progression, transmission and treatment	Uptake increased to 250 per 1000 PWID of:	2015–2027
			Current treatment	Current treatment: £23.4 million saved (£5.4 after discounting)
			New DAA (SVR90%)	SVR90%: £36.3 million saved (£8.4 million after discounting)
		Lifetime complication rates, costs of complications	N = 4240 individuals	
Hellard et al. 2015 [72]	Australia	Closed compartmental model of disease progression and treatment	IFN-free DAA at	Late treatment vs no treatment: $AUS5078
			Early stage (from F0)	Early treatment vs late treatment: $AUS17,090
		Fixed rate of re-infection	Late-stage (from F2/3)	
		Direct healthcare costs (2014 prices)	N = 1000 individuals	
Scott et al. 2016 [73]	Australia	Open compartmental model of progression, transmission and treatment	DAA treatment scale up necessary to achieve WHO goals of 65 % reduction in HCV-related deaths and 80 % reduction in HCV incidence by 2030 via two scenarios if DAA treatment for IDU-acquired HCV prioritised to: Patients with advanced liver disease (F ≥ 3) or Current PWID	Prioritising advanced liver disease: Mortality target required 5662 (95 % CI 5202–6901) courses/year (30/1000 IDU-acquired infections)
				Prioritising PWID:
				Incidence and mortality targets achieved with 4725 (95 % CI 3278–8420) courses per year (59/1000 PWID)
				Additional 5564 (1959–6917) treatments/year (30/1000 IDU-acquired infections) required for 5 years for patients with advanced liver disease to avoid excess HCV-related deaths
				ICER: $AUS25,121 ($AUS11,062–$AUS39,036)/QALY

DAA direct acting agents, *F0–3* METAVIR score, *ICER* incremental cost-effectiveness ratio, *pegIFN/RBV* peglyated interferon/ribavirin, *QALY* quality-adjusted life-years, *SVR* sustained virological response
[a]Calculated from data in published source

Recently, at least three further modelling studies have evaluated the impact and cost-effectiveness of interferon-free DAAs in PWID. One study, based on UK data and integrating disease progression and transmission according to a previous model [55], projected that an increase in uptake of conventional treatment with a 58 % SVR from 10 per 1000 PWID to 250 per 1000 PWID (among a modelled population of 4240 PWID with HCV prevalence of 25 %) would result in cost savings of £5.4 million between 2015 and 2027 after discounting at 3.5 % per annum [58]. Using newer treatments with a 90 % SVR was projected to increase the amount saved to £36.3 million, or £8.4 million after discounting [58].

In Australia, Hellard et al. modelled the expected healthcare costs and QALYs among newly HCV-infected PWID according to three scenarios: no treatment; 'early' treatment after initial infection; or 'late' treatment prior to developing compensated cirrhosis [72]. Compared with no treatment, early treatment and late treatment were associated with ICERs of AUS $10,272/QALY (95 % CI $5689–13,690) and AUS $5078/QALY (95 % confidence interval $2847–5295), respectively. Both of these values are well below the unofficial Australian willingness to pay threshold of AUS $50,000/QALY. Early treatment was the most effective option in terms of QALYs gained, while late treatment was associated with a lower ICER because of a lower likelihood of re-infection in patients treated later in the course of infection due to the cessation of injection drug use. These researchers acknowledged that their analysis may have underestimated the cost-effectiveness of treatment for two reasons: it did not take into account any benefits from reduced infection transmission, and the costs of care for cirrhosis and liver cancer were based on minimum requirements [72].

Most recently, these authors have used a model that includes HCV transmission as well as disease progression and treatment, to estimate the treatment scale up and cost-effectiveness of reaching WHO targets of an 80 % reduction in incidence and 65 % reduction in HCV-related deaths by 2030, specifically among PWID [73]. According to this analysis, achieving the mortality target would require treatment to be scaled up to 30/1000 injecting drug use-acquired infections per year among patients with advanced liver disease, while the incidence target required 59/1000 PWID to be treated each year. Prioritising treatment at this level only to PWID would achieve the mortality target with fewer treatment courses in total, but at the expense of a clinically unacceptable number of deaths among individuals with advanced disease. Hence, additional treatments (at the aforementioned rate, 30/1000/year) were required for patients with advanced liver disease for the first five years. Achieving both targets in this way was associated with an ICER of AUS $25 121 (AUS$11 062–AUS$39 036) per QALY gained, below the unofficial cost-effectiveness threshold [73].

Conclusion and recommendations

The hepatitis C pandemic is a pressing public health threat. Strategic action at the policy level is urgently needed to increase access to HCV prevention, testing and treatment among PWID, the group at highest risk of HCV infection. Such action has the potential to substantially reduce the number of infected persons, along with the disease burden.

The World Health Organization has called for a global movement to create generalized access to HCV treatment [13], as have civil society organisations and other stakeholders [74]. They have further called for national and European strategies on HCV that include specific measures for PWID [28, 75, 76]. In 2014, the 67th World Health Assembly approved a resolution urging Member States to develop and implement coordinated multi-sectoral national strategies for preventing, diagnosing and treating viral hepatitis based on the local epidemiological context [77]. The first-ever WHO Global Health Sector Strategy on Viral Hepatitis (2016–2021) was adopted by the 69th World Health Assembly on 28 May 2016 [78]. Aiming to contribute to the United Nations Sustainable Development Goals [79] and to eliminate viral hepatitis as a public health threat by 2030, the strategy highlights the opportunities available through investing in an essential, priority set of core interventions that include comprehensive integrated harm reduction services for PWID, linked with treatment [78]. This global strategy is complemented by a draft WHO European Region action plan for consideration by the Regional Committee in September 2016 [80]. Additionally, in the 2014–2016 EU Action Plan on HIV and Co-infections, the European Union has committed to work with Member States, neighbouring countries, civil society and the ECDC to implement risk and harm reduction measures for PWID and their partners for the prevention and treatment of HIV, co-infections and drug dependency in the community and prisons [81].

All policymakers responsible for health services in European Union countries should ensure that:

- National HCV action plans and strategies that include measures specifically to address HCV in PWID are developed and implemented across Europe;
- Evidence-based, comprehensive, multi-professional, community-led harm reduction and care/support programmes are provided and linked to HCV testing and treatment in the public and prison health systems;
- PWID have equitable access to effective HCV treatment, in line with published guidelines;

- Measures are undertaken to reduce stigma and discrimination against PWID at the provider and institutional levels;
- HCV awareness and prevention campaigns are undertaken for healthcare providers (doctors, nurses and allied health professionals) and the PWID community; and
- The PWID community is involved in HCV service planning and implementation, with consideration given to peer support and PWID 'champions' initiatives.

Abbreviations

DAA, direct-acting antivirals; ECDC, European Centre for Disease Prevention and Control; HCV, hepatitis C virus; ICER, incremental cost-effectiveness ratio; NSP, needle and syringe programme; OST, opioid substitution therapy; Peg-IFN/RBV, pegylated interferon/ribavirin; PWID, people who inject drugs; QALY, quality adjusted life-years; SVR, sustained virological response; WHO, World Health Organization.

Acknowledgements

The authors thank the following individuals for their review and endorsement of this paper: Prof. Cathy Matheï (Assistant Professor, Academic Center for General Practice, Dept of Public Health and Primary Care, Free Clinic Antwerp, Belgium); Dr João Goulão (Portuguese National Coordinator on Drugs, Drug Addictions and the Harmful Use of Alcohol, Lisbon, Portugal); Dr Juan Antonio Pineda (Associate Professor, Infectious Diseases and Microbiology Unit, Hospital Universitario de Valme, Seville, Spain); Lisa Power, MBE (former Policy Director at Terrence Higgins Trust and Consultant at Potestatis.com, Cardiff, UK); Eberhard Schatz (Project Coordinator, Correlation Network and Foundation De Regenboog Groep [FRG], Amsterdam, Netherlands).
The authors acknowledge editorial support from Lee Baker (Interel, UK), funded by Gilead Sciences Europe Ltd.

Authors' contributions

All authors contributed equally via participation in the aforementioned meeting as well as providing input into the concept, outline and all drafts. All authors approved the final draft.

Authors' information

JD is Professor of Hepatology & Gastroenterology at the School of Medicine, University of Dundee Ninewells Hospital and Medical School, Dundee, United Kingdom.
JVL is Editor-in-Chief of *Hepatology, Medicine and Policy* and Senior Researcher, the Centre for Health and Infectious Disease Research (CHIP), WHO Collaborating Centre on HIV and Viral Hepatitis Rigshospitalet, University of Copenhagen, Denmark.
HR is Managing Director, Center for Disease Analysis, Lafayette, Colorado, USA

Competing interests

This paper was born from discussions at a meeting of experts and patient advocates funded by Gilead Sciences Europe Ltd. The opinions expressed in this paper are the authors' own and the authors did not receive fees in respect of their roles in this publication. The contents of the paper do not necessarily reflect the view of Gilead Sciences Europe Ltd.

Author details

[1]Division of Molecular and Clinical Medicine, School of Medicine, University of Dundee, Ninewells Hospital, Dundee, UK. [2]Centre for Health and Infectious Disease Research (CHIP) and WHO Collaborating Centre on HIV and Viral Hepatitis, Rigshospitalet, University of Copenhagen, Copenhagen, Denmark. [3]Center for Disease Analysis, Louisville, Colorado, USA.

References

1. World Health Organization. Hepatitis C in the WHO European Region. WHO 2015. http://www.euro.who.int/__data/assets/pdf_file/0010/283357/fact-sheet-en-hep-c.pdf?ua=1. Accessed 2 Jun 2016.
2. Hatzakis A. Achieving WHO Recommendations for HCV in the European Union. Presented at the Polaris Symposium, Barcelona, Spain, April 13 2016. http://polarisobservatory.com/Barcelona2016/. Accessed 1 June 2016.
3. GBD 2013 Mortality and Causes of Death Collaborators. Global, regional, and national age-sex specific all-cause and cause-specific mortality for 240 causes of death, 1990-2013: a systematic analysis for the Global Burden of Disease Study 2013. Lancet. 2015;385:117–71.
4. Cramp ME, Rosenberg WM, Ryder SD1, Blach S, Parkes J. Modelling the impact of improving screening and treatment of chronic hepatitis C virus infection on future hepatocellular carcinoma rates and liver-related mortality. BMC Gastroenterol. 2014;14:137.
5. Müllhaupt B, Bruggmann P, Bihl F, Blach S, Lavanchy D, Razavi H, et al. Modeling the health and economic burden of hepatitis C virus in Switzerland. PLoS One. 2015;10:e0125214.
6. Sibley A, Han KH, Abourached A, Lesmana LA, Makara M, Jafri W, et al. The present and future disease burden of hepatitis C virus infections with today's treatment paradigm - volume 3. J Viral Hepat. 2015;22 Suppl 4:21–41.
7. European Centre for Disease Prevention and Control. Hepatitis C surveillance in Europe – 2013. ECDC; 2015. http://ecdc.europa.eu/en/publications/Publications/hepatitis-c-surveillance-in-europe-2013.pdf. Accessed 2 Jun 2016.
8. Nelson PK, Mathers BM, Cowie B, Hagan H, Des Jarlais D, Horyniak D, et al. Global epidemiology of hepatitis B and hepatitis C in people who inject drugs: results of systematic reviews. Lancet. 2011;378:571–83.
9. European Monitoring Centre for Drugs and Drug Addiction. Hepatitis C treatment for injecting drug users. EMCDDA, 2015. http://www.emcdda.europa.eu/attachements.cfm/att_212353_EN_EMCDDA_POD_2013_Hep%20C%20treatment.pdf. Accessed 2 Jun 2016.
10. Wiessing L, Ferri M, Grady B, Kantzanou M, Sperle I, Cullen KJ, et al. Hepatitis C virus infection epidemiology among people who inject drugs in Europe: a systematic review of data for scaling up treatment and prevention. PLoS One. 2014;9:e103345.
11. Rolls DA, Sacks-Davis R, Jenkinson R, McBryde E, Pattison P, Robins G, et al. Hepatitis C transmission and treatment in contact networks of people who inject drugs. PLoS One. 2013;8:e78286.
12. Aspinall EJ, Corson S, Doyle JS, Grebely J, Hutchinson SJ, Dore GJ, et al. Treatment of hepatitis C virus infection among people who are actively injecting drugs: a systematic review and meta-analysis. Clin Infect Dis. 2013;57 Suppl 2:S80–9.
13. World Health Organization. Guidelines for the screening, care and treatment of persons with hepatitis C infection. WHO. 2014. http://www.who.int/hiv/pub/hepatitis/hepatitis-c-guidelines/en/. Accessed 2 Jun 2016.
14. European Centre for Disease Prevention and Control and European Monitoring Centre for Drugs and Drug Addiction. Prevention and control of infectious diseases among people who inject drugs. ECDC; 2011. http://www.emcdda.europa.eu/publications/ecdc-emcdda-guidance. Accessed 2 Jun 2016.
15. European Association for the Study of the Liver. EASL Recommendations on Treatment of Hepatitis C 2015. J Hepatol. 2015;63:199–236.
16. Grebely J, Robaeys G, Bruggmann P, Aghemo A, Backmund M, Bruneau J, et al. Recommendations for the management of hepatitis C virus infection among people who inject drugs. Int J Drug Policy. 2015;26:1028–38.
17. Joint Action on HIV and co-infection prevention and harm reduction. www.HAREACT.eu, accessed 2 Jun 2016.
18. World Health Organization. Global policy report on the prevention and control of viral hepatitis in WHO Member States. WHO. 2013. http://apps.who.int/iris/bitstream/10665/85397/1/9789241564632_eng.pdf. Accessed 2 Jun 2016.
19. Maticic M, Videcnik Zorman J, Gregorcic S, Schatz E, Lazarus JV. Are there national strategies, plans and guidelines for the treatment of hepatitis C in people who inject drugs? A survey of 33 European countries. BMC Infect Dis. 2014;14 Suppl 6:S14.
20. Spina A, Eramova I, Lazarus JV. Policy responses to viral hepatitis B and C among people who inject drugs in Member States of the WHO European region: a sub-analysis of the WHO 2013 global hepatitis policy survey. BMC Infect Dis. 2014;14 Suppl 6:S15.
21. Lazarus JV, Sperle I, Maticic M, Wiessing L. A systematic review of hepatitis C virus treatment uptake among people who inject drugs in the European Region. BMC Infect Dis. 2014;14 Suppl 6:S16.

22. Martin NK, Foster GR, Vilar J, Ryder S, Cramp ME, Gordon F, et al. HCV treatment rates and sustained viral response among people who inject drugs in seven UK sites: real world results and modelling of treatment impact. J Viral Hepat. 2015;22:399–408.
23. Larney S, Kopinski H, Beckwith CG, Zaller ND, Jarlais DD, Hagan H, et al. Incidence and prevalence of hepatitis C in prisons and other closed settings: results of a systematic review and meta-analysis. Hepatology. 2013;58:1215–24.
24. Arain A, Robaeys G, Stöver H. Hepatitis C in European prisons: a call for an evidence-informed response. BMC Infect Dis. 2014;14 Suppl 6:S17.
25. Grebely J, Oser M, Taylor LE, Dore GJ. Breaking down the barriers to hepatitis C virus (HCV) treatment among individuals with HCV/HIV coinfection: action required at the system, provider, and patient levels. J Infect Dis. 2013;207:S19–25.
26. Harris M, Rhodes T. Hepatitis C treatment access and uptake for people who inject drugs: review mapping the role of social factors. Harm Reduct J. 2013;10:7.
27. Papatheodoridis GV, Tsochatzis E, Hardtke S, Wedemeyer H. Barriers to care and treatment for patients with chronic viral hepatitis in Europe: a systematic review. Liver Int. 2014;34:1452–63.
28. Papatheodoridis G, Thomas HC, Golna C, Bernardi M, Carballo M, Cornberg M, et al. Addressing barriers to the prevention, diagnosis and treatment of hepatitis B and C in the face of persisting fiscal constraints in Europe: report from a high level conference. J Viral Hepat. 2016;23 Suppl 1:1–12.
29. Alavi M, Micallef M, Fortier E, Dunlop AJ, Balcomb AC, Day CA, et al. Effect of treatment willingness on specialist assessment and treatment uptake for hepatitis C virus infection among people who use drugs: the ETHOS study. J Viral Hepat. 2015;22:914–25.
30. Treloar C, Rhodes T. The lived experience of hepatitis C and its treatment among injecting drug users: qualitative synthesis. Qual Health Res. 2009;19:1321–34.
31. Jordan AE, Masson CL, Mateu-Gelabert P, McKnight C, Pepper N, Bouche K, et al. Perceptions of drug users regarding hepatitis C screening and care: a qualitative study. Harm Reduct J. 2013;10:10.
32. National Institute for Health and Care Excellence. Drug misuse in over 16s: psychosocial interventions (CG51). National Institute for Health and Care Excellence. 2007. https://www.nice.org.uk/guidance/cg51. Accessed 2 Jun 2016.
33. Hutchinson SJ, Dillon JF, Fox R, McDonald SA, Innes HA, Weir A, et al. Expansion of HCV treatment access to people who have injected drugs through effective translation of research into public health policy: Scotland's experience. Int J Drug Policy. 2015;26:1041–9.
34. Hagan H, Pouget ER, Des Jarlais DC. A systematic review and meta-analysis of interventions to prevent hepatitis C virus infection in people who inject drug. J Infect Dis. 2011;204:74–83.
35. Joint United Nations Programme on HIV/AIDS (UNAIDS). Services for people who inject drugs. Guidance note. UNAIDS, 2014. http://www.unaids.org/sites/default/files/media_asset/2014_guidance_servicesforpeoplewhoinjectdrugs_en.pdf. Accessed 2 Jun 2016.
36. Goldberg D, Hutchison S. Hepatitis C — setting standards in a journey towards the eradication of infection and disease as a serious health issue in the EU. 2014. http://www.hcvaction.org.uk/resource/hepatitis-c-setting-standards-journey-towards-eradication-infection-and-disease-serious. Accessed 2 Jun 2016.
37. Crawford S, Bath N. Peer support models for people with a history of injecting drug use undertaking assessment and treatment for hepatitis C virus infection. Clin Infect Dis. 2013;57 Suppl 2:S75–9.
38. Grebely J, Knight E, Genoway KA, Viljoen M, Khara M, Elliott D, et al. Optimizing assessment and treatment for hepatitis C virus infection in illicit drug users: a novel model incorporating multidisciplinary care and peer support. Eur J Gastroenterol Hepatol. 2010;22:270–7.
39. Keats J, Micallef M, Grebely J, Hazelwood S, Everingham H, Shrestha N, et al. Assessment and delivery of treatment for hepatitis C virus infection in an opioid substitution treatment clinic with integrated peer-based support in Newcastle, Australia. Int J Drug Policy. 2015;26:999–1006.
40. Treloar C, Rance J, Bath N, Everingham H, Micallef M, Day C, et al. Evaluation of two community-controlled peer support services for assessment and treatment of hepatitis C virus infection in opioid substitution treatment clinics: The ETHOS study, Australia. Int J Drug Policy. 2015;26:992–8.
41. WHO, UNODC, UNAIDS technical guide for countries to set targets for universal access to HIV prevention, treatment and care for injecting drug users – 2012 revision. WHO. 2013. http://www.who.int/hiv/pub/idu/targets_universal_access/en/. Accessed 2 Jun 2016.
42. European Commission. Action Plan on Drugs 2013-2016 [2013/C 351/01]. Brussels, 2013. http://eur-lex.europa.eu/legal-content/EN/TXT/?uri=celex%3A52013XG1130(01). Accessed 2 Jun 2016.
43. Maticic M. A national multidisciplinary healthcare network for treatment of hepatitis C in people who inject drugs in Slovenia. BMC Infect Dis. 2014;14 Suppl 6:S6.
44. Stone S (ed). Global State of Harm Reduction 2014. Harm Reduction International. 2014. http://www.ihra.net/files/2015/02/16/GSHR2014.pdf. Accessed 2 Jun 2016.
45. Michel L, Lions C, Van Malderen S, Schitz J, Vanderplasschen W, Holm K, et al. Insufficient access to harm reduction measures in prisons in 5 countries (PRIDE Europe): a shared European public health concern. BMC Public Health. 2015;15:1093.
46. Moorman AC, Xing J, Ko S, Rupp LB, Xu F, Gordon SC, et al. Late diagnosis of hepatitis C virus infection in the Chronic Hepatitis Cohort Study (CHeCS): Missed opportunities for intervention. Hepatology. 2015;61:1479–84.
47. European Association for the Study of the Liver and HIV in Europe. New consensus definition of late presentation for viral hepatitis. http://www.easl.eu/medias/files/HiE_late%20present_Press%20release_new_2015OCT_final.pdf. Access 2 Jun 2016.
48. Aspinall EJ, Doyle JS, Corson S, Hellard ME, Hunt D, Goldberg D, et al. Targeted hepatitis C antibody testing interventions: a systematic review and meta-analysis. Eur J Epidemiol. 2015;30:115–29.
49. Hahné SJ, Veldhuijzen IK, Wiessing L, Lim TA, Salminen M, Laar M. Infection with hepatitis B and C virus in Europe: a systematic review of prevalence and cost-effectiveness of screening. BMC Infect Dis. 2013;13:181.
50. Coats JT, Dillon JF. The effect of introducing point-of-care or dried blood spot analysis on the uptake of hepatitis C virus testing in high-risk populations: A systematic review of the literature. Int J Drug Policy. 2015;26:1050–5.
51. Swain MG, Lai MY, Shiffman ML, Cooksley WG, Zeuzem S, Dieterich DT, et al. A sustained virologic response is durable in patients with chronic hepatitis C treated with peginterferon alfa-2a and ribavirin. Gastroenterology. 2010;139:1593–601.
52. van der Meer AJ, Veldt BJ, Feld JJ, Wedemeyer H, Dufour JF, Lammert F, et al. Association between sustained virological response and all-cause mortality among patients with chronic hepatitis C and advanced hepatic fibrosis. JAMA. 2012;308:2584–93.
53. Holmes JA, Thompson AJ. Interferon-free combination therapies for the treatment of hepatitis C: current insights. Hepat Med. 2015;7:51–70.
54. Sievert W, Razavi H, Estes C, Thompson AJ, Zekry A, Roberts SK, et al. Enhanced antiviral treatment efficacy and uptake in preventing the rising burden of hepatitis C-related liver disease and costs in Australia. J Gastroenterol Hepatol. 2014;29 Suppl 1:1–9.
55. Martin NK, Hickman M, Hutchinson SJ, Goldberg DJ, Vickerman P. Combination interventions to prevent HCV transmission among people who inject drugs: modeling the impact of antiviral treatment, needle and syringe programs, and opiate substitution therapy. Clin Infect Dis. 2013;57 Suppl 2:S39–45.
56. Martin NK, Vickerman P, Grebely J, Hellard M, Hutchinson SJ, Lima VD, et al. Hepatitis C virus treatment for prevention among people who inject drugs: Modeling treatment scale-up in the age of direct-acting antivirals. Hepatology. 2013;58:1598–609.
57. Alfaleh FZ, Nugrahini N, Matičič M, Tolmane I, Alzaabi M, Hajarizadeh B, et al. Strategies to manage hepatitis C virus infection disease burden - volume 3. J Viral Hepat. 2015;22 Suppl 4:42–65.
58. Bennett H, McEwan P, Sugrue D, Kalsekar A, Yuan Y. Assessing the long-term impact of treating hepatitis c virus (HCV)-infected people who inject drugs in the UK and the relationship between treatment uptake and efficacy on future infections. PLoS One. 2015;10:e0125846.
59. Duberg AS, Blach S, Falconer K, Kåberg M, Razavi H, Aleman S. The future disease burden of hepatitis C virus infection in Sweden and the impact of different treatment strategies. Scand J Gastroenterol. 2015;50:233–44.
60. Echevarria D, Gutfraind A, Boodram B, Major M, Del Valle S, Cotler SJ, et al. Mathematical modeling of hepatitis C prevalence reduction with antiviral treatment scale-up in persons who inject drugs in metropolitan Chicago. PLoS One. 2015;10:e0135901.
61. Innes H, Goldberg D, Dillon J, Hutchinson SJ. Strategies for the treatment of Hepatitis C in an era of interferon-free therapies: what public health outcomes do we value most? Gut. 2015;64:1800–9.
62. Martinez AD, Dimova R, Marks KM, Beeder AB, Zeremski M, Kreek MJ, et al. Integrated internist - addiction medicine - hepatology model for hepatitis C

management for individuals on methadone maintenance. J Viral Hepat. 2012;19:47–54.
63. Alavi M, Grebely J, Micallef M, Dunlop AJ, Balcomb AC, Day CA, et al. Assessment and treatment of hepatitis C virus infection among people who inject drugs in the opioid substitution setting: ETHOS study. Clin Infect Dis. 2013;57 Suppl 2:S62–9.
64. Wade AJ, Macdonald AM, Doyle JS, Gordon A, Roberts SK, Thompson AJ, et al. The cascade of care for an Australian community-cased hepatitis C treatment service. PLoS One. 2015;10:e0142770.
65. McDonald SA, Innes HA, Hayes PC, Dillon JF, Mills PR, Goldberg DJ, et al. What is the impact of a country-wide scale-up in antiviral therapy on the characteristics and sustained viral response rates of patients treated for hepatitis C? J Hepatol. 2015;62:262–8.
66. Cure S, Guerra I, Dusheiko G. Cost-effectiveness of sofosbuvir for the treatment of chronic hepatitis C-infected patients. J Viral Hepat. 2015;22:882–9.
67. Gissel C, Götz G, Mahlich J, Repp H. Cost-effectiveness of Interferon-free therapy for Hepatitis C in Germany–an application of the efficiency frontier approach. BMC Infect Dis. 2015;15:297.
68. Kim DD, Hutton DW, Raouf AA, Salama M, Hablas A, Seifeldin IA, et al. Cost-effectiveness model for hepatitis C screening and treatment: Implications for Egypt and other countries with high prevalence. Glob Public Health. 2015;10:296–317.
69. Leleu H, Blachier M, Rosa I. Cost-effectiveness of sofosbuvir in the treatment of patients with hepatitis C. J Viral Hepat. 2015;22:376–83.
70. Martin NK, Vickerman P, Miners A, Foster GR, Hutchinson SJ, Goldberg DJ, et al. Cost-effectiveness of hepatitis C virus antiviral treatment for injection drug user populations. Hepatology. 2012;55:49–57.
71. Visconti AJ, Doyle JS, Weir A, Shiell AM, Hellard ME. Assessing the cost-effectiveness of treating chronic hepatitis C virus in people who inject drugs in Australia. J Gastroenterol Hepatol. 2013;28:707–16.
72. Hellard M, Thompson A, Scott N, Iser D, Doyle JS. Cost-effectiveness of treating chronic hepatitis C virus with direct-acting antivirals in people who inject drugs in Australia. J Gastroenterol Hepatol. 2016;31:872–82.
73. Scott N, McBryde ES, Thompson A, Doyle JS, Hellard ME. Treatment scale-up to achieve global HCV incidence and mortality elimination targets: a cost-effectiveness model. Gut. 2016. doi: 10.1136/gutjnl-2016-311504. [Epub ahead of print].
74. NoHep website. www.nohep.org. Accessed 2 Jun 2016.
75. Hepatitis C Coalition. Defuse hepatitis C, the viral time bomb: test and treat hepatitis C Position Paper for the 67th World Health Assembly, May 19–24, 2014. http://www.hepcoalition.org/advocate/advocacy-tools/article/defuse-hepatitis-c-the-viral-time. Accessed 2 Jun 2016.
76. Hepatitis C Initiative. Manifesto - Berlin Declaration. 2014. www.hepatitis-c-initiative.eu. Accessed 2 Ju 2016.
77. World Health Assembly. Resolution on hepatitis. 67th World Health Assembly, 24 May 2014. http://www.who.int/mediacentre/news/releases/2014/WHA-20140522/en/. Accessed 2 Jun 2016.
78. World Health Organization. Draft global health sector strategy on viral hepatitis, 2016–2021 – the first of its kind. WHO. 2015. http://www.who.int/hiv/strategy2016-2021/en/. Accessed 2 Jun 2015.
79. United Nations. The Global Goals for Sustainable Development, 2015. UN. 20155. www.un.org/sustainabledevelopment/sustainable-development-goals). Accessed 2 Jun 2016.
80. World Health Organization Europe. Action plan for the health sector response to viral hepatitis in the WHO European Region (Draft 3.0). http://www.euro.who.int/en/health-topics/communicable-diseases/hepatitis/news/news/2016/05/consultation-for-action-plans-on-hiv-and-viral-hepatitis. Accessed 2 Jun 2016.
81. European Commission. Action Plan on HIV/AIDS in the EU and neighbouring countries: 2014-2016 [SWD(2014) 106 final]. Brussels, 2014. http://ec.europa.eu/health/sti_prevention/docs/ec_hiv_actionplan_2014_en.pdf. Accessed 11 Feb 2016.

5

Knowledge about hepatitis B and hepatitis C virus infection and consequences: a cross-sectional assessment of baseline knowledge among infected patients

Partha Sarathi Mukherjee*, Eliza Dutta, Dipesh Kr. Das, Shatabdi Ghosh, Suvadip Neogi and Arka Sarkar

Abstract

Background: India has a high burden of disease from hepatitis B virus (HBV), with 3.7 % point-prevalence, as well as from hepatitis C virus (HCV), with 1–1.5 % prevalence. Societal ignorance about HBV and HCV in India limits the potential for prevention and treatment efforts to bring these diseases under control. Since patients' own knowledge about their health condition may have important health consequences, this study sought to assess knowledge levels among HBV and HCV patients referred to the virology laboratory of the Liver Foundation, West Bengal.

Methods: Patients who had tested positive for HBsAg or anti-HCV at government specialty clinics were invited to enroll in the study when they presented for follow-up laboratory testing. Study participants completed a survey that contained three multiple-choice questions about viral hepatitis etiology and five multiple-choice questions about the consequences of HBV and HCV infection. Mean knowledge scores for male and female respondents were compared, and comparisons were also made across different places of residence, age groups, education levels and income levels. One-way ANOVA was used to test for significant differences.

Results: Among 520 study participants, the mean knowledge score was 4.76 on an eight-point scale. Approximately 40 % of the study sample scored less than 4.0. Almost three-quarters of respondents correctly responded to the question, "Which organ of the human body is affected by hepatitis?" while almost two-thirds knew how hepatitis B is transmitted. Regarding consequences of HBV and HCV infection, less than one-third of study participants answered correctly when asked, "What happens when one is infected with hepatitis B or C?" Slightly more than two-thirds of people correctly answered the question about how hepatitis B is prevented. The mean knowledge score varied across age groups ($P = 0.0009$), education levels ($P = 0.0001$) and monthly household income levels ($P = 0.0001$). With higher levels of schooling and higher household income, there were corresponding increases in knowledge scores.

Conclusion: There is room for improving knowledge of HBV and HCV etiology and consequences among patients as well as healthcare workers in India. More awareness activities should be organized, accompanied by further research to track whether knowledge scores improve over time.

Keywords: HBV, HCV, Patients, Knowledge, Awareness

* Correspondence: spartham@gmail.com; http://www.liverfoundation.in
Liver Foundation, West Bengal, 12, Kyd Street, Kolkata 7000016, India

Background

Viral hepatitis has emerged as a major health problem worldwide, including in India. Among the five main types of hepatitis viruses, hepatitis B virus (HBV) and hepatitis C virus (HCV) are of the greatest concern due to their burden of illness and death. HBV and HCV can cause both acute and chronic disease [1, 2]. An estimated 240 million people are chronically infected with HBV (defined as hepatitis B surface antigen-positive for at least 6 months) and more than 780,000 people die every year due to complications of HBV, including cirrhosis and liver cancer [1, 3–7]. Between 130 and 150 million people globally are thought to have chronic HCV infection. As with HBV, potential outcomes of chronic HCV infection include liver cirrhosis and liver cancer. Approximately 500,000 people die each year due to HCV-related liver ailments [2, 7].

An estimated 100 million chronic HBV and HCV carriers reside in Southeast Asia [8–10]. Home to almost one-fifth of the world's population, India accounts for a large proportion of the global HBV burden, with 10–15 % of the entire pool of HBV carriers. It is considered an intermediate endemic country, with a 3.7 % point-prevalence [11, 12]. More than 40 million HBV carriers live there; annually, one million Indians are at risk of getting HBV infection, and about 100,000 deaths occur due to HBV infection [3, 5]. Approximately one million infants in India live with the lifetime risk of developing chronic HBV infection [11, 13]. Due to its large population, the country also accounts for a significant share of the global HCV burden, with 1–1.5 % prevalence. An estimated 15 to 18 million people live with acute or chronic HCV infection in India [14, 15]. About 20 % of liver diseases in the country are associated with HCV infection, and HBV infection accounts for an even larger proportion of the burden of liver diseases [8].

HBV and HCV are bloodborne diseases, and knowledge about transmission pathways and preventive measures can help reduce the risk of acquiring both diseases. Furthermore, appropriate medical treatment can lessen the effects of HBV and can cure HCV. However, societal ignorance in India about HBV and HCV limits the potential for prevention and treatment efforts to bring both epidemics under control [16].

Low knowledge about HBV and HCV may have serious consequences for patients and their families and other contacts. Patients who lack adequate information or are misinformed about HBV and HCV may not be sufficiently prepared to make decisions that can protect their health, including adhering to prescribed medical treatments. Patients' poor knowledge might also lead them unknowingly to expose their family members and others to HBV or HCV. Therefore, dissemination of correct information to patients as part of a holistic approach to their health care might help them develop good disease management strategies and might also constitute an essential component of effective viral hepatitis prevention programs, ultimately helping to reduce the burden of disease and death in India.

Additional negative consequences might arise from prevailing misconceptions about HBV and HCV, according to field experiences reported by the Liver Foundation, West Bengal (LFWB), an Indian nongovernmental organization. These misconceptions may deter people from seeking proper medical advice and may prompt some of them to turn to folk medicines for treatment. In the case of HIV, patients' limited knowledge and wrong perceptions about that disease have been linked to poor treatment outcomes [17]. This finding raises the question of whether a similar dynamic may undermine efforts to treat HBV and HCV patients. Furthermore, these patients may experience shame associated with the stigmatized nature of these diseases, potentially leaving them isolated and afraid to seek appropriate medical care, particularly those with limited knowledge about their health. Knowledge of the etiology and consequences of HBV and HCV may thus empower them to take an active part in their own treatment.

The present study was undertaken to assess HBV- and HCV-infected Indian patients' knowledge regarding HBV and HCV etiology and consequences. The majority of studies assessing knowledge, attitudes and practices regarding HBV and HCV in low- and middle-income countries have been conducted among medical and laboratory technicians [18–21], while a few have focused specifically on HBV and HCV knowledge among the general population [22, 23]. To the best of our awareness, this is the first study to investigate Indian HBV and HCV patients' knowledge of the etiology and consequences of HBV and HCV infection. The purpose of the study was to acquire evidence that can help to inform the future direction of HBV and HCV control efforts in the study location, West Bengal, and in other settings with similar populations and similar disease control objectives.

Methods

Setting and participants

The Liver Foundation, West Bengal works to raise awareness about HBV and HCV, liver disease and general health issues. Since 2007, LFWB has been conducting awareness and health education meetings in schools, colleges and community settings. In addition to the general population, target audiences include patients, physicians and other healthcare workers.

With the support of the Bristol-Myers Squibb Foundation (BMSF), LFWB established a laboratory to provide low-cost molecular virology and metabolic diagnosis for patients with liver diseases. Patients typically make their first visit to the LFWB laboratory following a two-stage diagnostic process. When a general physician has diagnosed a patient with a liver problem, it is standard practice for the patient to be referred to the speciality clinic of a government hospital. A consultant at the specialty clinic may advise the patient to undergo serological testing for HBsAg and anti-HCV, and patients who do so are tested at the same clinic. Those patients who test positive for either disease marker are then referred to the LFWB molecular virology laboratory for further testing.

For the purpose of this study, HBsAg-positive patients referred to the LFWB laboratory from government hospitals were considered by investigators to have a diagnosis of HBV, and similarly, anti-HCV-positive patients were considered to have a diagnosis of HCV. Patients with a diagnosis of HBV or HCV were invited to participate in the study at the time of their visit to the LFWB laboratory if they also met the following study inclusion criteria: (1) the patient was at least 18 years old, (2) the patient had previously undergone no more than one liver-related consultation with a certified physician at a government hospital, and (3) the patient was visiting the LFWB laboratory for the first time.

Patients who met these criteria and agreed to participate in the study were asked to immediately complete a study survey at the central office of the LFWB, which is adjacent to the laboratory. Study enrollment and data collection took place between February 2014 and January 2015. To ensure that study participants fully comprehended all survey questions, study investigators verbally administered the survey instrument in face-to-face interviews and explained questions if required to do so. The interviews were conducted in participants' native languages. Although Hindi and English were used in some cases, Bengali, or "Bangla," was used more often as it is the native language of the province (West Bengal).

Table 1 Questions put to study participants about viral hepatitis

1. Which organ of the human body is affected by hepatitis?
   a. Kidney
   b. Liver
   c. Stomach
   d. Do not know
2. Which is the most severe disease affecting the liver?
   a. Jaundice
   b. Hepatitis B and C
   c. Hepatitis A and E
   d. Do not know
3. How is hepatitis B or C transmitted?
   a. Through contaminated food and water
   b. Through sneezing and coughing
   c. Through contaminated blood
   d. Do not know
4. What happens when one is infected with hepatitis B or C?
   a. Jaundice will occur
   b. Jaundice may not occur
   c. Jaundice will never occur
   d. Do not know
5. How is jaundice cured?
   a. Wear "garland" of jaundice
   b. Take complete bed rest
   c. Take only boiled food
   d. Take proper medical advice
6. What should be the diet during jaundice?
   a. Completely vegetarian food
   b. Completely boiled food (without oil and spices)
   c. Glucose, sugarcane juice and fruits
   d. Normal healthy diet (homemade)
7. What should one do when affected with jaundice?
   a. Take leave from job and have complete bed rest
   b. Do normal work
   c. Do excess work
   d. Do not know
8. How is hepatitis B or C prevented?
   a. By isolating the infected person
   b. By avoiding street food
   c. Through vaccination and proper advice
   d. Do not know

Survey instrument

Study data were collected using a two-part questionnaire developed by investigators. The survey instrument was validated by administering it to 20 randomly selected HBV or HCV patients who fulfilled the study criteria. In the first part of the survey instrument, the following patient profile information was collected: name, age, sex, address, education background and monthly household income. The second part of the survey instrument was composed of eight multiple-choice questions: three about viral hepatitis etiology and five about the consequences of HBV and HCV infection. There were four multiple-choice options for each question, among which one was correct (Table 1).

Several questions used the term "jaundice" instead of asking directly about HBV and HCV because most of the lay public in India, even paramedics, think of jaundice as a liver disease while not being aware of viral hepatitis.

Moreover, the questionnaire was categorized into two parts, an etiology section with fewer questions and a consequences section with more questions, as the survey was conducted among infected patients who had had one specialist consultation.

Scoring

When a respondent chose either an incorrect response, multiple responses or "do not know," the question was scored as nil. Each correct response was given a score of 1. A respondent's total score thus could range from 0 to 8.

Statistical analysis

Knowledge scores were calculated for individual study participants, and descriptive statistics were generated from these data. Knowledge scores then were considered in relation to five sociodemographic factors: place of residence, sex, age, education background and monthly household income. For place of residence, mean knowledge scores were compared across 19 districts and one other area. For sex, male and female study respondent scores were compared. Other comparisons were made using five age groups, five education levels and five income levels. One-way ANOVA was used to test for significant differences between mean knowledge scores for the categories associated with each sociodemographic factor [24].

Ethics

Participation in this study was voluntary. Written consent was obtained from all participants prior to study enrollment.

Results

Among 603 patients invited to participate in the study, 520 agreed and completed surveys, for a response rate of 86.2 %. Respondents resided in 19 districts in West Bengal, as well as in two neighboring states, Jharkhand and Bihar, and one neighboring country, Bangladesh. However, more than half were from three districts: Kolkata (23.5), North 24 Parganas (14.0) and South 24 Parganas (15.8 %) (Table 2). The study population was composed of 342 males and 178 females. The overall mean age was 36.7 years, ranging between 18 and 75 years of age (data not shown). Forty-two percent of study participants reported that the highest education level they had completed was middle school, while 11.7 of study participants had completed high school and 24.1 % had completed college or university. Almost 60 % of study participants belonged to households earning less than 5546 INR (approximately 81 USD) per month.

Table 3 shows the proportions of study participants providing correct, incorrect and "do not know" responses to the eight questionnaire items. Almost three-quarters of respondents correctly responded to the question, "Which organ of the human body is affected by hepatitis?" while almost two-thirds knew how hepatitis B is transmitted. Forty-six percent replied correctly when asked, "Which is the most severe disease affecting the liver?" Regarding consequences of HBV and HCV infection, less than one-third of study participants answered correctly when asked, "What happens when one is infected with hepatitis B or C?" Much larger proportions of respondents replied correctly when they were asked, "How is jaundice cured?" (72.1) and "What should be the diet during jaundice?" (61.9 %). Slightly more than two-thirds of participants correctly answered the question about how hepatitis B or hepatitis C is prevented.

The mean knowledge score reported in this study was 4.76 on an eight-point scale. Approximately 40 % of the study sample scored less than 4.0 (only half of the possible points). The mean score varied significantly across age groups ($P = 0.009$), with people aged 25–34 years scoring the highest (5.04) and people aged 55 years and older scoring the lowest (3.98). Mean scores also varied significantly across education levels ($P = 0.0001$) and monthly household income levels ($P = 0.0001$), increasing with higher education as well as higher income (Table 2).

When knowledge scores were disaggregated into etiology and consequences, significant differences were observed in both education ($P = 0.0001$) and household income ($P = 0.0001$) domains (Table 4). At higher levels of schooling and household income, knowledge scores in both domains improved. Regarding the relationship between knowledge scores and age, significant variation was found for knowledge about consequences of HBV and HCV infection ($p = 0.0001$) but not for knowledge about etiology. The highest knowledge score for the five "consequences" questions was 3.17 among people aged 35–44 years, while the lowest knowledge score was 2.28 among people aged 55 years and older.

Discussion

The purpose of this study was to investigate knowledge of HBV and HCV etiology and consequences among infected patients in West Bengal, India. The study population of 342 males and 178 females included a large proportion of people who had a high school education or less, and household income levels reported by study participants were fairly low overall. The mean knowledge score for all study participants was 4.76 on an eight-point scale. Although significantly different knowledge scores were seen across age groups, disaggregating the "etiology" and "consequences" questions indicated that age groups differed significantly only in regard to knowledge of HBV/HCV consequences. Positive correlations were seen between HBV/HCV knowledge scores and education levels, as well as between these scores and household income levels.

Studies that have examined the association of socioeconomic status with knowledge of lung cancer and knowledge of stroke suggest a positive relationship [25–27]. Another study showed that lower socioeconomic status was associated with lower awareness about the harmful effects of smoking [28]. The present study found similar results: lower monthly household income correlated with less knowledge of viral hepatitis etiology and disease consequences, and knowledge scores increased progressively across higher income strata. The same pattern was found for educational attainment, which is widely regarded as a proxy for socioeconomic status [29]. We speculate that study participants with lower socioeconomic status might have had less access to information about HBV and HCV, including fewer opportunities to visit healthcare facilities to obtain such

Table 2 Sociodemographic characteristics of the study population and mean knowledge scores

Variable	(%) N	Mean score on 8-point scale	*P*-value
District (*n* = 520)			
Bankura	1.5 (8)	3.50	0.122
Birbhum	2.3 (12)	4.92	
Burdwan	3.3 (17)	4.12	
Coochbehar	0.2 (1)	4.00	
Darjiling	0.2 (1)	4.00	
East Midnapore	4.2 (22)	5.45	
Hooghly	6.0 (31)	5.06	
Howrah	7.5 (39)	4.38	
Jalpaiguri	0.2 (1)	6.00	
Kolkata	23.5 (122)	5.14	
Malda	2.9 (15)	4.87	
Murshidabad	6.3 (33)	4.70	
Nadia	7.1 (37)	4.84	
North 24 Pargana	14.0 (73)	5.14	
North Dinajpur	0.6 (3)	3.00	
Purulia	0.4 (2)	4.50	
South 24 Pargana	15.8 (82)	4.02	
South Dinajpur	0.8 (4)	5.25	
West Midnapore	1.9 (10)	4.20	
Other	1.4 (7)	5.43	
Sex (*n* = 520)			
Male	65.8 (342)	4.73	0.574
Female	34.2 (178)	4.84	
Age (years) (*n* = 520)			
< 25	15.4 (80)	4.70	0.009
25 – 34	34.2 (178)	5.04	
35 – 44	23.7 (123)	4.98	
45 – 54	15.2 (79)	4.44	
55+	11.5 (60)	3.98	

Table 2 Sociodemographic characteristics of the study population and mean knowledge scores *(Continued)*

Education (*n* = 489)[a]			
No formal education[b]	3.1 (15)	2.80	0.0001
Completed primary education (4th standard)	19.6 (96)	3.56	
Completed middle school (8th standard)	41.5 (203)	4.78	
Completed high school (12th standard)	11.7 (57)	5.42	
Completed college/ university or above	24.1 (118)	6.18	
Total monthly household income (INR) (*n* = 399)[c]			
Less than 1865	17.3 (30)	3.57	0.0001
1866 – 5546	40.6 (203)	4.48	
5547 – 9248	25.3 (68)	5.13	
9249 – 13 873	5.3 (39)	5.41	
More than 13 873	11.5 (59)	6.10	

[a]31 respondents did not answer the question about education
[b]Respondents who reported that they had received less than 4th standard education were classified as "no formal education."
[c]121 respondents did not answer the question about income

Table 3 Proportions of correct and incorrect responses on eight-item questionnaire (*N* = 520)

Question	Responses (%)		
	Correct	Incorrect	Do not know
Etiology			
Which organ of the human body is affected by hepatitis?	74.2	1.9	23.8
Which is the most severe disease affecting the liver?	46.0	20.8	33.3
How is hepatitis B or C transmitted?	63.5	8.1	28.5
Consequences			
What happens when one is infected with hepatitis B or C?	32.7	40.4	26.9
How is jaundice cured?	72.1	23.3	4.6
What should be the diet during jaundice?	61.9	33.8	4.2
What should one do when affected with jaundice?	58.1	33.7	8.3
How is hepatitis B or C prevented?	67.9	10.8	21.3

Table 4 Mean scores for knowledge of etiology and consequenses of hepatitis B and C, disaggregated by sociodemographic factors

	Etiology Max score = 3 (95 % confidence interval)	*P* value	Consequences Max score = 5 (95 % confidence interval)	*P* value
District (*n* = 520)				
Bankura (*n* = 8)	1.25 (0.78 – 2.32)	0.517	2.25 (0.72 – 3.78)	0.089
Birbhum (*n* = 12)	2.00 (1.19 – 2.81)		2.92 (1.92 – 3.91)	
Burdwan (*n* = 17)	1.59 (1.01 – 2.16)		2.53 (1.78 – 3.28)	
Coochbehar (*n* = 1)	2.00		2.00	
Darjiling (*n* = 1)	2.00		2.00	
East Midnapore (*n* = 22)	2.00 (1.51 – 2.49)		3.45 (2.83 – 4.08)	
Hooghly (*n* = 31)	1.84 (1.45 – 2.23)		3.22 (2.76 – 3.69)	
Howrah (*n* = 39)	1.82 (1.49 – 2.14)		2.56 (2.056 – 3.07)	
Jalpaiguri (*n* = 1)	2.00		2.00	
Kolkata (*n* = 122)	1.99 (1.79 – 2.18)		3.14 (2.89 – 3.41)	
Malda (*n* = 15)	2.07 (1.49 – 2.64)		2.81 (2.01 – 3.59)	
Murshidabad (*n* = 33)	1.79 (1.37 – 2.21)		2.91 (2.43 – 3.38)	
Nadia (*n* = 37)	1.76 (1.38 – 2.13)		3.08 (2.58 – 3.58)	
North 24 Pargana (*n* = 73)	1.99 (1.74 – 2.23)		3.15 (2.88 – 3.42)	
North Dinajpur (*n* = 4)	1.00 (−1.48 – 3.48)		2.00 (−2.97 – 6.87)	
Purulia (*n* = 2)	2.00 (−10.71 – 14.71)		2.500 (−16.56 – 21.56)	
South 24 Pargana (*n* = 82)	1.54 (1.28 – 1.79)		2.49 (2.18 – 2.79)	
South Dinajpur (*n* = 4)	2.25 (0.73 – 3.77)		300 (1.16 – 4.84)	
West Midnapore (*n* = 10)	1.60 (0.99 – 2.20)		2.60 (1.91 – 3.29)	
Other (*n* = 7)	2.14 (1.02 – 3.27)		3.29 (2.13 – 4.45)	
Sex (*n* = 520)				
Male (*n* = 342)	1.79 (1.67 – 1.91)	0.200	2.93 (2.78 – 3.08)	0.895
Female (*n* = 178)	1.92 (1.76 – 2.08)		2.92 (2.71 – 3.12)	
Age (years) (*n* = 520)				
< 25 (*n* = 80)	2.02 (1.79 – 2.26)	0.151	2.68 (2.36 – 2.99)	0.0001
25 – 34 (*n* = 178)	1.90 (1.75 – 2.05)		3.14 (2.94 – 3.33)	
35 – 44 (*n* = 123)	1.81 (1.62 – 2.00)		3.17 (2.91 – 3.43)	
45 – 54 (*n* = 79)	1.63 (1.37 – 1.89)		2.81 (2.53 – 3.09)	
55+ (*n* = 60)	1.70 (1.38 – 2.02)		2.28 (1.89 – 2.68)	
Education (*n* = 489)[a]				
No formal education[b]	0.93 (0.29 – 1.58)	0.0001	1.87 (1.24 – 2.49)	0.0001
Completed primary education (4th standard)	1.31 (1.08 – 1.54)		2.25 (1.99 – 2.50)	
Completed middle school (8th standard)	1.79 (1.64 – 1.94)		2.99 (2.79 – 3.18)	
Completed high school (12th standard)	2.21 (1.95 – 2.47)		3.21 (2.93 – 3.49)	
Completed college/university or above	2.49 (2.37 – 2.61)		3.69 (3.49 – 3.89)	
Total monthly household income (INR) (*n* = 399)[c]				
Less than 1865 (*n* = 30)	1.53 (1.05 – 2.01)	0.0001	2.03 (1.51- 2.56)	0.0001
1866 – 5546 (*n* = 203)	1.61 (1.46 – 1.76)		2.87 (2.67 – 3.06)	
5547 – 9248 (*n* = 68)	1.99 (1.73 – 2.24)		3.15 (2.85 – 3.45)	
9249 – 13 873 (*n* = 39)	2.15 (1.88 – 2.43)		3.26 (2.86 – 3.65)	
More than 13 873 (*n* = 59)	2.36 (2.12 – 2.59)		3.75 (3.44 – 4.05)	

[a]31 respondents did not answer the question about education
[b]Respondents who reported that they had received less than 4th standard education were classified as "no formal education"
[c]121 respondents did not answer the question about income

information. Costs of medical care, distance from such facilities and a lack of transportation might be related reasons for low knowledge among these patients, who might benefit from health policies and programs that consider these factors when developing HBV and HCV awareness campaigns.

If patients from lower socioeconomic strata are more inclined than other patients to utilize traditional healing practices, this may also help to explain the differences in knowledge scores, since traditional healing practices have the potential to foster misconceptions about HBV and HCV. We observed that 15 % of study participants who responded incorrectly to a question about a cure for jaundice believed in such local folk remedies as wearing a "jaundice-garland" to cure it. Twenty-one percent of all respondents believed that glucose in either a commercially available powder form or in the form of sugar cane should be the only diet of a person with jaundice. More research is needed to determine whether such beliefs and practices negatively affect HBV and HCV patients' health outcomes, and to identify interventions that may improve the situation. There may be valuable guidance in other health fields; for example, research has been conducted on initiatives to train traditional healers in diabetes prevention and care in Cameroon, and to involve traditional healers in the scale-up of antiretroviral treatment for people living with HIV in Lesotho [30, 31].

With respect to age, we found that study participants aged 25–34 years had the highest overall mean knowledge score, and that study participants aged 35–44 years had the highest knowledge scores for HBV/HCV consequences, while those aged 55 years and older scored the lowest in both cases. The literacy rate in India increased from 12 % at the end of British rule in 1947 to 74 % in 2011, [32] which might partially explain our age-related study findings. However, there is still the question of why knowledge scores among study participants aged 18–24 years were also fairly low. There is a need for research that elucidates the relationship between age and HBV/HCV knowledge in India, as well as research that identifies key knowledge pathways for different age groups.

Provider-related factors should also be considered in relation to study participants' low overall knowledge scores. All study participants were newly diagnosed with HBV or HCV, and all of them had received only one consultation related to the diagnosis. The consultation might not have been sufficient to provide a patient with adequate HBV or HCV knowledge. Previous studies have reported that patients' inability to understand medical jargon, their fear of asking a medical practitioner for explanations about terminology, inadequate consultation time to address all queries due to over-burdened schedules, unfriendly healthcare staff and hospitality issues, patients' fears of verbal abuse by physicians and allied healthcare staff, and their anxiety about and fear of the disease are major barriers to effective communication between patients and healthcare staff [33–35]. These barriers could be presumed to affect patients' knowledge, potentially leading to misconceptions related to bloodborne viral hepatitis and increasing their health risks. A comprehensive disease prevention program should take such considerations into account.

Poor knowledge and misconceptions about HBV and HCV among general practitioners and other health workers might be another reason for low patient knowledge. Low levels of knowledge of bloodborne viral hepatitis among healthcare workers and medical students have been reported in studies conducted in developing countries. Setia et al., for instance, reported that 31 of medical practitioners, 38 of dental practitioners and 49 % of nurses claimed to have been vaccinated against hepatitis C, although no such vaccine exists [36]. Another study, conducted among students in four medical colleges in Pakistan, revealed that 73 % did not get screened for bloodborne hepatitis following a needlestick injury [37]. Studies have furthermore reported that discrimination and ostracism have originated from misinformation disseminated by healthcare personnel [38–41]. Informed doctors as well as other healthcare workers can play an important role in promoting accurate information about hepatitis and jaundice to patients. In doing so, health providers might also help reduce stigma for HBV and HCV patients across all settings, including operating rooms.

We suggest that these and other studies support the need to improve patients' hepatitis knowledge through more effective HBV and HCV education programs targeting patients, healthcare practitioners and the general population alike. Such programs are particularly important in a country such as India, where jaundice is reported as a disease along with hepatitis in the National Sample Survey report and it is common for general practitioners to address jaundice instead of hepatitis as a disease, resulting in a society where yellowing of the eyes and urine is equated with jaundice as a synonym for hepatitis [42]. The National Program for Prevention and Control of Viral Hepatitis in India is not in action, even now, only a committee that was formed in 2012 to formulate such a control program in viral hepatitis [43]. National Family Health Survey, India reports reveal that liver disease, including hepatitis, is not a national public health priority; therefore more clarity in thought is needed from policy-makers [44].

A 2013 review concluded that educational interventions have significant beneficial effects on persons who are at risk for or have been diagnosed with HBV or HCV. These effects extend to disease knowledge and behavior modification, including getting testing for the disease, receiving vaccinations, and being willing to commence and adhere to treatment [45]. It is recognized that there is limited knowledge about infectious diseases in general, including viral hepatitis, particularly among people with a low educational and socioeconomic level. Therefore, more current information locally can lead to focused action for knowledge empowerment,which is also mentioned in the World Health Organization's first-ever Global Health Sector Strategy on Viral Hepatitis [46]. Hence assessments of HBV and HCV patients' knowledge levels are the necessary starting point in the process of determining how to overcome knowledge-related barriers to treatment and the prevention of on-ward transmission. Our present study offers important insights in this regard, and is notable for not being preceded by any other published research of this kind relating to an Indian population. Further research is needed, as the full population of HBV and HCV patients in India is diverse, with patients representing a wide range of cultural, socioeconomic and other backgrounds that may inform their knowledge and perspectives regarding viral hepatitis.

Some of the limitations of this study may have implications for the generalizability of its findings. More than half of the individuals who made up the relatively small sample of 520 reported that they lived in the districts of Kolkata, North 24 Pargana and South 24 Pargana. The heavy representation of these districts may be related to the large number of referrals that the LFWB receives, mainly from speciality clinics of government hospitals in Kolkata. Furthermore, the study did not include many participants from higher-income households. Almost 60 % of study participants reported having a monthly household income under 5547 INR, while monthly per capita income for West Bengal is INR 6575, and the national monthly per capita income is INR 7378 [47]. A larger study population, more evenly distributed across districts might have contributed to a better understanding of knowledge among HBV and HCV patients.

Conclusion

The knowledge gaps observed among HBV and HCV patients in this study suggest a need for further research and for educational interventions that take into account the needs of diverse populations in India, including members of different age groups and socioeconomic strata. A country-wide focus on correct knowledge dissemination by healthcare professionals, improved physician-patient communication and the introduction of a positive health culture based on scientifically proven evidence can contribute to sustained viral hepatitis control in India.

Acknowledgments
The authors are thankful to all field staff who helped in collecting data and to Dr. Abhijit Chowdhury for his constructive input on the manuscript. The authors are also grateful to all LFWB patients who participated in this study.

Funding
The study was funded through a Bristol-Myers Squibb Foundation grant to the Liver Foundation, West Bengal as a part of 'Delivering Hope' program.

Authors' contributions
PSM conceptualized and designed the study, and also critically reviewed each draft of this paper. ED and DKD also took part in designing the study, analyzing data and drafting the manuscript. SG and AS were involved in designing and implementing the study. SN, the molecular virology laboratory's research assistant, was the first contact person for study participants. All authors read and approved the final manuscript.

Competing interests
The study was funded by the Bristol-Myers Squibb Foundation (BMSF).

References

1. World Health Organization. Hepatitis B. World Health Organization Fact Sheet No. 204. 2014. http://www.who.int/mediacentre/factsheets/fs204/en/. Accessed Jul 2014.
2. World Health Organization. Hepatitis C. World Health Organization Fact Sheet No. 164. 2014. http://www.who.int/mediacentre/factsheets/fs164/en/. Accessed Jul 2014.
3. Lavanchy D. Evolving epidemiology of hepatitis C virus. Clin Microbiol Infect. 2011;17:107–15.
4. Lok AS. Chronic hepatitis B. N Engl J Med. 2002;346:1682–83.
5. Te HS, Jensen DM. Epidemiology of hepatitis B and C viruses: a global overview. Clin Liver Dis. 2010;14:1–21.
6. Goldstein ST, Zhou F, Hadler SC, Bell BP, Mast EE, Margolis HS. A mathematical model to estimate global hepatitis B disease burden and vaccination impact. Int J Epidemiol. 2005;34:1329–39.
7. Lozano R, Naghavi M, Foreman K, Lim S, Shibuya K, Aboyans V, Abraham J, et al. Global and regional mortality from 235 causes of death for 20 age groups in 1990 and 2010: a systematic analysis for the Global Burden of Disease Study 2010. Lancet. 2012;380:2095–128.
8. National Centre for Disease Control (NCDC) Newsletter. 2014;3(1). http://www.ncdc.gov.in/writereaddata/linkimages/NewsLtr0103_20146480274026.pdf. Accessed Jan 2014.
9. Hwang EW, Cheung R. Global epidemiology of hepatitis B virus (HBV) infection. N Am J Med Sci. 2011;4:7–13.
10. Messina JP, Humphreys I, Flaxman A, Brown A, Cooke GS, Pybus OG, Barnes E. Global Distribution and Prevalence of Hepatitis C Virus Genotypes. Hepatology. 2015;61:77–87.
11. Puri P. Tackling hepatitis B disease burden in India. J Clin Exp Hepatol. 2014; 4:312–9.
12. Dutta S. An overview of molecular epidemiology of hepatitis B virus (HBV) in India. Virol J. 2008;5:156.
13. World Health Organization on behalf of Ministry of health and family welfare, Government of India: operational guidelines for hepatitis B vaccine introduction in the universal immunization program. 2011. http://www.searo.who.int/india/topics/routine_immunization/Operational_Guidelines_for_HepatitisB_vaccine_introduction_in_UIP_2011.pdf?ua=1. Accessed 7 Dec 2014 .
14. Mohd Hanafiah K, Groeger J, Flaxman AD, Wiersma ST. Global epidemiology of hepatitis C virus infection: new estimates of age-specific antibody to HCV seroprevalence. Hepatology. 2013;57:1333–42.
15. Jayasekera CR, Barry M, Roberts LR, Nguyen MH. Treating hepatitis C in lower-income countries. N Engl J Med. 2014;370:1869–71.
16. World Health Organization. Towards a comprehensive national hepatitis prevention and control programme, India. 2014. http://www.searo.who.int/india/publications/technical_consultation_world_hepatitis-day2014.pdf. Accessed 28 Jul 2014.
17. Fawzi MCS, Jagannathan P, Cabral J, Banares R, Salazar J, Farmer P, Behforouz H. Limitations in knowledge of HIV transmission among HIV-

positive patients accessing case management services in a resource-poor setting. AIDS Care. 2006;18:764–71.
18. Khan N, Ahmed SM, Khalid MM, Siddiqui SH, Merchant AA. Effect of gender and age on knowledge, attitude and practice regarding hepatitis B and C and vaccination status of hepatitis B among medical students of Karachi, Pakistan. J Pak Med Assoc. 2010;60:450–55.
19. Omuemu VO, Omuemu CO, Agboghoroma OF, Akofu AN, Benka-Coker AO. A KAP study of hepatitis B virus (HBV) infection among medical students in University of Benin. Annals of Biomedical Sciences. 2008;7:1–2.
20. Mesfin YM, Kibret KT. Assessment of knowledge and practice towards hepatitis B among medical and health science students in Haramaya University. Ethiopia PLoS One. 2013;8(11):e9642.
21. Singh A, Jain S. Prevention of hepatitis B-knowledge and practices among medical students. Indian Med Gazette. 2012. http://medind.nic.in/ice/t12/i2/icet12i2p52.pdf. Accessed Feb 2012.
22. ul Haq N, Hassali MA, Shafie AA, Saleem F, Farooqui M, Ajadhey H. A cross sectional assessment of knowledge, attitude and practice towards hepatitis B among healthy population of Quetta, Pakistan. BMC Public Health. 2012;12:692.
23. Razi A, ur Rehman R, Naz S, Ghafoor F, Aman M. Attitude and practices of university students regarding hepatitis B and C. ARPN. J Agricultural and Biol Sci. 2010;4:38–43.
24. Oberoi SS. Updating income ranges for Kuppuswamy's socio-economic status scale for the year 2014. Indian J Public Health. 2015;59:156–7.
25. Price JH, Everett SA. Perception of lung cancer and smoking in an economically disadvantaged population. J Community Health. 1994;9:361–75.
26. Nobile CGA, Anfosso R, Pavia M, Angelillo IF. Cigarette smoking: knowledge, attitudes and behaviour in an adult population in Italy. Public Health. 2000; 114:348–52.
27. Reeves MJ, Hogan JG, Rafferty AP. Knowledge of stroke risk factors and warning signs among Michigan adults. Neurology. 2002;59:1547–57.
28. Siahpush M, McNeill A, Hammond D, Fong GT. Socioeconomic and country variations in knowledge of health risks of tobacco smoking and toxic constituents of smoke: results from the 2002 International Tobacco Control (ITC) Four Country Survey. Tob Control. 2006;15 suppl 3:iii65–70.
29. Shavers VL. Measurement of socioeconomic status in health disparities research. J Natl Med Assoc. 2007;99:1013–23.
30. Mbeh GN, Edwards R, Ngufor G, Assah F, Fezeu L, Mbanya J-C. Traditional healers and diabetes: results from a pilot project to train traditional healers to provide health education and appropriate health care practices for diabetes patients in Cameroon. Glob Health Promot. 2010;17(2 Suppl):17–26.
31. Furin J. The role of traditional healers in community-based HIV care in rural Lesotho. J Community Health. 2011;36:849–56.
32. Government of India, Ministry of Home Affairs. http://censusindia.gov.in. Accessed 2011.
33. Fong Ha J, Anat DS, Longnecker N. Doctor-patient communication: a review. Ochsner J. 2010;10:38–43.
34. Ong LM, de Haes JCJM, Hoos AM, Lammes FB. Doctor-patient communication: a review of literature. Soc Sci Med. 1995;40:903–18.
35. Basu S, Andrews J, Kishore S, Panjabi R, Stuckler D. Comparative performance of private and public healthcare systems in low- and middle-income countries: a systematic review. PLoS Med. 2012;9:6.
36. Setia S, Gambhir RS, Kapoor G, Garg S, Setia S. Attitudes and awareness regarding hepatitis B and hepatitis C amongst health-care workers of a tertiary hospital in India. Ann Med Health Sci Res. 2013;3:551–8.
37. Raza W, Tariq W, Zafar Z, Ali I, Khar MU, Khurram M. Knowledge, attitude and practices (KAP) of medical students towards hepatitis B and C. Ann Pak Inst Med Sci. 2008;4:116–20.
38. Khalil T. Willingness of Saudi dental professionals to treat hepatitis B virus-infected patients. Niger J Clin Pract. 2015;18:247–50.
39. Mahboobi N, Agha-Hosseini F, Mahboobi N, Safari S, Lavanchy D, Alavian SM. Hepatitis B virus infection in dentistry: a forgotten topic. J Viral Hepat. 2010;17:307–16.
40. World Health Organization Western Pacific Region. Hepatitis B infection in Philippines: do something! 2013. http://www.wpro.who.int/hepatitis/hepatitis_WHD_feature_stories/en/. Accessed 26 Aug 2015.
41. Ellard J, Wallace J. Stigma, discrimination and hepatitis B: a review of current research (ARCSHS Monograph Series No. 93). Melbourne: Australian Research Centre in Sex, Health and Society, La Trobe University; 2013. ISBN 9781921915468.
42. National Sample Survey Organization, Ministry of Statistics and Programme Implementation, Government of India. Morbidity, Health care and conditions of the aged. Report No –507. NSSO 60th round. March 2006. http://mospi.nic.in/rept%20_%20pubn/507_final.pdf.
43. National Centre for Disease Control, Directorate General of Health Services, Ministry of Health and Family Welfare, Govt. of India. National Programme on Prevention and Control of Viral Hepatitis in India 12th Five Year Plan (2012–2017). http://www.ncdc.gov.in/.
44. National Family Health Survey, India (2015–2016). http://rchiips.org/nfhs/nfhs4.shtml.
45. Shah HA, Abu-Amara M. Education provides significant benefits to patients with hepatitis B virus or hepatitis C virus infection: a systematic review. Clin Gastroenterol Hepatol. 2013;11:922–33.
46. World Health Organization. Sixty-ninth world health assembly. Provisional agenda 15.1. Draft global health sector strategies, Viral hepatitis- 2016–2021 http://apps.who.int/gb/ebwha/pdf_files/WHA69/A69_32-en.pdf?ua=1. Accessed 22 Apr 2016.
47. Press Information Bureau, Government of India. 2015. http://pib.nic.in/newsite/erelease.aspx. Accessed 22 Jul 2015.

6

Hepatitis B knowledge among key stakeholders in Haimen City, China: Implications for addressing chronic HBV infection

Chari Cohen[1*], Alison A. Evans[1,2], Peixin Huang[3], W. Thomas London[1,4], Joan M. Block[1] and Gang Chen[1]

Abstract

Background: This article describes hepatitis B-related knowledge, attitudes and practices after completion of the Gateway to Care campaign, a citywide public health education program that targeted city residents, health care providers and individuals chronically infected with hepatitis B virus in Haimen City, China.

Methods: Pre/post questionnaires assessed hepatitis B knowledge change among health care providers and post-campaign surveys evaluated hepatitis B knowledge, attitudes and behaviors (including stigma-related beliefs and practices) among health care providers, city residents and chronically infected individuals. Focus groups were conducted to gain a more in-depth understanding of the needs of the target communities, and to identify future intervention strategies to improve hepatitis B testing and linkage to care and treatment.

Results: Results indicate high levels of hepatitis B knowledge among multiple stakeholders in Haimen City, with significant knowledge improvement among health care providers. Stigma-related beliefs and myths regarding separation of infected individuals from certain aspects of family life were common among all stakeholder groups, despite high levels of accurate knowledge about hepatitis B transmission and prevention. Self-report of hepatitis B screening was low among city residents, as was awareness of hepatitis B treatment.

Conclusions: More efforts are needed to improve awareness of HBV treatment, decrease HBV-related stigma, improve screening rates, and reduce cost of antiviral treatment. Future interventions in Haimen City should be driven by behavioral change theory, to not only improve knowledge, but to improve screening behaviors and address hepatitis B-related stigma and discrimination.

Keywords: Chronic hepatitis B infection, Hepatitis B knowledge and behaviors, Hepatocellular carcinoma, Gateway to Care campaign, Haimen City, China

Background

An estimated 248 million individuals worldwide are chronically infected with the hepatitis B virus (HBV) [1]. Approximately 40 % live in China, where an estimated 100 million people are chronically infected, and where up to 500,000 people die annually from HBV-related complications, including primary liver cancer (hepatocellular carcinoma [HCC]) [2-5]. In China, most infection occurs at birth (perinatal transmission) or during early childhood, leading to high rates of chronic infection [4, 5]. The high prevalence of chronic HBV infection in China has yielded a high burden of HBV-related HCC incidence and mortality, with 55 % of liver cancer deaths worldwide occurring in China [6]. HBV immunization programs administered by the Chinese Ministry of Health and the World Health Organization (WHO), including the universal vaccination of newborns program begun in 1992, have improved HBV vaccine coverage in parts of China, which is reflected in a recent decline of prevalence rates [7, 8]. However, HBV vaccination does not help those who are already

* Correspondence: chari.cohen@hepb.org
[1]Hepatitis B Foundation, Doylestown, PA, USA
Full list of author information is available at the end of the article

infected, and chronic HBV infection is still a considerable health issue in China with a serious public health impact.

The key to reducing morbidity and mortality associated with chronic HBV infection is improving rates of HBV screening and ensuring that infected individuals receive appropriate medical management [9, 10]. This is especially needed in areas that have high HBV prevalence and HCC incidence. However, multiple barriers result in low levels of screening, diagnosis, care and treatment for HBV. Key barriers to screening and vaccination include geography (i.e. rural areas), limited knowledge among the general population and health care providers, and HBV-related stigma [7, 9, 11, 12-14]. Treatment uptake is also low, primarily due to under-diagnosis and cost of antiviral treatment [15]. To help overcome barriers to HBV screening, the Hepatitis B Foundation (HBF) implemented the "Gateway to Care Campaign: Haimen City Project" in August 2010, in collaboration with the Haimen City Center for Disease Control and Prevention (HCCDC) [16]. This 3-year project is described in detail in a previous publication [16]. Briefly, the project consisted of a targeted citywide public health information and awareness campaign, specialized education and training for key constituencies (including health care providers, government officials and infected individuals), and expansions in health care infrastructure to increase screening, vaccination, treatment, and care management services.

This article describes HBV-related knowledge, attitudes and practices among key Haimen City constituencies (city residents, health care providers and infected individuals), as well as knowledge change among health care providers after implementation of the Gateway to Care program. The study also identifies potentially effective strategies that could be implemented in the future to improve HBV screening and care rates in Haimen City. Thus, these findings may guide the design of future interventions.

Methods

Haimen City, China

Haimen City, which has a population of 1.03 million, is located in Jiangsu Province, approximately 60 miles northwest of Shanghai. HCC has been the leading cause of cancer death in Haimen City since death registration began in 1970, and the incidence and mortality of HCC in Haimen City are among the highest in China, and in the world (Haimen City CDC Vital Statistics, unpublished data). City public health officials estimate that there are currently 80,000 residents aged 25 to 64 living with chronic HBV infection [16]. A population-based prospective cohort study enrolling more than 90,000 Haimen City residents found a 13.7 % chronic HBV infection rate. This study, which has been following infected individuals since 1992, established a direct link between viral load and liver cancer in chronically infected individuals [17]. The Gateway to Care campaign, designed by the HBF and HCCDC, grew out of the need for improved knowledge, screening and access to care in Haimen City. HBF, founded in 1991, is a United States-based non-profit organization engaged in scientific and public health research, education and patient advocacy.

Gateway to care awareness and education program methodology

A multi-platform education and awareness campaign for the general public consisted of print media (newspapers, brochures, direct home mailings), community awareness events, and free educational giveaway products such as playing cards, drinking cups and calendars. All platforms provided information on HBV transmission, prevention, testing and treatment, as well as healthy lifestyle behaviors. In addition, educational messages highlighted the importance of being tested for HBV and the need for chronically infected individuals to receive regular check-ups to monitor liver disease progression. Another educational aim was to debunk common myths about HBV transmission, for example by explaining that HBV is not transmitted through casual contact or sharing eating utensils.

In addition to the public information and awareness campaign, 52 in-person educational seminars were provided for key constituencies. The seminars targeted citywide township government officials, village community leaders, township and village doctors, and chronically infected HBV patients hospitalized in the Haimen City People's Hospital. The seminars were led by trained educators from HCCDC and infectious disease specialists from the People's Hospital. Each seminar lasted for at least 1 h and focused on increasing knowledge about HBV transmission, prevention, testing, and appropriate medical management and treatment (including screening for early detection of HCC). A primary goal of the seminars was to encourage appropriate testing and referral to care, as per published clinical guidelines [18]. More than 90 % of targeted health care providers (1441) attended these educational seminars, including medical doctors, obstetricians, nurse assistants, school nurses, and public health officials from the 23 townships and 239 villages that comprise Haimen City.

Program evaluation focused on HBV-related knowledge, attitudes and practices of health care providers, city residents, and infected individuals. Due to logistical constraints, government officials were not a focus of the evaluation. There were two components to the evaluation: an assessment of change in knowledge, attitudes and behaviors among health care providers who attended in-person educational seminars; and an assessment of post-campaign knowledge, attitudes and behaviors among random samples of health care providers, city residents and chronically infected individuals.

Data collection and analysis

To assess changes in knowledge before and after in-person seminars, health care providers were asked to complete a seven-item self-administered pre/post questionnaire. The pre/post questionnaire measured baseline knowledge and knowledge change immediately after seminar attendance in the following HBV-related domains: transmission, prevention, diagnosis, symptomology, epidemiology and treatment (Table 1, Additional file 1). A total of 710 providers completed the pre-questionnaire and 680 completed the post-questionnaire. To protect privacy and encourage participation, the pre- and post-questionnaires for individual participants were not linked. Results were analyzed using SAS v. 9.3 (Cary, NC). Poisson regression was used to examine stratum-specific differences in frequency of correct answers to the pre- and post-questionnaires by sex, age group, and educational level.

Additionally, a post-campaign survey was conducted among random samples of health care providers ($n = 227$), Haimen City residents ($n = 249$), and chronically infected individuals ($n = 20$). These self-administered paper surveys evaluated HBV-related knowledge, attitudes and behaviors, including stigma-related beliefs and practices (Table 1, Additional file 1). Health care provider survey participants were recruited throughout the city, and city residents were recruited from two randomly selected villages. Chronically HBV-infected individuals were recruited from the Haimen City People's Hospital. The surveys were analyzed using Microsoft Excel to calculate the percentage of correct responses on the HBV knowledge questions and the percentages of similar responses, by group, on the attitude and practice questions.

Six focus groups were conducted to gain a more in-depth understanding of how well the Gateway to Care campaign had met the needs of the target communities and to identify future intervention strategies for improving HBV testing, care and treatment. Focus groups were led by trained facilitators from HCCDC, and participants were recruited by HCCDC project staff.

Two focus groups were conducted with a total of 14 health care providers from two randomly selected townships. The providers were asked to comment on their preferred methods for receiving HBV education, strategies for improving HBV testing among community members, and strategies for promoting routine check-ups and antiviral treatment for chronically HBV-infected individuals. Two focus groups were conducted with a total of 15 city residents from two villages. These focus groups addressed methods for improving HBV awareness and HBV screening at the community level. Two focus groups were conducted with a total of 20 chronic HBV patients at the People's Hospital, with patients asked for their perspectives on strategies for encouraging completion of check-ups and uptake of oral antiviral treatment. All focus groups were conducted in Chinese. All sessions were recorded, and notes were taken by the facilitators. Transcripts were translated into English for analysis.

Focus group data were analyzed by study team members from both HBF and HCCDC, using thematic analysis methodology as a guide to in-depth engagement with the text [19]. The process included multiple readings of the focus group transcripts to become familiar with the domains and themes of the text. A coding table was created to separate questions and responses into distinct domains for each of the three types of participants (providers, city residents and HBV-infected individuals) (Table 2). Coding of the text took place in two phases: open and selective coding. Open coding helped to identify themes and summarize the data generally. Selective coding was then used to code data related to the identified domains/variables. Memo-writing was used throughout the coding process to highlight key themes and relationships that were being identified within the text.

Table 1 Domains and variables of self-administered questionnaires

Domains of pre/post health care provider survey	HBV knowledge • Transmission • Prevention • Diagnosis • Symptomology • Epidemiology (local, national) • Treatment (when to treat, how to treat)
Domains of post-campaign self-administered surveys for health care providers, residents, and HBV-infected individuals	HBV knowledge • Transmission • Prevention • Diagnosis • Treatment
	Attitudes towards HBV • Transmission • Vaccination • Treatment • Importance of seeing a doctor • Importance of being tested
	HBV-related behaviors • Seeking HBV knowledge • Distancing from an infected individual • Getting tested for HBV • Getting vaccinated against HBV • Seeing a doctor if infected

Table 2 Domains and primary questions for focus groups conducted with health care providers ($n = 14$), Haimen City residents ($n = 15$) and chronically HBV-infected individuals ($n = 20$)

Domains	Primary Questions
HBV knowledge	Providers and City Residents
Effective/preferred means of gaining knowledge	• What is the most effective way to gain knowledge about prevention and control of hepatitis B and liver cancer? • What is the best way for you to receive health education and promotion?
	Infected Individuals
	• What is the most effective way to gain knowledge about prevention and control of hepatitis B and liver cancer?
Attitudes towards HBV	Providers and City Residents
Necessary tools to fight the hepatitis B epidemic in Haimen City	• What is the most important help the community and patients need in fighting hepatitis B?
	Infected Individuals
	• What is the most important help you need in addressing hepatitis B?
HBV-related behaviors	Providers and City Residents
• Effective ways to encourage routine check-ups for infected individuals • Effective ways to encourage antiviral treatment for infected individuals who are candidates	• What is the best way to encourage hepatitis B testing for people unaware of their infection status? • What is the best way to encourage routine check-ups for asymptomatic hepatitis B patients? • What is the best way to encourage asymptomatic hepatitis B treatment candidates to receive appropriate antiviral treatment?
	Infected Individuals
	• What is the best way to encourage routine check-ups for asymptomatic hepatitis B patients? • What is the best way to encourage asymptomatic hepatitis B treatment candidates to receive appropriate antiviral treatment?

Data anonymity and ethics statement

The program that this study is based on was reviewed and approved in 2010 by the Medical Ethics Review Committee of Haimen City. All data from the surveys and focus groups were collected anonymously, with no identifying information recorded.

Results

HBV-related knowledge change among health care providers who attended seminars

A total of 710 health care providers completed the HBV knowledge pre-test, 50.8 % of whom were male. The median age of the pre-test group was 45 (range 24–68). A total of 680 providers completed the HBV knowledge post-test, of whom 51.2 % were male. The median age of the post-test group was 46 (range 24–68). Neither age nor gender differed significantly between the pre- and post-test groups.

Respondents correctly answered 67.3 % of the pre-test questions and 85.9 % of the post-test questions, indicating an overall knowledge increase of 18.6 % ($p < 0.0001$) (Table 3). Male providers correctly answered 68.1 % of the pre-test questions and 85.6 % of the post-test questions, indicating a knowledge increase of 17.4 % ($p < 0.0001$) (Table 4). Female providers correctly answered 66.4 % of the pre-test questions and 86.3 % of the post-test questions, indicating a knowledge increase of 19.9 % ($p < 0.01$). There were significant knowledge increases for all age groups except the group aged 65 and older. Additionally, there were significant knowledge increases for those who had completed high school or less (14.4 %, $p < 0.01$) and those who had completed junior college (20.8 %, $p < 0.0001$). There was an 18.3 % knowledge increase among the small number of providers who had completed college ($p = 0.06$). Results of the Poisson regression indicate that controlling for age, gender and education (individually and together) did not change the estimate of the pre/post effect on HBV knowledge overall.

Post-campaign knowledge, attitudes and practices among health care providers

Of the 226 health care providers who completed the post-campaign questionnaire, 46.5 % were female and the mean age was 41 (age range 22–68). Nineteen percent had a high school education or less, 32.7 % had completed junior college, 20.8 % had completed college and 27.4 % had post-college secondary education. A total of 93.4 % of providers stated that they had received HBV education within the past 2 years. A total of 94.7 % correctly answered the questionnaire's transmission question, 100 % correctly answered the HBV testing/diagnosis question, 88.5 % correctly answered the prevention question, and 93.8 % correctly answered the treatment question (Table 5).

Most providers (75.2 %) responded that it is necessary to test patients for HBV regardless of symptoms, while 24.3 % felt that it is important to test only patients who are symptomatic. Eighty percent reported that they tested their patients for HBV, 76.1 % reported suggesting to their patients that they be tested, and 85.8 % stated that they provide HBV education to their patients.

Table 3 Percent change in correct responses by health care providers completing pre/post HBV knowledge surveys

	Pre-Test % Correct	Post-Test % Correct	% Change	*P* value
Question 1	89.3	98.5	+9.2	<.0001
Question 2	79.2	94.4	+15.2	<.0001
Question 3	30.7	64.7	+34.0	<.0001
Question 4	58.5	74.1	+15.6	<.0001
Question 5	75.9	87.1	+11.2	<.0001
Question 6	65.5	87.8	+22.3	<.0001
Question 7	71.8	94.7	+22.9	<.0001

Ninety-six percent of providers believed that infected individuals need regular check-ups, and 95.0 % advised their asymptomatic patients to get regular check-ups. While 97.8 % of providers agreed that it was important for treatment candidates to receive treatment, only 65.5 % of them reported suggesting treatment to their asymptomatic treatment candidates. Almost all providers (97.0 %) felt that individuals who are susceptible to HBV should be vaccinated, particularly if they have an infected family member, and 95.1 % reported recommending HBV vaccination to susceptible persons.

Health care providers participating in focus groups indicated that individualized, in-person, small group educational sessions were an effective way to acquire knowledge about HBV prevention and control. Providers also felt that a multi-platform strategy was the best way to improve HBV knowledge and awareness among members of the public. Suggested strategies for building public awareness included delivering HBV messages through mass media (potentially TV, newspapers and social media), community seminars, and in-person education by village doctors. Providers stressed the importance of repetitive messaging. Reducing the cost of laboratory tests was seen as the most important strategy for encouraging routine check-ups among HBV-infected individuals. Offering free treatment as well as educating infected patients about the consequences of HBV and about available treatment options were noted as ways to encourage treatment candidates to seek HBV treatment.

Table 5 Percentages of HBV knowledge questions answered correctly in post-campaign surveys

	Health Care Providers	City Residents	Infected Individuals
HBV Transmission	94.7 %	85.9 %	95 %
HBV Diagnosis	100 %	84.3 %	100 %
HBV Prevention	88.5 %	80.7 %	95 %
HBV Treatment	93.8 %	57.8 %	80 %

Table 4 Results of Poisson regression examining stratum-specific differences in frequency of correct answers to pre/post knowledge surveys among health care providers by sex, age group and educational level

Percent Correct by Group	Pre-test (*N* = 710)	(*n*)	Post-test (*N* = 680)	(*n*)	Change	Univariate *p*-value	After Controlling for Pre/post Survey
Total	67.3 %	710	85.9 %	680	+18.6 %	<0.0001	
Gender							
Male	68.1 %	362	85.6 %	349	+17.4 %	<0.0001	0.24
Female	66.4 %	348	86.3 %	331	+19.9 %	<0.001	
Age Group							
< 35	66.9 %	117	87.6 %	107	+20.7 %	<0.001	0.13
35–39	61.4 %	144	85.3 %	131	+23.9 %	<0.001	
40–44	66.2 %	124	86.2 %	120	+20.0 %	<0.001	
45–49	68.6 %	66	87.3 %	63	+18.7 %	<0.01	
50–54	71.0 %	63	85.7 %	63	+14.7 %	0.05	
55–59	71.6 %	16	85.7 %	76	+14.1 %	0.03	
60–64	71.3 %	81	85.5 %	81	+14.3 %	0.03	
≥ 65	68.1 %	39	81.7 %	39	+13.6 %	0.17	
Educational Level							
≤ High School	70.5 %	213	84.9 %	213	+14.4 %	<.001	0.05
Jr/Tech Coll	65.1 %	429	85.9 %	408	+20.8 %	<.0001	
≥ College	71.0 %	68	89.3 %	59	+18.3 %	0.06	

Post-campaign knowledge, attitudes and practices among city residents

Of the 249 city residents who completed the post-campaign questionnaire, 55.8 % were female and the mean age was 48 (age range 18–88). Forty-nine percent had a middle-school education or less, 15.7 % had completed high school, 8.8 % had completed junior college or college, 2.0 % had post-secondary education, and 1.6 % had no formal education. About half (47.8 %) indicated that they had received some type of HBV education/information in the previous 2 years. A total of 85.9 % people correctly answered the questionnaire's transmission question, 84.3 % correctly answered the HBV diagnosis question, 80.7 % correctly answered the prevention question, and 57.8 % correctly answered the treatment question (Table 5). Just over half of respondents (56.6 %) felt that it is either better, or necessary, for an HBV-infected individual to use separate utensils, and 24.9 % stated that they have tried to keep their distance from infected individuals because of fear of getting infected. The majority (67.5 %) believed that it is necessary to be tested for HBV, but only 35.3 % reported that they had ever been tested. Sixty-four percent of respondents felt that individuals who are susceptible to HBV should be vaccinated, and 42.2 % stated that they had been vaccinated. Eight percent did not know their HBV vaccination status. More than two-thirds of people (67.5 %) felt that infected individuals should have regular check-ups, and 75.9 % felt that treatment candidates should receive treatment even if they are asymptomatic.

The city residents who participated in the focus groups preferred to receive HBV health messaging through repetitive television seminars and face-to-face talks with their doctors. They believed that there was a need for people to have repeated exposure to HBV education rather than just hearing the messages once. They thought that improving HBV knowledge through education would encourage people to get tested, especially if free testing was available. Providing free or subsidized HBV treatment and educating people about the consequences of untreated HBV infection were thought to be effective strategies for encouraging infected individuals (including those who are asymptomatic) to seek treatment.

Post-campaign knowledge, attitudes and practices among chronically infected individuals

Of the 20 HBV-infected individuals who completed the post-campaign questionnaire, 65.0 % were female and the mean age was 58 (age range 44–68). Thirty-five percent had completed elementary school, 55.0 % had completed middle school, and 10.0 % had completed high school. All (100 %) correctly answered the questionnaire's HBV testing/diagnosis question, 88.5 % correctly answered the prevention question, and 93.8 % correctly answered the treatment question (Table 5). Almost all (95.0 %) correctly identified HBV transmission routes, while all (100.0 %) knew that a blood test was the only way to diagnose an HBV infection. Ninety-five percent were aware that the HBV vaccine could prevent transmission of HBV. Eighty percent knew that HBV-infected individuals might need treatment even if they had no symptoms. Eighty percent responded that they had received some type of HBV education in the past 2 years, and 95 % percent reported that they received a regular check-up at least once a year. All respondents stated that they had received HBV treatment at some point (55.0 % were on treatment and 45.0 % had taken treatment in the past). Thirty percent felt that it was necessary to separate their eating utensils from those of non-infected family members, and 65.0 % felt that while this was not necessary, it was advisable.

Discussion

According to study results, HBV knowledge among health care providers significantly improved after attendance at an educational seminar. The results also indicate high levels of HBV knowledge among city residents and chronically infected individuals. However, city residents were less aware of the availability of treatment for HBV. For all three groups of study participants, having accurate knowledge was not necessarily enough to dispel stigma-related myths or foster behavior change regarding HBV screening or treatment. While 85.9 % of city residents correctly identified HBV transmission routes, more than half still felt that it was better to keep eating utensils of infected family members separate. One-quarter of these residents reported maintaining a distance from HBV-infected individuals for fear of becoming infected themselves. There were similar results among HBV-infected individuals who responded to the survey: virtually all correctly identified HBV transmission routes, but 65 % felt that it was better to not share their eating utensils with family members. Among providers, another gap between knowledge and practice was observed. While providers had high levels of knowledge regarding HBV transmission and diagnosis, almost 25 % reported that they only screen patients if they display symptoms of HBV. There also appeared to be discordance between providers and residents regarding testing, as only 35 % of residents recalled being tested for HBV.

While almost all providers agreed that it was important for treatment candidates to receive treatment, only 65.5 % of them suggested treatment to their asymptomatic treatment candidates. Results from the focus groups suggest that the high cost of antiviral treatment might play a role in this. Interestingly, among the 20 HBV-infected individuals who completed the post-campaign survey, almost all indicated that they underwent annual check-ups and had received treatment for their chronic HBV infection. However, it is not known if the respondents were referring to approved antiviral drug therapies for chronic HBV infection or to all types of treatment, including traditional Chinese medicine. The focus groups indicated that treatment was cost-prohibitive, and it has been documented that the proportion of HBV-infected individuals who receive antiviral treatment remains low in China [19]. More studies are needed in Haimen City to ascertain the percentage of infected individuals who routinely receive medical check-ups as per published guidelines and who receive appropriate antiviral treatment for their chronic HBV infection.

Additional research would be helpful in identifying strategies that could be used to enhance future educational/awareness interventions. Strategies should not only foster knowledge improvements, but also promote changes in beliefs and attitudes that can ultimately play a role in stigma reduction and behavior change. This could help to increase screening for all residents, improve treatment for some treatment candidates, and reduce discriminatory practices directed at infected individuals. Such strategies could be based upon behavioral change theories such as the Heath Belief Model, Health Behavior Framework and Transtheoretical Stages of Change [20]. These theories focus on multiple constructs that can be targeted for change, including knowledge, risk perception, beliefs, attitudes, and self-efficacy [20]. In doing so, they can guide the development of future interventions to improve effectiveness in changing HBV-related behaviors. Both the Health Belief Model and Transtheoretical Stages of Change theories have been used successfully to improve HBV screening behavior and similar types of cancer screening behaviors such as pap tests and colorectal screening [21, 14]. A study drawing on the constructs of the Health Behavior Framework looked at awareness of HBV, knowledge of transmission routes, perceived susceptibility, perceived severity, doctor recommendation, stigma of HBV infection, and perceived efficacy of testing among diverse ethnic groups in the United States (including Koreans, Vietnamese, Hmong, Chinese, Cambodians, and Taiwanese). Results indicate that it could prove to be a valid model for designing interventions aimed at overcoming challenges to HBV screening [22].

Stigma and discrimination surrounding hepatitis B in China and in other parts of the world has been well documented [23, 24, 11]. A study among Chinese Canadians found that perceptions of HBV-related stigma were associated with a decreased likelihood of undergoing HBV screening [11]. Strategies to overcome stigma have focused primarily on improving HBV-related knowledge, but little research has been done to assess the efficacy of this approach. A recent study conducted in rural China found that fear of HBV infection rather than lack of knowledge was what led to HBV-related stigma and discrimination [14]. Our results add evidence to the finding that knowledge by itself is not enough to overcome stigma and discrimination. Even with high levels of HBV knowledge, large proportions of those surveyed indicated a preference for separating themselves and/or their eating utensils from infected individuals, for fear of becoming infected. Studying this phenomenon further may lead to a better understanding of the pathway leading to HBV-related stigma and discrimination, which may in turn inform the design of appropriate theory-based interventions to reduce stigma and discrimination.

In terms of developing future HBV education and awareness efforts in China, focus group results across all groups of study participants suggest that repetitive educational interventions are advisable and that seminar-style education sessions should be supplemented with face-to-face (one-on-one) education by health care providers and with media-based communication. Additionally, since the costs of screening and treatment were thought to be prohibitive, future initiatives should address how these costs can be reduced.

It is necessary for key stakeholders, including health care providers, infected individuals and city residents, to have awareness and knowledge of HBV in order to address chronic HBV infection in China. Educational campaigns, such as the Gateway to Care, can play an important role. However, educational/awareness campaigns remain limited in their ability to improve HBV screening and care without seeing a change in access to HBV treatment. In China, cost seems to play a prohibitive role in both treatment recommendations by providers (as seen in this study) and treatment uptake by patients [19]. Improved access to treatment must be a necessary component in addressing chronic HBV infection in China into the future.

This study faced certain limitations. Pre-test data were not available from all groups, which limits the conclusions that can be drawn regarding the impact of the Gateway to Care campaign on knowledge change of city residents and chronically infected individuals. The pre- and post-intervention questionnaires measuring knowledge change among health care providers were not linked for individual study participants, so a matched analysis could not be conducted. A matched analysis might have yielded a better understanding of knowledge improvement as it relates to provider type or demographic factors. However, the pre-post analysis confirmed that the Gateway to Care campaign significantly improved HBV-related knowledge among participating providers who completed the pre/post surveys. Long-term follow-up was not completed, so we do not know if HBV-related knowledge change among providers was sustainable.

All questionnaires were specifically designed for use in this study, and while they were piloted tested, no formal psychometric testing was done to evaluate instrument validity and reliability (although low percentages of missing responses may indicate that questions were well understood by respondents). Additionally, while focus group participants were randomly selected, they are not necessarily representative of the greater population in Haimen City. This could limit the generalizability of conclusions that could be made from focus group data.

Conclusions

The Gateway to Care education and awareness campaign was successful in fostering high levels of accurate HBV knowledge among health care providers in Haimen City, China. Additionally, city residents and chronically infected individuals were knowledgeable about HBV transmission, prevention and symptomology. City residents were less aware of the availability of treatment for chronic HBV infection, and results indicate that cost of treatment can serve as an additional barrier to care. Even with accurate HBV knowledge, all study groups indicated a preference for separating infected individuals in certain social situations. More research is needed to better understand and address the complexities associated with these stigma-related beliefs and practices. Future HBV programs in Haimen City should focus on reducing cost of antiviral treatment, and should continue to improve awareness and knowledge, but should also include the use of theoretically driven behavior change interventions to improve rates of HBV screening for city residents, as well as to increase the provision of appropriate care for infected individuals and treatment for treatment candidates.

Abbreviations

HBF: Hepatitis B Foundation; HBV: Hepatitis B virus; HCC: Hepatocellular carcinoma.

Competing interests

The authors declare that they have no competing interests.

Authors' contributions

All authors contributed significantly to the study. CC participated in study design, led qualitative data analysis of focus groups and participated in quantitative analysis and interpretation, and led manuscript development/writing. GC participated in study design, served as U.S.-based project director, participated in data analysis and interpretation, and provided manuscript content and edits. JMB participated in study design, and provided substantial manuscript content and edits. AAE participated in study design, led data analysis and interpretation, and provided substantial manuscript content and edits. WTL participated in study design and provided substantial manuscript content and edits. PH participated in study design, served as Haimen City-based project director, and provided manuscript review/edits. All authors gave final approval of the manuscript, and agree with the manuscript results and conclusions. The criteria for authorship has been read and met by all authors.

Authors' information

CC, DrPH, MPH, is Director of Public Health at the Hepatitis B Foundation. She serves as senior advisor for Hep B United and director of Hep B United Philadelphia—both national and local coalitions, respectively, to improve hepatitis B screening, vaccination and linkage to care among high-risk groups in the U.S. She also serves as chair of the Coalition Against Hepatitis for People of African Origin (CHIPO), policy director for the Asian Pacific Islander Caucus for Public Health (APIC), and steering committee member of the National Viral Hepatitis Roundtable (NVHR). GC, MD, PhD, serves as director of China Programs at the Hepatitis B Foundation and was the project director for the original Haimen City Cohort project that began in 1992. AAE, ScD, is an associate professor at Drexel University School of Public Health, serves as senior public health advisor to the Hepatitis B Foundation, and served on the 2010 Academy of Sciences Institute of Medicine committee on Viral Hepatitis and Liver Cancer. JMB, RN, BSN, is co-founder and executive director of the Hepatitis B Foundation, co-chair of Hep B United, and served on the World Health Organization's Committee for the Development of Guidelines for the Management of Hepatitis B. WTL, MD, is an emeritus professor of Fox Chase Cancer Center, serves on the Board of Directors of the Hepatitis B Foundation, and is the senior medical advisor for the Foundation. PH serves as a public health scientist with the Haimen City Center for Disease Control and Prevention (HCCDC), Haimen City, China.

Acknowledgements

The authors would like to thank John Kim, MPH, for assistance with SAS analysis of the pre-post data collection instruments. The authors acknowledge funding support for the Gateway to Care Haimen City project from the Bristol-Myers Squibb Foundation. This funder had no role in study design, data collection, data analysis, decision to publish, or preparation of the manuscript. The authors also thank the Haimen City Centers for Disease Control and Prevention for their contribution of funds to cover some of the programmatic costs associated with the Gateway to Care campaign. (Author P. Huang is on staff at HCCDC)

Author details

[1]Hepatitis B Foundation, Doylestown, PA, USA. [2]Drexel University School of Public Health, Philadelphia, PA, USA. [3]Haimen City Center for Disease Control and Prevention, Haimen City, China. [4]Fox Chase Cancer Center, Philadelphia, PA, USA.

References

1. Schweitzer A, Horn J, Mikolajczyk RT, Krause G, Ott JJ. Estimations of worldwide prevalence of chronic hepatitis B virus infection: a systematic review of data published between 1965 and 2013. Lancet. 2015;386(10003):1546–55.
2. He J, Gu DF, Wu XG, Kristi R, Duan XF, et al. Major causes of death among men and women in China. N Engl J Med. 2005;353:1124–34.
3. Liang X, Bi S, Yang W, Wang L, Cui G, et al. Epidemiological serosurvey of hepatitis B in China–declining HBV prevalence due to hepatitis B vaccination. Vaccine. 2009;264 7(47):6550–7.
4. Xia GL, Liu CB, Cao HL, Bi SL, Zhan MY, et al. Prevalence of hepatitis B and C virus infections in the general Chinese population. Results from a nationwide cross sectional seroepidemiologic study of hepatitis A, B, C, D and E virus infections in China, 1992. Int Hepatol Commun. 1996;5:62–73.
5. Zhuang H. Epidemiology of hepatitis. Chin J Vaccines Immun. 2004;10:180–1.
6. McGlynn KA, London WT. Epidemiology and natural history of hepatocellular carcinoma. Best Pract Res Clin Gastroenterol. 2005;19(1):3–23.

Table 2 Results of univariate analysis of factors associated with HCV monoinfection and HCV/HIV coinfection

	p[d]	HCV monoinfected[a] vs. Uninfected[c]				HCV/HIV coinfected[b] vs. Uninfected				n
		RRR[e]	95 % CI[f]		p	RRR	95 % CI		p	
			Lower limit	Upper limit			Lower limit	Upper limit		
Male (vs. Female)[g]	0.164	0.6	0.3	1.1	0.083	0.8	0.4	1.8	0.589	541
Aged ≥35 years (vs. Aged <35 years)	0.015	1.4	0.9	2.2	0.114	0.7	0.4	1.3	0.265	541
Greek nationality (vs. Non-Greek nationality)	0.224	0.4	0.1	1.6	0.174	0.3	0.1	1.5	0.133	541
Lived in urban area in the past 5 years (vs. Lived in semi-urban/rural area)	0.019	1.1	0.7	1.9	0.701	3.0	1.2	7.4	0.016	522
Living alone or with spouse/partner without children (vs. With family[h])	0.012	2.0	1.2	3.3	0.007	2.3	1.2	4.3	0.013	541
Homeless ≥1 night in the past 12 months (vs. Never in the past 12 months)	<0.001	1.5	0.9	2.4	0.119	3.7	2.0	6.9	<0.001	533
Did not graduate high school (12th grade) (vs. Graduated high school)	0.022	1.3	0.8	2.0	0.225	2.4	1.3	4.5	0.007	536
Unemployed / student / other (vs. Employed)	0.013	1.2	0.7	2.0	0.425	3.0	1.3	6.8	0.009	539
Economically inactive[i] (vs. Employed)		1.1	0.5	2.2	0.859	4.3	1.6	11.7	0.005	
Incarcerated at least once in lifetime (vs. Never)	0.001	2.2	1.4	3.4	<0.001	2.5	1.4	4.7	0.003	536
Use of primary substance ≥ 4 days a week (vs. <4 days a week)	0.086	0.7	0.4	1.2	0.203	1.4	0.6	3.2	0.454	540
Use of ≥3 substances of abuse (vs. Use of <3 substances of abuse)[j]	0.690	1.1	0.7	1.8	0.534	1.3	0.7	2.3	0.400	541
2–4 years of injection (vs. 0–1 year)	<0.001	1.6	0.5	4.8	0.404	8.8	1.0	78.1	0.051	535
5–9 years of injection (vs. 0–1 year)		2.8	1.0	7.7	0.040	7.8	0.9	66.6	0.060	
≥10 years of injection (vs. 0–1 year)		6.1	2.4	15.1	<0.001	11.0	1.4	87.3	0.023	
Injected on average 2–3 times per day in the past 30 days (vs. <2 times/day)	<0.001	0.7	0.3	1.7	0.472	2.2	0.8	6.1	0.128	529
Injected on average >3 times per day in the past 30 days (vs. <2 times/day)		1.1	0.5	2.4	0.824	5.0	2.1	11.7	<0.001	
Non-sterile syringe in last injection (vs. Sterile syringe in last injection)	0.149	1.6	0.6	4.3	0.342	2.9	0.9	8.9	0.062	519
Shared syringes in the past 12 months (vs. Never in the past 12 months)	<0.001	1.7	0.9	3.1	0.080	4.5	2.2	9.1	<0.001	504
Shared other injection equipment in the past 12 months (vs. Never in the past 12 months)	0.024	1.0	0.6	1.6	0.989	2.0	1.1	3.6	0.026	506
Two or more sexual partners in the past 12 months (vs. <2 sexual partners)	0.300	0.8	0.5	1.3	0.404	1.2	0.7	2.1	0.550	537
Sex in exchange for money etc. in the past 12 months (vs. Never in the past 12 months/non-active)	0.218	1.8	0.6	5.2	0.306	2.9	0.8	10.0	0.092	529
No condom use in last intercourse (vs. Use of condom use or non-active)	0.005	0.9	0.6	1.4	0.654	0.4	0.2	0.7	0.004	529
Ever entered treatment for drug-related problems before (vs. Never before)	0.275	1.4	0.9	2.2	0.157	1.0	0.6	1.9	0.874	536
Never tested for HCV before (vs. Tested for HCV before)	<0.001	0.4	0.3	0.7	<0.001	0.1	0.1	0.3	<0.001	528
Never tested for HIV before (vs. Tested for HIV before)	<0.001	0.5	0.3	0.8	0.001	0.2	0.1	0.4	<0.001	533

[a]Diagnosed HCV positive and HIV negative. [b]Diagnosed HCV positive and HIV positive. [c]Diagnosed HCV negative and HIV negative. [d]Overall p-value for this covariate. [e]RRR: relative risk ratios. [f]95 % confidence intervals. [g]Gender was measured by the following item: "What is your gender?" Response options included "male", "female", "other (transgender)". No person responded "other" in the sample used in the present analysis. [h]Includes children and or parents. [i]The category "economically inactive" includes the long-term sick, unpaid carers and persons living on pensions or benefits, but excludes students. In the present analysis, the status "student" was collapsed with the category "unemployed" under the assumption that, like people who are unemployed, students may be motivated to improve their physical and socioeconomic conditions and therefore are ready to undertake fewer health risks. [j]Tobacco use was not measured. Possible abuse of alcohol or non-medical use of prescription drugs is included

Table 3 Results of the multinomial logistic regression analysis of factors associated with HCV monoinfection and HCV/HIV coinfection (final model comprising only the significant – $p < 0.10$ – variables from the previous model, $n = 450$)

Correlate (vs. Reference category)		HCV monoinfected[a] vs. Uninfected[c]				HCV/HIV coinfected[b] vs. Uninfected			
	p^d	RRR[e]	95 % CI[f]		p	RRR	95 % CI		p
			Lower limit	Upper limit			Lower limit	Upper limit	
Male (vs. Female)[g]	0.023	0.4	0.2	0.9	0.018	0.7	0.2	2.0	0.499
Aged ≥35 years (vs. Aged <35 years)	0.015	1.2	0.7	2.1	0.493	0.5	0.2	1.0	0.066
Lived in urban area in the last 5 years (vs. Lived in semi-urban/rural area)	0.006	1.4	0.8	2.6	0.255	4.8	1.7	13.7	0.004
Living alone or with a spouse/partner without children (vs. With family[h])	0.007	2.6	1.3	4.9	0.005	3.1	1.3	7.3	0.010
Incarcerated at least once in lifetime (vs. Never)	0.018	2.0	1.2	3.4	0.008	2.5	1.1	5.3	0.021
5–9 years of injection (vs. 0–1 year)	0.002	2.4	0.8	7.2	0.134	6.0	0.6	60.6	0.129
2–4 years of injection (vs. 0–1 year)		1.5	0.4	5.6	0.529	8.2	0.7	92.2	0.088
≥10 years of injection (vs. 0–1 year)		5.5	1.9	15.9	0.002	14.1	1.5	133.8	0.021
Injected on average 2–3 times per day in the past 30 days (vs. <2 times/day)	0.003	1.1	0.3	3.4	0.916	2.6	0.6	10.5	0.186
Injected on average >3 times per day in the past 30 days (vs. <2 times/day)		1.1	0.4	2.9	0.805	4.5	1.6	12.8	0.005
Shared syringes in the past 12 months (vs. No syringe sharing in the past 12 months)	0.002	2.5	1.2	5.2	0.014	4.7	1.9	11.5	0.001
No condom use in last intercourse (vs. Use of condom or non-active)	0.043	0.8	0.5	1.4	0.424	0.4	0.2	0.9	0.018
Never tested for HCV before (vs. Tested for HCV before)	0.001	0.6	0.3	0.9	0.028	0.2	0.1	0.5	<0.001

[a]Diagnosed HCV positive and HIV negative. [b]Diagnosed HCV positive and HIV positive. [c]Diagnosed HCV negative and HIV negative. [d]Overall p-value for this covariate. [e]RRR: relative risk ratios. [f]95 % confidence intervals. [g]Gender was measured by the following item: "What is your gender?" Response options included "male", "female", "other (transgender)". No person responded "other" in the sample used in the present analysis. [h]Includes children and / or parents

reduction of HIV incidence [46, 63]. However, these programs have not proved financially sustainable [64]. Furthermore, under the austerity policies imposed from 2010 up to the present, public spending allotted to harm reduction has been minimal.

Living alone or only with a spouse/partner (without children or other family members, e.g., parents) trebled in our study the risk of HCV infection with or without HIV. Previous research has shown that higher-risk drug use is positively associated with intimacy among friendship networks [65]. At the same time, pockets of social support may reduce HCV and HIV related morbidity and mortality [66]. Taking care of children and living with a member of one's (biological) family is an often overlooked yet potentially important aspect of social support, especially in countries like Greece where the family retains its pivotal role in the lives of drug users [67]. The latter may influence health behaviors through self-regulation in conformity to norms or through others' health promoting behaviors and expectations [68]. In our study the likely absence of social support may have nurtured the adoption of risky behaviors in relation to HIV.

Our findings also suggest that those who have been incarcerated have twice as high a risk of HCV infection with or without HIV, suggesting that prison environments foster high-risk injection and sexual behavior and hence the acquisition of infection. The cross-sectional nature of our data does not allow us to make inferences about causality, but the independent association between incarceration and HCV, HIV, and HCV/HIV coinfection in this population is well documented [51, 69]. In Greece, no administrative alternatives to imprisonment are implemented for drug users. As of 2016, prisoners in Greece do not have access to sterile injection equipment or condoms, while screening, HIV counseling, and ART are not routinely available [70]. Since 2015, OST and drug-related health care has been available in only two of the eighteen prison units in operation in the country. Furthermore, following incarceration, low coverage of services and other structural barriers (e.g., lack of essential documents, language restrictions, poverty, stigma or fear) may have promoted behaviors with higher health risk in this population.

HCV/HIV coinfection (but not HCV monoinfection) was independently associated with frequent injection and residing in metropolitan areas. More specifically, living in an urban area and averaging more than 3 injections a day increased the risk by almost five. Living in an urban area represents a marker for high-risk factors.

These factors include barriers in access to health services coupled with relatively easy access to multiple and novel substances of unknown composition and adverse effects, participation in larger, unknown and changing injection and sexual networks, and exposure to sex work (e.g. [5]). In addition, fear of arrest or punishment may displace or lead drug injectors to avoid using outreach programs, or to hurried injections and injection practices that increase opportunities for parenteral exposures to HIV.

Theoretically, having a test for infectious diseases is an indicator of health-protecting attitude [50], leading to the assumption that drug users who have been tested in the past will more likely be uninfected. Counterintuitively, our study showed that the risk of being infected was negatively associated with previous HCV testing. Unfortunately, the cross-sectional nature of the present study and the fact that we did not measure the time at which both the infection and previous testing occurred, or whether the test result was known to the participant, prevent us from being able to interpret these findings.

There was also a negative association between having used a condom in the last sexual intercourse and the risk of HCV/HIV coinfection (but not of HCV monoinfection). Again, lack of additional data (e.g., frequency of sexual activity, partner's sexual orientation etc.) or more relevant variables (e.g., overall consistency of condom use) prevent us from fully explaining these findings. However, a number of hypotheses may be proposed: first, it may be that those who responded that they *did* use a condom in their last sexual intercourse had been – prior to the last occasion– largely reckless in their sexual behavior. Second, the category included people who had no sex in the last 12 months, who possibly knew their positive serological status and abstained from sex. Third, the present data were collected in a period in which the HIV epidemic and the corresponding health-risk awareness and HIV counselling programs were at their greatest extent, reaching a substantial number of injection drug users (especially in Athens) [41, 46, 62]. Against this background it may be that those who reported that they *did* use a condom in the last sexual intercourse were giving the socially desired response. Finally, it may also be that those who responded that they *did not* use a condom in the last sexual intercourse were more cautious with other high-risk behaviors.

The findings of our study should be seen in the light of several limitations. First, the study participants were recruited only from OST outpatient clinics and only from central and southern Greece. In theory this affects the generalizability of our findings. However, clinics and participants in the present study comprised about 70 % of national totals that year (2013). Second, we focused only on injection drug users and injection practices in general among heroin and other opioid users. Using stimulants (e.g., in the case of Greece, 'shisha,' a variant of methamphetamine) also has destabilizing effects [5, 71]. However, only a small proportion of study participants reported primary use of stimulants, including cocaine (2.4 %), and therefore this behavior was not included as a correlate in the analysis. Third, the cross-sectional design of the study does not allow the establishment of a causal relationship or a direction of causality between empirically related variables. Furthermore, as we did not measure whether HIV and HCV seropositives were known positives prior to the data collection, or whether they had already received specialised infectious diseases treatment, we could not check for possible interactions with other variables examined in the study. Finally, although data collection protocols have been employed for years in ways that elicit valid responses, possible misreporting associated with recall and social desirability biases [72] during the interview cannot be overlooked.

Conclusions

The positive association observed between infection and lengthy injection histories points to the need for scaling-up OST programmes and retaining people in treatment. The positive association between HCV/HIV coinfection and, independently, frequent daily injection and living in urban areas suggests that more injection equipment, screening and brief advice are required in order to reach out to more injection drug users, especially in the inner city areas of all major cities in the country. Prior incarceration increases the risk of infection, and this alone highlights the need to provide routine testing and harm reduction services in all detention centres in the country. Importantly, keeping in contact with their family (i.e., parents and/or children) may reduce the risk of infection for people who inject drugs, and this element could guide counselling that takes place at the treatment centre level and relies on building up family support systems.

Acknowledgements

The Drug Related Infectious Diseases (DRID) Medical Doctors Group of the Greek Organisation Against Drugs (OKANA) consists of the following people: Konstantina Alexakou; Olga Anagnostou; Giorgos Androulakis; Emmanuel Chalkiadakis; Ioanna Detsi; Anastasia Drimousi; Dimitra Frontzou; Melpomeni Gargoulaki; Maria Iosifidou; Katerina Kaliva; Anna Katsilli; Stavroula Kollia; Maria Kollitsida; Argyrios Kotsalis; Spiroula Makristathi; Theodoros Papadopoulos; Eleftheria Petroulaki; Vasilis Pinakas; Michael Spirellis; Konstantinos Stamatopoulos; Victoria Stavridou; Yolanda-Irena Stepen-Topalidi; Christos Tanis; Anastasios Tsantilas; Panayiota Tsekoura; Efrosini Tsirogianni. The present study relies on data routinely collected in the context of the implementation of the nationwide epidemiological surveillance system pertaining to the characteristics of the persons entering drug-related treatment and testing for infectious diseases in Greece. The authors would like to acknowledge the significant role of OKANA, the OKANA Directors and especially the Heads and the personnel of the opioid substitution treatment clinics for collecting and making these data available to the Greek REITOX Focal Point of the European Monitoring Centre for Drugs and Drug Addiction. Dr. Evaggelos Kafetzopoulos is the present OKANA Director and Professor Melpomeni-Minerva (Meni) Malliori was the Director when the data for the present study were collected (2013).

Funding

The authors certify that no funding has been received for the conduct of this study and/or preparation of this manuscript.

Authors' contributions

The Group of Drug Related Infectious Diseases (DRID) medical doctors of OKANA were responsible for the acquisition of the data. AF and MT directed the data collection and management process. AF designed the study and wrote the manuscript. EK and AA prepared the data and conducted all statistical analyses. CR overviewed the statistical analyses and contributed substantially to the writing of the manuscript. MT and AK read and critically revising the paper. All authors reviewed the data, contributed to their interpretation, and approved the final manuscript.

Competing interests

The authors declare that they have no competing interests.

Author details

[1]Epidemiology Unit, Greek Reitox Focal Point of the EMCDDA, University Mental Health Research Institute, 2 Soranou tou Efesiou St., Athens 11527, Greece. [2]Panteion University of Social and Political Sciences, 136, Leoforos A. Siggrou, Kallithea, Athens 17671, Greece. [3]University Mental Health Research Institute, 2 Soranou tou Efesiou St., Athens 11527, Greece. [4]Greek Organisation Against Drugs, Athens Greece, 21, Averof st., 10433 Athens, Greece.

References

1. Aceijas C, Rhodes T. Global estimates of prevalence of HCV infection among injecting drug users. Int J Drug Policy. 2007;18(5):352–8.
2. Hagan H, Thiede H, Des Jarlais DC. HIV/hepatitis C virus co-infection in drug users: risk behavior and prevention. AIDS. 2005;19 Suppl 3:S199–207.
3. Strader DB. Coinfection with HIV and hepatitis C virus in injection drug users and minority populations. Clin Infect Dis. 2005;41 Suppl 1:S7–13.
4. Hope VD, Eramova I, Capurro D, Donoghoe MC. Prevalence and estimation of hepatitis B and C infections in the WHO European Region: a review of data focusing on the countries outside the European Union and the European Free Trade Association. Epidemiol Infect. 2013;FirstView:1–17.
5. Miller CL, Wood E, Spittal PM, Li K, Frankish JC, Braitstein P, Montaner JS, Schechter MT. The future face of coinfection: prevalence and incidence of HIV and hepatitis C virus coinfection among young injection drug users. J Acquir Immune Defic Syndr. 2004;36(2):743–9.
6. Rhodes T, Platt L, Judd A, Mikhailova LA, Sarang A, Wallis N, Alpatova T, Hickman M, Parry JV. Hepatitis C virus infection, HIV co-infection, and associated risk among injecting drug users in Togliatti, Russia. Int J STD AIDS. 2005;16(11):749–54.
7. Vickerman P, Martin NK, Roy A, Beattie T, Group EC, Des Jarlais D, Strathdee S, Wiessing L, Hickman M. Is the HCV–HIV co-infection prevalence amongst injecting drug users a marker for the level of sexual and injection related HIV transmission? Drug Alcohol Depend. 2013;132(1):172–81.
8. Alter MJ. Epidemiology of viral hepatitis and HIV co-infection. J Hepatol. 2006;44(1 Suppl):S6–9.
9. Lumbreras B, Jarrin I, del Amo J, Perez-Hoyos S, Muga R. Garcia-de la Hera M, Ferreros I, Sanvisens A, Hurtado I, Hernandez-Aguado I: Impact of hepatitis C infection on long-term mortality of injecting drug users from 1990 to 2002: differences before and after HAART. AIDS. 2006;20(1):111–6.
10. Smit C, van den Berg C, Geskus R, Berkhout B, Coutinho R, Prins M. Risk of hepatitis-related mortality increased among hepatitis C virus/HIV-coinfected drug users compared with drug users infected only with hepatitis C virus: a 20-year prospective study. J Acquir Immune Defic Syndr. 2008;47(2):221–5.
11. Smith DJ, Combellick J, Jordan AE, Hagan H. Hepatitis C virus (HCV) disease progression in people who inject drugs (PWID): A systematic review and meta-analysis. Int J Drug Policy. 2015;26(10):911–21.
12. Di Martino V, Rufat P, Boyer N, Renard P, Degos F, Martinot-Peignoux M, Matheron S, Le Moing V, Vachon F, Degott C, et al. The influence of human immunodeficiency virus coinfection on chronic hepatitis C in injection drug users: a long-term retrospective cohort study. Hepatology. 2001;34(6):1193–9.
13. Monto A, Currie S, Wright TL. Liver disease in injection drug users with hepatitis C, with and without HIV coinfection. J Addict Dis. 2008;27(2):49–59.
14. Sanvisens A, Fuster D, Serra I, Tor J, Tural C, Rey-Joly C, Muga R. Estimated liver fibrosis and its impact on all-cause mortality of HCV-monoinfected and HCV/HIV-coinfected drug users. Curr HIV Res. 2011;9(4):256–62.
15. Altice FL, Kamarulzaman A, Soriano V, Schechter M, Friedland GH. Treatment of medical, psychiatric, and substance-use comorbidities in people infected with HIV who use drugs. Lancet. 2010;376(9738):367–87.
16. Taylor LE, Swan T, Matthews GV. Management of Hepatitis C Virus/HIV Coinfection Among People Who Use Drugs in the Era of Direct-Acting Antiviral–Based Therapy. Clin Infect Dis. 2013;57 suppl 2:S118–24.
17. Khalsa JH, Kresina T, Sherman K, Vocci F. Medical management of HIV-hepatitis C virus coinfection in injection drug users. Clin Infect Dis. 2005;41 Suppl 1:S1–6.
18. Kresina TF, Bruce RD, Cargill VA, Cheever LW. Integrating care for hepatitis C virus (HCV) and primary care for HIV for injection drug users coinfected with HIV and HCV. Clin Infect Dis. 2005;41 Suppl 1:S83–8.
19. McCance-Katz EF. Treatment of opioid dependence and coinfection with HIV and hepatitis C virus in opioid-dependent patients: the importance of drug interactions between opioids and antiretroviral agents. Clin Infect Dis. 2005;41 Suppl 1:S89–95.
20. Baum MK, Jayaweera DT, Duan R, Sales S, Lai S, Rafie C, Regev A, Page JB, Berkman R, Campa A. Quality of life, symptomatology and healthcare utilization in HIV/HCV co-infected drug users in Miami. J Addict Dis. 2008;27(2):37–48.
21. Scheft H, Fontenette DC. Psychiatric barriers to readiness for treatment for hepatitis C Virus (HCV) infection among injection drug users: clinical experience of an addiction psychiatrist in the HIV-HCV coinfection clinic of a public health hospital. Clin Infect Dis. 2005;40 Suppl 5:S292–6.
22. Graham CS, Wells A, Edwards EM, Herren T, Tumilty S, Stuver SO, Samet JH, Nunes D, Horsburgh Jr CR, Koziel MJ. Effect of exposure to injection drugs or alcohol on antigen-specific immune responses in HIV and hepatitis C virus coinfection. J Infect Dis. 2007;195(6):847–56.
23. Cescon A, Chan K, Raboud JM, Burchell AN, Forrest JI, Klein MB, Loutfy MR, Machouf N, Montaner JS, Tsoukas C, et al. Significant differences in clinical outcomes between HIV-hepatitis C virus coinfected individuals with and without injection drug use history. AIDS. 2014;28(1):121–7.
24. Mehta SH, Thomas DL, Sulkowski MS, Safaein M, Vlahov D, Strathdee SA. A framework for understanding factors that affect access and utilization of treatment for hepatitis C virus infection among HCV-mono-infected and HIV/HCV-co-infected injection drug users. AIDS. 2005;19 Suppl 3:S179–89.
25. Rey D, Carrieri MP, Spire B, Loubiere S, Dellamonica P, Gallais H, Cassuto GP, Gastaut JA, Obadia Y. Factors associated with liver biopsy performance in HCV-HIV coinfected injecting drug users with HCV viremia: results from a five-year longitudinal assessment. J Urban Health. 2004;81(1):48–57.
26. Beyrer C, Malinowska-Sempruch K, Kamarulzaman A, Strathdee SA. 12 myths about HIV/AIDS and people who use drugs. Lancet. 2010;376(9737):208–11.
27. Graham CS. Hepatitis C and HIV Co-infection: Closing the Gaps. JAMA. 2015;313(12):1217–8.

28. Akselrod H, Grau LE, Barbour R, Heimer R. Seroprevalence of HIV, hepatitis B virus, and HCV among injection drug users in Connecticut: understanding infection and coinfection risks in a nonurban population. Am J Public Health. 2014;104(9):1713–21.
29. Fisher DG, Reynolds GL, Jaffe A, Perez MJ. Hepatitis and human immunodeficiency virus co-infection among injection drug users in Los Angeles County. California J Addict Dis. 2006;25(2):25–32.
30. Garten RJ, Zhang J, Lai S, Liu W, Chen J, Yu XF. Coinfection with HIV and hepatitis C virus among injection drug users in southern China. Clin Infect Dis. 2005;41 Suppl 1:S18–24.
31. Del Fava E, Kasim A, Usman M, Shkedy Z, Hens N, Aerts M, Bollaerts K, Scalia Tomba G, Vickerman P, Sutton AJ. Joint modeling of HCV and HIV infections among injecting drug users in italy using repeated cross-sectional prevalence data. Stat Commun Infect Dis. 2011. http://dx.doi.org/10.2202/1948-4690.1009.
32. Solomon SS, Srikrishnan AK, Mehta SH, Vasudevan CK, Murugavel KG, Thamburaj E, Anand S, Kumar MS, Latkin C, Solomon S, et al. High prevalence of HIV, HIV/hepatitis C virus coinfection, and risk behaviors among injection drug users in Chennai, India: a cause for concern. J Acquir Immune Defic Syndr. 2008;49(3):327–32.
33. Marmor M, Des Jarlais DC, Cohen H, Friedman SR, Beatrice ST, Dubin N, el-Sadr W, Mildvan D, Yancovitz S, Mathur U, et al. Risk factors for infection with human immunodeficiency virus among intravenous drug abusers in New York City. AIDS. 1987;1(1):39–44.
34. Mathei C, Shkedy Z, Denis B, Kabali C, Aerts M, Molenberghs G, Van Damme P, Buntinx F. Evidence for a substantial role of sharing of injecting paraphernalia other than syringes/needles to the spread of hepatitis C among injecting drug users. J Viral Hepat. 2006;13(8):560–70.
35. Zocratto KB, Caiaffa WT, Proietti FA, Carneiro-Proietti AB, Mingoti SA, Ribeiro GJ. HCV and HIV infection and co-infection: injecting drug use and sexual behavior, AjUDE-Brasil I Project. Cad Saude Publica. 2006;22(4):839–48.
36. Dumchev KV, Soldyshev R, Qian HZ, Zezyulin OO, Chandler SD, Slobodyanyuk P, Moroz L, Schumacher JE. HIV and hepatitis C virus infections among hanka injection drug users in central Ukraine: a cross-sectional survey. Harm Reduct J. 2009;6:23.
37. Bollepalli S, Mathieson K, Jasiurkowski B, Hillier A, Post J, Bhanu S, Martin D, Van Thiel DH, Nadir A. A comparison of risk factors for HCV-mono-infection, HIV-mono-infection, and HCV/HIV-co-infection in a community setting. Dig Dis Sci. 2008;53(2):517–21.
38. Bollepalli S, Mathieson K, Bay C, Hillier A, Post J, Van Thiel DH, Nadir A. Prevalence of risk factors for hepatitis C virus in HIV-infected and HIV/hepatitis C virus-coinfected patients. Sex Transm Dis. 2007;34(6):367–70.
39. Hosseini M, SeyedAlinaghi S, Kheirandish P, Esmaeli Javid G, Shirzad H, Karami N, Jahani M, Seyed Ahmadian M, Payvarmehr F, Mohraz M, et al. Prevalence and correlates of co-infection with human immunodeficiency virus and hepatitis C virus in male injection drug users in Iran. Arch Iran Med. 2010;13(4):318–23.
40. European Monitoring Centre for Drugs and Drug Addiction [EMCDDA]. European drug report: trends and developments. Luxembourg: Publications Office of the European Union; 2015.
41. University Mental Health Research Institute [UMHRI]. National Report to the EMCDDA: "Greece: New Developments, Trends". Athens: Greek Reitox Focal Point of the EMCDDA; 2014.
42. Hellenic Center for Disease Control and Prevention [HCDCP]. HIV/AIDS Surveillance Report in Greece, 31-12-2014 (Issue 29). Athens: Hellenic Center for Disease Control and Prevention; 2014.
43. Kokkevi A, Alevizou S, Arvanitis Y, Liappas J, Stefanis C. AIDS-related behavior and attitudes among i.v. drug users in Greece. Int J Addict. 1992;27(1):37–50.
44. Pharris A, Wiessing L, Sfetcu O, Hedrich D, Botescu A, Fotiou A, Nikolopoulos GK, Malliori M, Salminen M, Suk JE, et al. Human immunodeficiency virus in injecting drug users in Europe following a reported increase of cases in Greece and Romania, 2011. Euro Surveill. 2011;16(48). Available online: http://www.eurosurveillance.org/ViewArticle.aspx?ArticleId=20032.
45. Paraskevis D, Nikolopoulos G, Tsiara C, Paraskeva D, Antoniadou A, Lazanas M, Gargalianos P, Psychogiou M, Malliori M, Kremastinou J et al. HIV-1 outbreak among injecting drug users in Greece, 2011: a preliminary report. Euro Surveill. 2011;16(36). Available online: http://www.eurosurveillance.org/ViewArticle.aspx?ArticleId=19962.
46. Hatzakis A, Sypsa V, Paraskevis D, Nikolopoulos G, Tsiara C, Micha K, Panopoulos A, Malliori M, Psichogiou M, Pharris A, et al. Design and baseline findings of a large-scale rapid response to an HIV outbreak in people who inject drugs in Athens, Greece: the ARISTOTLE programme. Addiction. 2015;110(9):1453–67.
47. Sypsa V, Paraskevis D, Malliori M, Nikolopoulos GK, Panopoulos A, Kantzanou M, Katsoulidou A, Psichogiou M, Fotiou A, Pharris A, et al. Homelessness and other risk factors for HIV infection in the current outbreak among injection drug users in Athens, Greece. Am J Public Health. 2015;105(1):196–204.
48. Malliori M, Sypsa V, Psichogiou M, Touloumi G, Skoutelis A, Tassopoulos N, Hatzakis A, Stefanis C. A survey of bloodborne viruses and associated risk behaviours in Greek prisons. Addiction. 1998;93(2):243–51.
49. Simon R, Donmall M, Hartnoll R, Kokkevi A, Ouwehand AW, Stauffacher M, Vicente J. The EMCDDA/Pompidou Group treatment demand indicator protocol: a European core item set for treatment monitoring and reporting. Eur Addict Res. 1999;5(4):197–207.
50. European Monitoring Centre for Drugs and Drug Addiction [EMCDDA]. DRID Guidance Module: behavioural indicators for people who inject drugs. Lisbon: EMCDDA; 2013.
51. Yen YF, Yen MY, Su LW, Li LH, Chuang P, Jiang XR, Deng CY. Prevalences and associated risk factors of HCV/HIV co-infection and HCV mono-infection among injecting drug users in a methadone maintenance treatment program in Taipei, Taiwan. BMC Public Health. 2012;12:1066.
52. Hagan H, Pouget ER, Des Jarlais DC. A systematic review and meta-analysis of interventions to prevent hepatitis C virus infection in people who inject drugs. J Infect Dis. 2011;204(1):74–83.
53. Wodak A, Cooney A. Do needle syringe programs reduce HIV infection among injecting drug users: a comprehensive review of the international evidence. Subst Use Misuse. 2006;41(6–7):777–813.
54. Des Jarlais DC, Marmor M, Paone D, Titus S, Shi Q, Perlis T, Jose B, Friedman SR. HIV incidence among injecting drug users in New York City syringe-exchange programmes. Lancet. 1996;348(9033):987–91.
55. Hurley SF, Jolley DJ, Kaldor JM. Effectiveness of needle-exchange programmes for prevention of HIV infection. Lancet. 1997;349(9068):1797–800.
56. Gibson DR, Brand R, Anderson K, Kahn JG, Perales D, Guydish J. Two- to sixfold decreased odds of HIV risk behavior associated with use of syringe exchange. J Acquir Immune Defic Syndr. 2002;31(2):237–42.
57. Des Jarlais DC, Hagan H, Friedman SR, Friedmann P, Goldberg D, Frischer M, Green S, Tunving K, Ljungberg B, Wodak A, et al. Maintaining low HIV seroprevalence in populations of injecting drug users. JAMA. 1995;274(15):1226–31.
58. Strathdee SA, van Ameijden EJ, Mesquita F, Wodak A, Rana S, Vlahov D. Can HIV epidemics among injection drug users be prevented? AIDS. 1998;12(Suppl A):S71–9.
59. MacDonald M, Law M, Kaldor J, Hales JJ, Dore G. Effectiveness of needle and syringe programmes for preventing HIV transmission. Int J Drug Policy. 2003;14(5):353–7.
60. WHO. Effectiveness of Sterile Needle and Syringe Programming in Reducing HIV/AIDS Among Injecting Drug Users. Evidence for Action. Technical Paper. Geneva: WHO; 2004.
61. Hedrich D, Kalamara E, Sfetcu O, Pharris A, Noor A, Wiessing L, Hope V, Van de Laar M. Human immunodeficiency virus among people who inject drugs: Is risk increasing in Europe? Euro Surveill. 2013;18(48):20648.
62. Terzidou M, Fotiou A. Explosion de VIH chez les consommateurs de drogues en Grèce pendant la crise économique [HIV outbreak among people who inject drugs in Greece during the economic crisis]. SWAPS. 2015;78:19–23.
63. Nikolopoulos GK, Sypsa V, Bonovas S, Paraskevis D, Malliori-Minerva M, Hatzakis A, Friedman SR. Big Events in Greece and HIV infection among people who inject drugs. Subst Use Misuse. 2015;50(7):1–14.
64. Nikolopoulos GK, Fotiou A. "Integrated interventions are dead. Long live sustainable integrated interventions!"—Austerity Challenges the Continuation of Effective Interventions in the Field of Drug Use-Related Harm Reduction. Subst Use Misuse. 2015;50(8–9):1220–2.
65. Friedman SR, Aral S. Social networks, risk-potential networks, health, and disease. J Urban Health. 2001;78(3):411–8.
66. Uchino BN. Social support and health: a review of physiological processes potentially underlying links to disease outcomes. J Behav Med. 2006;29(4):377–87.
67. Fotopoulou M. Reasons behind Greek problem drug users' decisions to quit using drugs and engage in treatment of their own volition: sense of self and the Greek filotimo. Addiction. 2014;109(4):627–34.
68. Lloyd JJ, Ricketts EP, Strathdee SA, Cornelius LJ, Bishai D, Huettner S, Havens JR, Latkin C. Social contextual factors associated with entry into opiate

agonist treatment among injection drug users. Am J Drug Alcohol Abuse. 2005;31(4):555–70.
69. Burris S, Chiu J. Punitive Drug Law and the Risk Environment for Injecting Drug Users: Understanding the Connections. In: Working paper prepared for the Third Meeting of the Technical Advisory Group of the Global Commission on HIV and the Law, 7–9 July 2011. 2011.
70. Zurhold H, Stöver H. Inventory of harm reduction measures in European prisons. Frankfurt: Frankfurt University of Applied Sciences; 2013.
71. Degenhardt L, Mathers B, Guarinieri M, Panda S, Phillips B, Strathdee SA, Tyndall M, Wiessing L, Wodak A, Howard J. Meth/amphetamine use and associated HIV: implications for global policy and public health. Int J Drug Policy. 2010;21(5):347–58.
72. Johnson T, Fendrich M. Modeling sources of self-report bias in a survey of drug use epidemiology. Ann Epidemiol. 2005;15(5):381–9.

8

National alliance for Wilson's disease: health policy

Francisco Hevia-Urrutia[1], Ileana Alvarado-Echeverría[1], Alfredo Sanabria-Castro[1], Marta Sánchez-Molina[1], Luis Meza-Sierra[1], Alexander Parajeles-Vindas[1], Oscar Méndez-Blanca[1], Álvaro Sánchez-Siles[2], Manuel Saborío-Rocafort[3], Marcela Barguil-Gallardo[1], Iliana Chavarría-Quirós[1] and Cecilia Monge-Bonilla[1*]

Abstract

Wilson's disease is an inherited disorder in which defective biliary excretion of copper leads to its accumulation, particularly in the liver and brain. Mutations in the ATP7B gene on chromosome 13 cause Wilson's disease. If left untreated it will cause liver failure, neurological damage, and will be life threatening. It is considered a rare disease afflicting approximately 1 in 30,000 persons worldwide, although this rate is similar in the different countries some places show higher incidence rates. Since Costa Rica reports the highest number of cases per population, essential public health initiatives that promote wellbeing, prevent disease complications, and prolong life among the affected population have been carried out during the last decades. The most recent lead in this matter is the conformation of the Costa Rica's National Alliance for Wilson's disease whose main objective is to provide practical, operational, timely and relevant guidance to patients, families, and healthcare professionals in the region for early diagnosis and treatment. The development and implementation of the National Alliance for Wilson's disease activities is crucial because it will reaffirm that early intervention and appropriate treatment, will reduce if not eliminate the burden of Wilson's disease.

Keywords: Wilson's disease, Ceruloplasmin, Hepatolenticular degeneration, Fulminant liver failure Costa Rica, National Alliance

Background

Wilson's disease (WD) also named hepatolenticular degeneration is a rare genetic disorder that causes excessive copper accumulation in the liver and brain and is fatal if not detected and treated [1]. The disease was named after Samuel Alexander Kinnier Wilson, M.D., who in 1912 reported pathologic findings of lenticular degeneration in the brain associated with cirrhosis of the liver [2]. The epidemiology of WD varies worldwide it is estimated that the pathology affects approximately 1 in 30,000 people [3] and one in 90–150 individuals carry a single abnormal Wilson's disease gene. Countries like Costa Rica and Japan show the highest prevalence; 1 in 60 per million people; almost doubling world's reports [4]; aspect that has become a health issue. The elevated number of cases in Costa Rica could be explained because: the high rates of consanguinity in the country, in which a small number of founding families date back to the eighteenth century [5] and low migration rates.

Despite the high incidence of WD in Costa Rica currently the relation between the number of deaths caused by hepatolenticular degeneration and the mortality by other liver diseases is not certain. Therefore a group of pioneers have been working together in the last years with the objective of studying profusely this disease and creating specific treatment and diagnosis guidelines for the region.

Axiom of Wilson's disease in Costa Rica:

"When approaching liver disease in Costa Rica; in patients under 30 years of age with chronic liver disease not secondary to alcohol consumption; the most likely diagnosis is Wilson's disease." Hevia-Urrutia M.D.

* Correspondence: ceciliamonge4@yahoo.com
[1]Hospital San Juan de Dios, Caja Costarricense del Seguro Social, 4917-1000 San José, Costa Rica
Full list of author information is available at the end of the article

History of Wilson's disease in Costa Rica

In 1970 Antillón-Salazar M.D. reported the first patient with WD in Costa Rica, a 17 year old man [6]. Around the same time, in Canada, Karl Schosinsky a Costa Rican M.D. contributed in the development of a precise, quantitative, enzymatic method for serum ceruloplasmin determination [7]. About thirteen years later Hevia-Urritia M.D., treated two young female patients (approximately 16 years old) with fulminant hepatic failure on the same month (Fig. 1), a rare condition at the time also described by McCullough et al. [8] In 1989, the incidence of WD in Costa Rica was reported as 4.9 per 100000 inhabitants, the highest in the world. Since the determination varies greatly upon location, Costa Rican regions with high incidence were identified and located in the central part of the country, showing close similarity to colonization cores (Fig. 2).

On 1990, Herra et al., reported that between 1972 and 1989, 150 cases of WD were diagnosed in Costa Rica; of these 120 were treated at Hospital San Juan de Dios. Seven patients died of acute liver failure, hemolytic anemia, encephalopathy, gastrointestinal bleeding or kidney insufficiency [9].

At the same moment, because of the high prevalence of WD in Costa Rica nationwide-inter-hospital working groups, consisting of medical microbiologists and pathologists, were established to analyze different diagnostic methods of copper metabolism for accuracy and effectiveness.

Hevia-Urrutia M.D and a group of patients founded in 1989 the Costa Rican Association of Patients with Wilson's Disease (A.C.O.P.A.W.) [10]. The goal of this association is to bring WD patients and their families together to inform, educate, and discuss valuable information regarding medications, health care, research, family screening, and support. Since its early days, A.C.O.P.A.W has had an annual meeting the first week of October, led and coordinated entirely by WD patients.

A major achievement was also obtained in 1989, during Oscar Arias Sanchez's government. The Costa Rican congress declared WD a "National Interest Disease", this ensure the adequate treatment (penicillamine, zinc and trientine) and management of patients by the Costa Rican Social Security National Health System (CCSS) (Fig. 1).

During 1997 the determination of the specific genetic mutations for Costa Rican WD patients proved different from mutations in US patients and most parts of Europe [11]; however the mutations observed in these patients (AsnSer 1270) were the same as those found in patients with WD in Sicily, Italy [12, 13]. Since then, Wilson's disease familial genetic mapping has been an important research line and has identify other genetic mutations that affect the population as well the most affected families in the country.

In 2009, the clinical presentation and demographic characteristics of the Costa Rican pediatric WD patients were described and showed similar characteristics to that in children diagnosed in other countries [14].

As worldwide in Costa Rica WD patients with fulminant hepatic failure are priority for liver transplant, nevertheless when this is not an option, innovative medical treatment with prostaglandins, vitamin E and haemoperfusion is administered [15]. In Costa Rica this management protocol has been used in the last 10 years and has shown positive outcomes in at least four patients (all women under 20 years of age) (Fig. 1).

In 2015 a collaborative alliance that includes gastroenterologists, researchers, neurologists, psychologists, psychiatrists, surgeons, geneticists, as well as other healthcare providers was created. The main purpose of this national alliance is to modify the way healthcare is delivered to WD patients, assuring that all Costa Rican

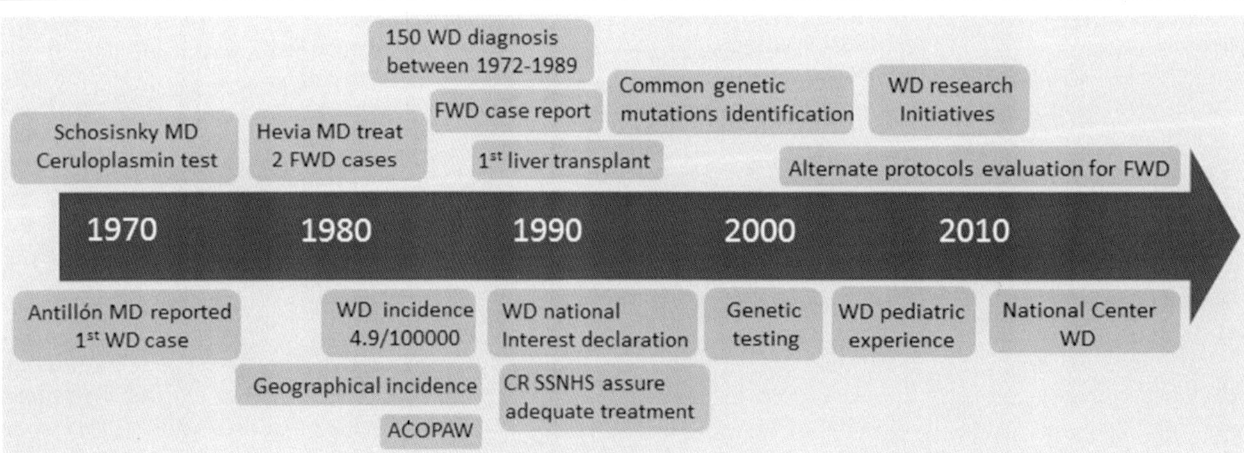

Fig. 1 Timeline of Wilson's Disease Events in Costa Rica. WD: Wilson's disease, MD: Medical doctor, FWD: fulminant Wilson's disease, ACOPAW: Costa Rican Wilson's disease Patient Association, CR: Costa Rica, SSNHS: Social Security National Health System

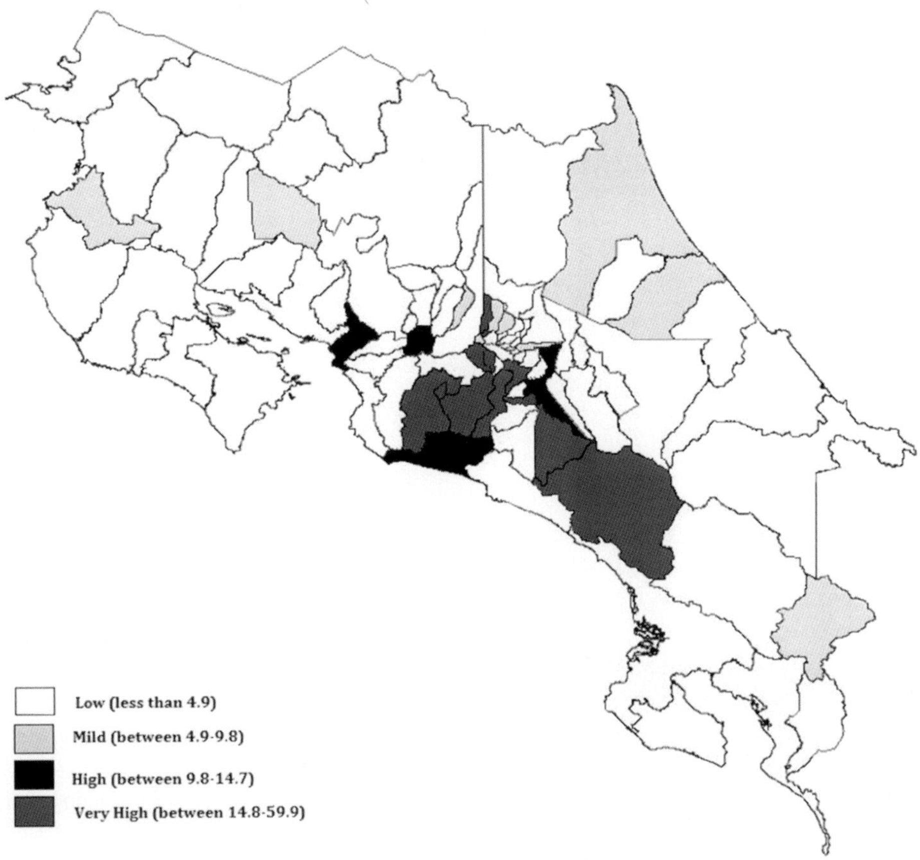

Fig. 2 Incidence of Wilson's disease in Costa Rica by canton from 1970 to 1989. Data is presented in cases per 100000 inhabitants

hospitals diagnose, treat and manage WD accurately, effectively, rapidly and in a homogenous manner. The National Alliance for WD based at the San Juan de Dios Hospital includes healthcare professionals from other centers like the Hospital Mexico (hepatic transplant team) and the National Children's Hospital (genetic screening).

In order to achieve its objectives the National Alliance for WD has establish a network that activates upon new possible WD diagnoses. Each member of this coalition has different roles but work in collaboration during the whole process which starts with diagnosis confirmation. Once the diagnosis is established members become fully involve in the family screening, best treatment option determination and disease management. The members also determine in conjunction priority research projects related to WD, and develop educational activities like workshops, exercise prescription and referral and other decision-making tools; addressed for healthcare professionals. These precise and effective mechanisms of interaction and communication have shown great results in approaching and solving urgent cases of WD, particularly in cases of fulminant hepatic failure.

The National Alliance for WD in Costa Rica aims to establish a Latin American Wilson's disease network through the Latin American Hepatology Association (ALEH). This network will assist in the establishment of additional national alliances, centers and committees in other Latin American countries, to collaborate in the training of diagnostic, management and treatment protocols, along with providing educational and scientific support regarding WD.

Currently the National Alliance for WD in Costa Rica considers the possible establishment of collaboration with a research group in Pamplona, Spain; that has developed a successful gene therapy for WD in animal models. For the future the creation of joint collaborations and programs with other organizations outside Costa Rica that perform similar actions as the National Alliance for Wilson's Disease are in scope. These institutions include: Medlineplus [16], National Library of Medicine Genetics Home Reference [17], NCBI Genes and Disease, Wilson's Disease Association (WDA), American Association for the Study of Liver Diseases (AASLD), American Liver Foundation [18], European Society for Liver diseases (EASL), Canadian Liver Foundation (CLF) [19] and Euro Wilson Registry [20].

Because of the high prevalence of WD in Costa Rica current research is being conducted to improve diagnosis, management and treatment of WD patients. Some of the research initiatives include: new variations of D-penicillamine load tests to achieve earlier diagnosis, the significance of free copper levels in patients after diagnosis and during treatment, the use of medications such as tetrathiomolibdate in patients with neurological symptoms [21], long term results and impact of immediate physiotherapy in patients with neurological symptoms, programs for early detection of cognitive and psychological abnormalities during childhood in undiagnosed patients, WD screen training for school teachers, zinc as a possible treatment for pregnant patients and medical management of fulminant hepatitis secondary to WD with prostaglandins, haemoperfusion and vitamin E.

Symptoms of Wilson's disease

The liver is the first organ to be affected by the buildup of copper due to WD; however, patients are often misdiagnosed with infectious hepatitis. Excess copper can also produce psychiatric or neurologic symptoms [22, 23] which may cause the patient to present tremors, difficulty walking, talking and swallowing, along with various degrees of mental illness. Other signs and symptoms of WD include fatigue, lack of appetite, abdominal pain, jaundice, bruising, edema in the lower extremities, ascites and Kayser-Fleischer rings on ophthalmological examination [24]. In Costa Rica, the majority of WD patients exhibit liver disease and in more than 5% the pathology presents as fulminant hepatic failure. So it is crucial to test patients for WD if they have unexplained steatosis, liver failure, cirrhosis, cholestasis, and neurological impairment, specifically because of the high incidence of Wilson's disease in the country.

Specific guidelines for diagnosing Wilson's disease

Early diagnosis and family screening of WD is fundamental, so treatment can be initiated before liver failure or neurological damage ensues. The 2001 International Meeting of Wilson's disease, held in Leipzig, concluded that when evaluating a potential WD patient, these fundamental diagnostic elements should be included [25, 26]:

- Ceruloplasmin (ferroxidase enzyme) which is normally lower than 200 mg/L. When ceruloplasmin is low, deficiency disorders may occur, including neurological symptoms like Menkes disease [27]. Serum ceruloplasmin has also been related, since 1975, to the detection of problems during early gestation [28].
- Serum free copper, which is normally greater than 200 mcg/L.
- Hepatic copper, which is normally greater than 250 mcg/g dry weight.
- The presence of Kayser-Fleischer rings on slit-lamp examination. However rings may be absent in up to 50 % of patients with hepatic WD and most asymptomatic siblings, but present in other hepatic diseases such as primary biliary cirrhosis. In contrast, Kayser-Fleischer rings are present almost invariably in neurological WD [29] and in neurodegenerative diseases like Alzheimer's disease [30].

While often the criteria of the Leipzig score are met [25], the combination of Kayser-Fleischer rings and a low serum ceruloplasmin (<0.1 g/L) level can be sufficient to establish a diagnosis of Wilson's disease [26].

Nowadays, the genetic diagnosis is also a feasible option, especially for family screening. The sequence analysis of ATP7B gene is clinically available to identify the mutations in the ATP7B gene on chromosome 13. However, the existence of more than 500 mutants makes the genetic testing laborious and expensive [31] and in approximately 17 % of clinically confirmed WD cases, no mutation is identified [32]. Nevertheless significant genotype-phenotype correlation exists. ATP7B mutations result in absent or totally nonfunctional Wilson ATPase and are associated with severe hepatic disease [33, 34] (Table 1).

In Costa Rica, after a patient has been diagnosed it is essential that family members also get tested. The most successful WD detection and diagnostic method for family members of patients diagnosed with WD is as follows:

- Once a patient is identified with WD, their first and second degree relatives should undergo screening for WD through ceruloplasmin determination at the nephrology laboratory, which specializes in diagnosing copper metabolism abnormalities, including WD. Test results are available in a timely manner (less than 7 days).
- If ceruloplasmin level is low or normal-low, the result is reported to Hevia-Urrutia M.D. team and the individual will undergo 24-h urinary copper screening.
- In cases where both tests are abnormal or positive for WD, further diagnostic procedures such as a 24-h D-penicillamine challenge, liver biopsy, and genetic testing may take place.

Guidelines for treatment of Wilson's disease

Patients in Costa Rica diagnosed with WD (symptomatic and asymptomatic) are referred to a tertiary care level hospital and followed by specialists in gastroenterology and hepatology. Patients diagnosed with fulminant WD undergo an inter-hospital protocol for treatment of fulminant hepatic failure and liver transplant.

Several drugs are available for the treatment of Wilson's disease, including D-penicillamine, trientine,

Table 1 Scoring system on Wilson's disease [26]

Typical clinical symptoms and signs		Other tests	
Kayser-Fleischer Rings		Liver Copper (in the absence of cholestasis)	
Present	2	>5x ULN (>4 μmol/g)	2
Absent	0	0.8-4 μmol/g	1
Neurologic Symptoms[b]		Normal (<0.8 μmol/g)	-1
Severe	2	Rhodamine -positive granules[a]	1
Mild	1	Urinary copper (in absence of acute hepatitis)	
Absent	0	Normal	0
Serum Ceruloplasmin		1-2x ULN	1
Normal (>0.2 g/L)	0	>2x ULN	2
0.1-0.2 g/L	1	Normal but >5x ULN after D penicilamine	2
<0.1 g/L	2	Mutation analysis	
Coombs-negative hemolytic anemia		On both chromosomes detected	4
Present	1	On 1 chromosome detected	1
Absent	0	No mutations detected	0
TOTAL SCORE EVALUATION			
4 or more Diagnosis established			
3 Diagnosis possible, more tests needed			
2 or less Diagnosis very unlikely			

Scoring System on Wilson's disease. 8th International Meeting on Wilson's disease. Leipzig, 2001
[a]If no quantitative liver copper available, [b]or typical abnormalities at brain magnetic resonance imaging. ULN, upper limit of normal

zinc, tetrathiomolybdate, and dimercaprol. These drugs are designed to remove excess copper and to prevent its accumulation. If treatment is initiated immediately after diagnosis, for both presymptomatic and symptomatic patients, deterioration can be avoided and life expectancy can be comparable to healthy subjects; of course, a patient must be compliant with their therapy. In Costa Rica, treatment with zinc during pregnancy and nursing is considered because of the teratogenic effects of chelating agents like D-penicillamine and trientine.

Diet is an additional consideration and WD patients should avoid foods naturally high in copper including: chocolate, nuts, mushrooms, crustaceans, soy and gelatin, along with the use of cooking utensils containing copper. To ensure the safety of water flowing through copper pipes, water should run for a few minutes before drinking [29]. The fact that in Costa Rica rural areas, from where many WD patients come from, have a high copper diet constitutes an aspect that must be taken into account (Table 2).

Table 2 Treatment recommendations for Wilson's disease [26]

• Initial treatment for symptomatic patients with Wilson's disease should include a chelating agent (D-penicillamine or trientine). Trientine may be better tolerated	• Patients with acute liver failure due to Wilson's disease should be treated with liver transplantation when the revised King's score is 11 or higher
GRADE II-1, B, 1	GRADE II-2, B, 1
AASLD Class I, Level B	AASLD Class I, Level B
• Zinc may have a role as a line therapy in neurological patients	• Patients with decompensated cirrhosis, unresponsive to chelation treatment, should be evaluated promptly for liver transplantation
GRADE II-2, C, 2	GRADE II-2, B, 1
AASLD Class II, Level C	AASLD Class I, Level B
• Treatment of presymptomatic patients or those with neurological disease on maintenance therapy can be accomplished with a chelating agent or with zinc	• Treatment for Wilson's disease should be continued during pregnancy, but dosage reduction is advisable for D-penicillamine and trientine
GRADE II-1, B, 1	GRADE II-3, B, 1
AASLD Class I, Level B	AASLD Class I, Level C
• Treatment is lifelong and should not be discontinued, unless liver transplantation is performed	• For routine monitoring, serum copper and ceruloplasmin, liver enzymes and international normalized ratio, functional parameters, complete blood count and urine analysis as well as physical and neurological examinations should be performed regularly, at least twice annually
GRADE II-1, B, 1	GRADE II-2, B, 1
AASLD Class I, Level B	AASLD Class I, Level C
• If zinc is used, careful monitoring of transaminases is needed, with changing to chelators if these laboratory parameters are increasing	• The 24-h urinary copper excretion on medication and after 2 days of cessation of therapy should be measured at least yearly. The estimated serum non ceruloplasmin bound copper may be another useful parameter to control therapy
GRADE C1	
AASLD Class I, Level B	
• Patients should avoid intake of foods and water with high concentrations of copper, especially during the year of treatment	
GRADE II-3, B, 2	GRADE II-3, B, 1
AASLD Class I, Level C	AASLD Class I, Level C

8th International Meeting on Wilson's disease. Leipzig, 2001

Conclusion

While hepatolenticular degeneration is a rare disease worldwide, it is much more common in Costa Rica. Important advances relating the pathology have being made in the last decades through a series of actions and efforts in health policy, politics, and multidisciplinary work. One of the latest interventions is the foundation in 2015 of the National Alliance for Wilson's disease.

The ultimate goal of the Costa Rica's National Alliance for Wilson's disease is to promote awareness and early intervention of WD in a country un-proportionally afflicted with this deadly disease. Currently this initiative has begun implementing actions by evaluating guidelines for early diagnosis and adequate treatments, dissemination of relevant information on current research, legal issues and the support for WD patients and families; that have proof substantial reduction on Wilson's disease affliction.

The future prospects of the Costa Rican WD National Alliance is the establishment of international clinical and research collaborations with other Latin American countries, Europe and Japan. As well the development of relations with similar organizations like the Wilson Disease Centers of Excellence. These mutual benefit collaborative initiatives are the cornerstone for future diagnosis, treatment and management of WD.

Abbreviations

AASLD, American Association for the Study of Liver Diseases; ACOPAW, Costa Rican Wilson's Disease Patient Association; ALEH, Latin American Hepatology Association; CCSS, Costa Rican Social Security National Health System; EASL, European Society for Liver Diseases; CLF, Canadian Liver Foundation; WD, Wilson's disease; WDA, Wilson's Disease Association

Acknowledgement

Non applicable. Funding for the development of this manuscript is own from the authors.

Authors' contributions

All authors contributed equally in the design, data analysis and writing of this manuscripts. As well, all authors read and approved the final paper.

Competing interests

The authors declare that they have no competing interests.

Author details

[1]Hospital San Juan de Dios, Caja Costarricense del Seguro Social, 4917-1000 San José, Costa Rica. [2]Hospital México, Caja Costarricense del Seguro Social, San José, Costa Rica. [3]Hospital Nacional de Niños, Caja Costarricense del Seguro Social, San José, Costa Rica.

References

1. Clinic M. Wilson's Disease: Diseases and Conditions. 2014. Available from: http://www.mayoclinic.org/diseases-conditions/wilsons-disease/basics/definition/con-20043499.
2. Kinnier Wilson SA. Progressive Lenticular Degeneration: a familial nervous disease associated with cirrhosis of the liver. Lancet Elsevier. 1912;179(4626):1115–9.
3. Huster D. Wilson disease. Best Pract Res Clin Gastroenterol. 2010;24(5):531–9.
4. Herra SA, Hevia FJ, Vargas M, Schosinsky K. Fulminant Wilson's disease in Costa Rica. Clinico-pathological study of 7 cases. G E N. 1990;44(1):9–14.
5. Freimer NB, Reus VI, Escamilla MA, McInnes LA, Spesny M, Leon P, et al. Genetic mapping using haplotype, association and linkage methods suggests a locus for severe bipolar disorder (BPI) at 18q22-q23. Nat Genet. 1996;12(4):436–41.
6. Antillón-Salazar A, Aguilar-Alvarez J. Degeneracion Hepatolenticular de Wilson: Reporte del primer caso en Costa Rica. Acta Medica Cost San José. 1970;13(1):19–22.
7. Schosinsky KH, Lehmann HP, Beeler MF. Measurement of ceruloplasmin from its oxidase activity in serum by use of o-dianisidine dihydrochloride. Clin Chem. 1974;20(12):1556–63.
8. McCullough AJ, Fleming CR, Thistle JL, Baldus WP, Ludwig J, McCall JT, et al. Diagnosis of Wilson's disease presenting as fulminant hepatic failure. Gastroenterology. 1983;84(1):161–7.
9. Hevia F, Miranda M. The special problem of Wilson's Disease in Costa Rica. Gastroenterol Int. 1989;1:228.
10. Asociación Costarricense de Pacientes con Enfermedad de Wilson. Available from: https://www.facebook.com/ACOPAW1912/.
11. Shah AB, Chernov I, Zhang HT, Ross BM, Das K, Lutsenko S, Parano E, Pavone L, Evgrafov O, Ivanova-Smolenskaya I, Annerén G, Westermark K, Urrutia F, Penchaszadeh G, et al. Identification and analysis of mutations in the Wilson disease gene (ATP7B): population frequencies, genotype-phenotype correlation, and functional analyses. Am J Hum Genet. 1997;61(2):317–28.
12. Bull PC, Thomas GR, Rommens JM, Forbes JR, Cox DW. The Wilson disease gene is a putative copper transporting P-type ATPase similar to the Menkes gene. Nat Genet. 1993;5(4):327–37.
13. Petrukhin K, Fischer SG, Pirastu M, Tanzi RE, Chernov I, Devoto M, et al. Mapping, cloning and genetic characterization of the region containing the Wilson disease gene. Nat Genet. 1993;5(4):338–43.
14. Jiménez G, Cambronero V, Morales C, Mora A, Guzmán C, Jiménez-Rivera C. Wilson's disease: pediatric experience in Costa Rica. Gastroenterol Hepatol. 2009;32(4):274–8.
15. Pham HP, Schwartz J, Cooling L, Hofmann JC, Kim HC, Morgan S, et al. Report of the ASFA apheresis registry study on Wilson's disease. J Clin Apher. 2016;31(1):11–5.
16. NIH U.S National library of Medicine. MedlinePlus Wilson Disease Also called: Copper storage disease, Hepatolenticular degeneration. Available from: https://www.nlm.nih.gov/medlineplus/wilsondisease.html.
17. U.S National Library of Medicine Genetics Home Reference. Wilson Disease. Available from: https://ghr.nlm.nih.gov/condition/wilson-disease.
18. American Liver Foundation. Available from: http://www.liverfoundation.org/
19. Canadian Liver Foundation. Available from: http://www.liver.ca/.
20. EuroWilson. Available from: www.eurowilson.org.
21. Brewer GJ, Hedera P, Kluin KJ, Carlson M, Askari F, Dick RB, et al. Treatment of Wilson disease with ammonium tetrathiomolybdate: III. Initial therapy in a total of 55 neurologically affected patients and follow-up with zinc therapy. Arch Neurol. 2003;60(3):379–85.
22. Sahoo MK, Avasthi A, Sahoo M, Modi M, Biswas P. Psychiatric manifestations of Wilson's disease and treatment with electroconvulsive therapy. Indian J Psychiatry. 2010;52(1):66–8.
23. Benhamla T, Tirouche YD, Abaoub-Germain A, Theodore F. The onset of psychiatric disorders and Wilson's disease. L'Encéphale. 2007;33(6):924–32.
24. Stremmel W, Meyerrose KW, Niederau C, Hefter H, Kreuzpaintner G, Strohmeyer G. Wilson disease: clinical presentation, treatment, and survival. Ann Intern Med. 1991;115(9):720–6.
25. Ferenci P, Caca K, Loudianos G, Mieli-Vergani G, Tanner S, Sternlieb I, et al. Diagnosis and phenotypic classification of Wilson disease. Liver Int. 2003; 23(3):139–42.
26. Clinical Practice Guidelines EASL. Wilson's disease. J Hepatol. 2012;56(3):671–85.
27. Aoki T. Genetic disorders of copper transport–diagnosis and new treatment for the patients of Wilson's disease. No To Hattatsu. 2005;37(2):99–109.
28. Schosinsky KH, Lehmann HP, Beeler MF. Automated determination of serum ceruloplasmin activity with o-dianisidine dihydrochloride as substrate. Clin Chem. 1975;21(6):757–9.
29. Rodriguez-Castro KI, Hevia-Urrutia FJ, Sturniolo GC. Wilson's disease: A review of what we have learned. World J Hepatol. 2015;7(29):2859–70.
30. Rembach A, Doecke JD, Roberts BR, Watt AD, Faux NG, Volitakis I, et al. Longitudinal analysis of serum copper and ceruloplasmin in Alzheimer's disease. J Alzheimers Dis. 2013;34(1):171–82.
31. Schilsky ML, Ala A. Genetic testing for Wilson disease: availability and utility. Curr Gastroenterol Rep. 2010;12(1):57–61.
32. Durand F. Wilson's disease: an old disease keeps its old secrets. Eur J Gastroenterol Hepatol. 2007;19(2):97–9.
33. Wilson DC, Phillips MJ, Cox DW, Roberts EA. Severe hepatic Wilson's disease in preschool-aged children. J Pediatr. 2000;137(5):719–22.
34. Thomas GR, Forbes JR, Roberts EA, Walshe JM, Cox DW. The Wilson disease gene: spectrum of mutations and their consequences. Nat Genet. 1995;9(2):210–7.

9

Insights on the Russian HCV care cascade: minimal HCV treatment for HIV/HCV co-infected PWID

Judith I. Tsui[1*], Stephen C. Ko[2], Evgeny Krupitsky[3,4], Dmitry Lioznov[4,5], Christine E. Chaisson[6], Natalia Gnatienko[7] and Jeffrey H. Samet[8,9]

Abstract

Background: The human immunodeficiency virus (HIV) epidemic in Russia, driven by injection drug use, has seen a steady rise in the past two decades. Hepatitis C virus (HCV) infection is highly prevalent in people who inject drugs (PWID). The study aimed to describe the current frequency of HCV testing and treatment among HIV-infected PWID in St. Petersburg, Russia.

Methods: This study examined baseline data from the "Linking Infectious and Narcology Care" (LINC) and "Russia Alcohol Research Collaboration on HIV/AIDS" (Russia ARCH) studies. Participants included in this analysis were HIV-infected with a history of injection drug use. Descriptive statistics were performed to assess frequency of HCV testing and treatment.

Results: Participants ($n = 349$ [LINC], 207 [Russia ARCH]) had a mean age of 33.8 years (IQR: 31–37) in LINC and 33.0 (IQR: 30–36) in Russia ARCH; 26.6 % (LINC) and 29.0 % (Russia ARCH) were female; 100 % were Caucasian. Nearly all participants had been tested for HCV (98.9 % in LINC, 97.1 % in Russia ARCH). Almost all reported being diagnosed HCV positive (98.9 % in LINC, 97.1 % in Russia ARCH). Only 2.3 % of LINC and 5.0 % of Russia ARCH participants reported ever receiving HCV treatment.

Conclusions: Among these cohorts of HIV-infected PWID in St. Petersburg, Russia, as of 2015 nearly all reported being tested for HCV and testing positive, while only 3.3 % received any HCV treatment. In this new era of effective HCV pharmacotherapy, an enormous chasm in the HCV treatment cascade in Russia exists providing substantial opportunities for curing HCV in HIV-infected Russians with a history of injection drug use.

Keywords: HIV, HCV, PWID, Russia

* Correspondence: tsuij@uw.edu
[1]Department of Medicine, Section of General Internal Medicine, University of Washington School of Medicine and Harborview Hospital, 325 9th Ave, Box 359780, Seattle, WA 98104, USA
Full list of author information is available at the end of the article

Background

Worldwide, hepatitis C virus (HCV) infection is estimated to affect 80 million people [1], placing them at risk for liver cirrhosis, hepatocellular carcinoma, and associated morbidity and mortality [2]. In most parts of the world, HCV transmission occurs through parenteral exposure, including via injection drug use (IDU) [3]. HCV is highly prevalent among people who inject drugs (PWID) through the sharing of contaminated injection paraphernalia [4].

Following the collapse of the former Soviet Union in the 1990s and the Afghan war, Russia experienced increased access to heroin and an upsurge in injection drug use among young adults along with subsequent risk for related viral infections [5]. Harm reduction programs exist in Russia, but are inadequate [6]. Access to needle exchange programs is limited and fear of law enforcement leads to reluctance to carry needles. Currently, opioid agonist treatments are illegal in Russia and thus unavailable for those persons with opioid use disorders [7, 8]. As a result, the prevalence of HIV and HCV among Russian PWID is among the highest in the world. It is estimated that a quarter of PWID in Russia have HIV [9], while the vast majority have HCV [4]. A recent study of HCV prevalence in eight Russian cities reported that PWID in St. Petersburg had the highest prevalence of HCV (90 %) [10]. Recent estimates of HCV prevalence in Russia suggest that 3–4 % of the population is infected [1, 11–13].

With new, direct-acting HCV agents offering attainable sustained virologic response (SVR) or cure, understanding the HCV cascade of care is paramount. The HCV cascade of care describes successive steps of healthcare specific to HCV that result in optimal health outcomes. Areas of the HCV cascade of care include initial screening, confirmatory viral load testing, linkage to care, staging of disease, initiation of therapy, and receipt and adherence to therapy [14]. Deficits along the care continuum have been reported in numerous countries including the U.S., Canada, Australia, and India, particularly among PWID [15–19]. Less is known about gaps in other countries, including Russia, which has one of the largest populations of HIV-infected PWID [20].

Given the confluence of the ongoing Russian epidemic of HCV and HIV co-infection and the new effective HCV treatments, we investigated care for HCV among HIV-infected Russian PWID in St. Petersburg, Russia. Specifically, we evaluated the frequency of HCV screening and treatment, hypothesizing that screening would far exceed treatment in this population.

Methods

This analysis is a descriptive, observational study on self-reported HCV testing and treatment among HIV-infected Russian PWID. We analyzed data collected from two studies in St. Petersburg, Russia: LINC and Russia ARCH, for which study methods have been previously published [21, 22]. Linking Infectious and Narcology Care (LINC), is a randomized controlled trial testing a peer-led strengths-based case management intervention to link HIV-infected PWID hospitalized at a narcology (addiction) hospital to HIV medical care in St. Petersburg, Russia. Participants were recruited from inpatient wards at the City Addiction Hospital (CAH) in St. Petersburg, Russia from July 2012 through May 2014. Russia Alcohol Research Collaboration on HIV/AIDS (Russia ARCH) is an observational cohort that aims to evaluate the longitudinal association between alcohol consumption and biomarkers of microbial translocation and inflammation. Participants were recruited between November 2012 and June 2015 from clinical HIV and addiction sites, non-clinical sites and snowball sampling in St. Petersburg, Russia. Eligibility criteria for both studies included the following: 1) 18–70 years of age; 2) HIV-infection; 3) having two contacts to assist with follow-up; 4) living within 100 km of St. Petersburg and 5) having a telephone. For LINC, additional criteria included being hospitalized at the narcology hospital, history of injection drug use, and not currently being on antiretroviral therapy (ART) (prior history of ART was not an exclusion). For Russia ARCH being ART-naïve (i.e. never having been on ART) was an eligibility criteria. All study participants provided informed consent and Institutional Review Boards of Boston University Medical Campus and First St. Petersburg Pavlov State Medical University approved the LINC and Russia ARCH studies.

For this analysis, the Russia ARCH sample was limited to participants who were not previously enrolled in the LINC study and who were categorized as PWID (i.e., participant reported at least one of the following: used needles to inject drugs prior to HIV diagnosis or past 30-day IDU). Using responses from the baseline questionnaire, we assessed the following: previous testing of HCV [23], location of HCV testing [23], date of HCV testing [23], physician reported HCV status [23], prior treatment for HCV [23], and date of HCV treatment initiation [23], demographics, HIV risk behaviors [24] and substance use [24–29]. Questions about HCV testing were worded in the following manner: "Have you ever been tested for the hepatitis C virus?", and "Has a doctor ever told you that you had the hepatitis C virus?" As such, questions did not refer to the specific diagnostic test done (i.e. screening antibody or HCV viral load). Not all questions were asked in both surveys.

Results

The total sample included 556 HIV-infected Russian adult PWID (n = 349 [LINC], 207 [Russia ARCH]). Details of enrollment are presented in Additional file 1: Figure S1 and Additional file 2: Figure S2. In LINC 382 potential participants were assessed, and of those, 349 were found to be eligible and were enrolled and included in the analysis. In Russia ARCH 556 persons were assessed, and of those 365 were found to be eligible and 364 were enrolled. Of those, 90 were also participants in LINC, 13 subsequently disenrolled from the study, and 54 were not known to be injection drug users, and were therefore excluded from this analysis, leaving 207 in the sample. Only 1 % of persons screened for LINC were excluded for current ART use, and 13 % of Russia ARCH persons screened were excluded for past or current ART.

Baseline demographic and other characteristics of each sample, and both samples combined, are shown in Table 1. Participants in these two studies were relatively young, the majority were men, and as is expected for this population, all were Caucasian. The vast majority completed secondary education, and approximately half reported being unemployed. Median time since HIV diagnosis was 7.1 years (IQR = 4-12), and median CD4 cell count was 349 (IQR = 201-550). All in Russia ARCH and the vast majority in LINC were HIV ART-naïve. Current substance use disorders were common in both cohorts (Table 1).

Almost all HIV-infected PWID in LINC (345 [98.9 %]) and Russia ARCH (201 [97.1 %]) reported past HCV testing; similarly nearly all participants in LINC (345 [98.9 %]) and Russia ARCH (201 [97.1 %]) reported past physician diagnosis of HCV. In most cases (328 [95.1 %]), the time since HCV diagnosis was ≥ 12 months in LINC. Of 345 reporting HCV testing in LINC, testing occurred in hospitals (193 [55.9 %]), outpatient clinics (107 [31.0 %]), and prisons (37 [10.7 %]) (Table 2). Almost all were HCV treatment-naïve in both LINC (336 [97.4 %]) and Russia ARCH (191 [95.0 %]) (Table 3).

Among eight reporting prior HCV treatment in LINC, 7 (87.5 %) initiated treatment ≥ 12 months prior. Of 10 with prior HCV treatment in Russia ARCH, 5 (50.0 %) reported achieving SVR and 3 (30.0 %) had unknown outcomes (Table 3). The median age of the 8 HIV-HCV co-infected PWID in LINC receiving HCV treatment was 32.6 (IQR 31.15-34.4), 5 (62.5 %) were never married, all 8 (100 %) were male, 1 (12.5 %) was working part-time, and 5 (62.5 %) completed secondary education or lower. Among ten Russia ARCH participants who reported receiving HCV treatment, the median age was 31.5 (IQR 29-35), 4 (40 %) were married or living with a partner, 6 (60 %) were male, 3 (30 %) were working part-time or full-time, and 9 (90 %) completed secondary education or lower.

Discussion

This study of two St. Petersburg Russian cohorts of HIV-infected PWID found an enormous gap between testing and receipt of HCV treatment, revealing a "chasm" in the hepatitis C virus (HCV) care cascade. This study found that nearly all participants reported being screened and informed that they had been HCV-infected, suggesting that screening efforts are robust in this population of PWID with HIV. In contrast to nearly ubiquitous rates of screening, few patients (LINC = 2.3 %, Russia ARCH = 5.0 %) reported ever receiving treatment. This points to a chasm with regard to not meeting European Association for the Study of the Liver (EASL) guidelines for prioritizing HCV treatment for PWID [30] and recommendations set forth by Grebely et al. [31]. Based on these results it appears that there is a substantial opportunity to improve care, and corresponding health outcomes, among HIV/HCV co-infected PWID in Russia.

The finding that HCV infection was nearly universal among these HIV-infected PWID in St. Petersburg is consistent with prior literature. Globally, Russia has among the highest burdens of HCV co-infection among PWID with HIV [32]. The HIV epidemic in Russia is primarily driven through parenteral drug use, and in this context, the prevalence of HCV infection, which almost invariably precedes infection with HIV, will be extremely high to omnipresent [33]. Indeed, modeling studies suggest that in countries where HIV is driven by injecting behavior, the prevalence of HCV can be used as a measure of HIV risk [34], and Russia has a high prevalence of HCV among PWID (50–90 %) [4, 10]. Therefore, it is not surprising that nearly all (97–99 %) of these HIV-infected PWID reported being told that they had HCV. However, it is unlikely that in all cases the diagnosis was confirmed with HCV RNA testing. Due to cost constraints, and the fact that patients frequently have to pay out of pocket for these tests, HCV RNA and genotype testing are uncommonly performed in Russia [35]. Given that approximately 25 % of HCV-infected people will spontaneously clear their infection [36], the true prevalence of current HCV infection, rather than past infection with HCV, in this sample was likely lower than reported.

This study demonstrates a large discrepancy between rates of testing and treatment among this population of HIV-infected PWID, many of whom were being treated for their opioid use disorders, which may explain their high testing rates. It appears that efforts to test these high risk patients for HCV infection are successful and thorough. However, despite these high rates of HCV

Table 1 Baseline demographic characteristics of HIV-infected Russian PWID in LINC ($n = 349$) and Russia ARCH ($n = 207$)

	LINC		Russia ARCH		Total	
Characteristic	No.	(%)	No.	(%)	No.	(%)
Median Age (IQR)	33.8 (31–37)		33.0 (30–36)		33.5 (31–37)	
Sex						
Male	256	73.4	147	71.0	403	72.5
Female	93	26.6	60	29.0	153	27.5
Race						
Caucasian	349	100	207	100	556	100
Other	0	0	0	0	0	0
Education						
Secondary Education or lower	314	90.0	179	86.5	493	88.7
Higher education	35	10.0	28	13.5	63	11.3
Marital Status						
Married or living with partner	105	30.1	96	46.4	201	36.2
Other	244	69.9	111	53.6	355	63.8
Employment						
Full-time	83	23.8	69	33.3	152	27.3
Part-time	41	11.7	22	10.6	63	11.3
Disability	11	3.2	3	1.4	14	2.5
Unemployed	190	54.4	106	51.2	296	53.2
Other (includes retired, homemaker)	24	6.9	7	3.4	31	5.6
Median Monthly Income (IQR)	35000 (20000–50000)		15000 (5000–30000)		28000 (10000–40000)	
Median Years Since HIV Diagnosis (IQR)	6.6 (4–12)		7.4 (4–12)		7.1 (4–12)	
Median CD4 Cell Count (IQR)	$n = 329$ 311 (163–492)		$n = 143$ 448 (294–639)		$N = 472$ 349 (201–550)	
ART (current or past)						
Yes	43	12.3	0	0	43	7.7
No	306	87.7	207	100	513	92.3
Past 12-month drug dependence	$n = 344$					
Yes	326	94.8	127	61.4	453	82.2
No	18	5.2	80	38.6	98	17.8
Past 30-day injection drug use	$n = 198$[a]					
Yes	183	92.4	94	45.4	277	68.4
No	15	7.6	113	54.6	128	31.6
Past 12-month alcohol dependence						
Yes			138	67.0		
No			68	33.0		

Abbreviations: *HCV* hepatitis C virus, *HIV* human immunodeficiency virus, *PWID* people who inject drugs, *ART* antiretroviral treatment, *IQR* interquartile range
[a]Available on a smaller sample due to data collection error

testing, it appears that only a very small fraction (3.3 %) of these HIV-infected PWID can access treatment. In contrast, another study not focused on HIV-infected persons reported lower rates of HCV diagnosis in Russia (40 %), but also low rates of treatment (< 0.1 %) [11]. Similarly, in other countries, such as the U.S., Canada, Australia, and India, it appears that HCV testing efforts often fall short, with many persons, including PWID, being unaware of their infection [17–19, 37–40]. The estimated proportion of persons treated for HCV in the U.S. is also low, 9 % reported in a recent meta-analysis [15], and HIV/HCV co-infected are often not referred for treatment [41]. It may be worth questioning the rationale for such an aggressive HCV testing program, given the limited effort to provide HCV treatment. The potential that awareness of HCV diagnosis positively

Table 2 HCV testing among HIV-infected Russian PWID in LINC ($n = 349$) and Russia ARCH ($n = 207$)

	LINC		Russia ARCH		Total	
Category	No.	(%)	No.	(%)	No.	(%)
HCV testing						
Yes	345	98.9	201	97.1	546	98.2
No	2	0.6	3	1.4	5	0.9
Unknown	2	0.6	3	1.4	5	0.9
HCV Diagnosis (Physician Notified)						
Yes	345	98.9	201	97.1	546	98.2
No	4	1.1	5	2.4	9	1.6
Unknown	0	0	1	0.5	1	0.2
Time since HCV diagnosis	$n = 345$					
≤ 6 months	6	1.7				
6–12 months	11	3.2				
≥ 12 months	328	95.1				
Location of HCV testing	$n = 345$					
Prison	37	10.7				
Outpatient clinic	107	31.0				
Hospital inpatient	193	55.9				
Needle exchange program	1	0.3				
Drug treatment program	6	3.4				
Family planning	2	0.6				
Other	2	0.6				

Abbreviations: *HCV* hepatitis C virus, *HIV* human immunodeficiency virus, *PWID* people who inject drugs

Table 3 HCV Treatment among HCV/HIV-co-infected Russian PWID in LINC ($n = 345$) and Russia ARCH ($n = 201$)

	LINC		Russia ARCH		Total	
Category	No.	(%)	No.	(%)	No.	(%)
HCV treatment status						
Current HCV treatment	3	0.9	1	0.5	4	0.7
Past HCV treatment	5	1.4	9	4.5	14	2.6
Never treated	336	97.4	191	95.0	527	96.5
Refused to answer	1	0.3	0	0.0	1	0.2
Time of HCV treatment initiation	$n = 8$					
≤ 6 months	1	12.5				
≥ 12 months	7	87.5				
Was SVR achieved			$n = 10$			
Yes			5	50.0		
No			2	20.0		
Don't know			3	30.0		

Abbreviations: *HCV* hepatitis C virus, *HIV* human immunodeficiency virus, *PWID* people who inject drugs, *SVR* sustained virologic response

impacts an individual's risk behaviors is another rationale for testing; however the evidence for this impact is mixed [38, 42, 43].

A limitation of this study is that HCV status was based on self-report. Also, we did not specify the nature of prior HCV testing in the questionnaire, nor ask about confirmatory viral load or genotype testing. Given the expense of confirmatory HCV viral load testing, it is likely that most participants only had an antibody test. Another limitation is that this study is based on secondary analysis of existing data from two other studies, which included eligibility criteria that participants could not be on ART. Therefore, the sample may not be fully representative of all co-infected PWID in St. Petersburg. The sample might potentially be biased toward patients who are difficult to link to care. However, there were relatively small numbers of participants who were ineligible because of ART use: in LINC 1 %, and in Russia ARCH 13 %. It is likely the sample may be potentially biased toward younger, newly diagnosed HIV-infected PWID with higher CD4 cell counts not meeting criteria for treatment. Russian guidelines at the time of study stated that ART should be initiated for any patients with CD4 cell counts below 350 cells/mm^3. At baseline, approximately half of the participants in the combined sample had baseline counts below that threshold, and over time we have observed that nearly one quarter of the sample has initiated ART. Another limitation is that we did not ask participants about specific treatments received; therefore, we cannot be sure that the few patients who reported being treated had actually received standard treatment (as opposed to vitamins or other supplements). However, the exact wording of the question ("Have you taken medication to treat hepatitis C, like Interferon and Ribavirin?") implied anti-HCV treatment that was the standard at the time.

This study was conducted largely before the arrival of direct-acting antiviral (DAA) therapies, when interferon based therapies were used. Of concern is that countries like Russia, which are transitioning from the classification of middle to high income (and thus restricted from generic medications), may be particularly challenged to afford new therapies for HCV. However, the study result speaks to a great need for treatment among co-infected PWID in Russia, particularly given the challenge of meeting WHO's targets for the goal of "elimination of viral hepatitis as a major public health threat by 2030" [44]. Given that persons who are co-infected with HIV/HCV are at greater risk for having progression of their HCV-related liver disease to cirrhosis and hepatocellular carcinoma, the need is more urgent to address treatment in this population in order to mitigate morbidity and avoid downstream costs [45–47]. Furthermore, treatment of HCV in this PWID population holds the potential to prevent HCV transmission ("treatment as prevention") [47–49]. Study results also indicate a need for expanded ART as an important initial step in engagement of care.

Conclusion

Among HIV-infected PWID in St. Petersburg, Russia, nearly all persons reported having been tested and found to have been infected with HCV, yet few (3.3 %) had ever been treated for their HCV infection. As such, the treatment chasm in the Russian HCV cascade of care among these HIV-infected PWID points to the great need for expanded HCV treatment in this population.

Abbreviations

ART: Antiretroviral therapy; CAH: City Addiction Hospital; DAA: Direct-acting antiviral; HCV: Hepatitis c virus; HIV: Human immunodeficiency virus; IDU: Injection drug use; IQR: Interquartile range; LINC: Linking Infectious and Narcology Care; PWID: People Who Inject Drugs; Russia ARCH: Russia Alcohol Research Collaboration on HIV/AIDS; SVR: Sustained virologic response

Acknowledgements

The project described was supported by grants R01DA032082 from the National Institute on Drug Abuse, U01AA020780, U01AA021989, U24AA020778, and U24AA020779 from the National Institute on Alcohol Abuse and Alcoholism. The authors wish to thank Sally Bendiks for her help in the submission, as well as the study participants for their contributions to research.

Funding

The project described was supported by grants R01DA032082 from the National Institute on Drug Abuse, U01AA020780, U01AA021989, U24AA020778, and U24AA020779 from the National Institute on Alcohol Abuse and Alcoholism. The content is solely the responsibility of the authors and does not necessarily represent the official views of the National Institute on Drug Abuse, National Institute on Alcohol Abuse and Alcoholism or the National Institutes of Health.

Authors' contributions

JIT and SCK conceived the study question, led the analytic planning and wrote the first draft of the manuscript. EK led the Russian team and was the principal investigator in Russia. DL was the infectionist and co-investigator on the study. CEC provided data management and conducted the analyses. NG was the project manager in the United States. JHS was the principal investigator of the parent study. All authors contributed to developing the analytic plan, reviewed, revised, and approved the submitted manuscript.

Competing interests

The authors declare that they have no competing interests.

Author details

[1]Department of Medicine, Section of General Internal Medicine, University of Washington School of Medicine and Harborview Hospital, 325 9th Ave, Box 359780, Seattle, WA 98104, USA. [2]Department of Global Health, Boston University School of Public Health, 801 Massachusetts Avenue, 3nd Floor, Boston, MA 02118, USA. [3]St. Petersburg Bekhterev Research Psychoneurological Institute, Bekhtereva St., 3, St. Petersburg 192019, Russian Federation. [4]First St. Petersburg Pavlov State Medical University, Lev Tolstoy St. 6/8, St. Petersburg 197022, Russian Federation. [5]Pasteur Research Institute of Epidemiology and Microbiology, St. Petersburg, Russian Federation, Mira St. 14, St. Petersburg 197101, Russian Federation. [6]Data Coordinating Center, Boston University School of Public Health, 85 East Newton Street, 9th Floor, Boston, MA 02118, USA. [7]Department of Medicine, Section of General Internal Medicine, Clinical Addiction Research and Education Unit, Boston Medical Center, 801 Massachusetts Avenue, 2nd Floor, Boston, MA 02118, USA. [8]Department of Medicine, Section of General Internal Medicine, Clinical Addiction Research and Education Unit, Boston University School of Medicine/Boston Medical Center, 801 Massachusetts Avenue, 2nd Floor, Boston, MA 02118, USA. [9]Department of Community Health Sciences, Boston University School of Public Health, 801 Massachusetts Avenue, 2nd Floor, Boston, MA 02118, USA.

References

1. Gower E, Estes C, Blach S, Razavi-Shearer K, Razavi H. Global epidemiology and genotype distribution of the hepatitis C virus infection. J Hepatol. 2014; 61:S45–57.
2. Di Bisceglie AM. Natural history of hepatitis C: its impact on clinical management. Hepatology. 2000;31:1014–8.
3. Alter MJ. Epidemiology of hepatitis C virus infection. World J Gastroenterol. 2007;13:2436–41.
4. Nelson PK, Mathers BM, Cowie B, Hagan H, Des JD, Horyniak D, et al. Global epidemiology of hepatitis B and hepatitis C in people who inject drugs: results of systematic reviews. Lancet. 2011;378:571–83.
5. Kalichman SC, Kelly JA, Sikkema KJ, Koslov AP, Shaboltas A, Granskaya J. The emerging AIDS crisis in Russia: review of enabling factors and prevention needs. Int J STD AIDS. 2000;11:71–5.
6. Samet JH. Russia and human immunodeficiency virus–beyond crime and punishment. Addiction. 2011;106:1883–5.
7. Sarang A, Rhodes T, Platt L. Access to syringes in three Russian cities: implications for syringe distribution and coverage. Int J Drug Policy. 2008;19 Suppl 1:S25–36.
8. Krupitsky E, Zvartau E, Woody G. Use of naltrexone to treat opioid addiction in a country in which methadone and buprenorphine are not available. Curr Psychiatry Rep. 2010;12:448–53.
9. Jolley E, Rhodes T, Platt L, Hope V, Latypov A, Donoghoe M, et al. HIV among people who inject drugs in Central and Eastern Europe and Central Asia: a systematic review with implications for policy. BMJ Open. 2012;2: e001465.
10. Heimer R, Eritsyan K, Barbour R, Levina OS. Hepatitis C virus seroprevalence among people who inject drugs and factors associated with infection in eight Russian cities. BMC Infect Dis. 2014;14 Suppl 6:S12.
11. Wedemeyer H, Dore GJ, Ward JW. Estimates on HCV disease burden worldwide - filling the gaps. J Viral Hepat. 2015;22 Suppl 1:1–5.
12. Pimenov N, Chulanov V, Komarova S, Karandashova I, Neverov A. Hepatitis C in Russia: current epidemiology and approaches to improving diagnosis and surveillance. Epidemiol Infect Dis. 2012;4:4–10.
13. Mukomolov S, Trifonova G, Levakova I, Bolsun D, Krivanogova E. Hepatitis C in the Russian Federation: challenges and future directions. Hepat Med. 2016;8:51–60.
14. Linas BP, Barter DM, Leff JA, Assoumou SA, Salomon JA, Weinstein MC, et al. The hepatitis C cascade of care: identifying priorities to improve clinical outcomes. PLoS One. 2014;9:e97317.
15. Yehia BR, Schranz AJ, Umscheid CA, Lo Re 3rd V. The treatment cascade for chronic hepatitis C virus infection in the United States: a systematic review and meta-analysis. PLoS One. 2014;9:e101554.
16. Mehta SH, Genberg BL, Astemborski J, Kavasery R, Kirk GD, Vlahov D, et al. Limited uptake of hepatitis C treatment among injection drug users. J Community Health. 2008;33:126–33.

17. Socias ME, Shannon K, Montaner JS, Guillemi S, Dobrer S, Nguyen P, et al. Gaps in the hepatitis C continuum of care among sex workers in Vancouver, British Columbia: Implications for voluntary hepatitis C virus testing, treatment and care. Can J Gastroenterol Hepatol. 2015;29:411–6.
18. Hajarizadeh B, Grebely J, McManus H, Estes C., Razavi H, Gray RT, et al. Chronic hepatitis C burden and care cascade in Australia in the era of interferon-based treatment. J Gastroenterol Hepatol. 2016. doi:10.1111/jgh.13453
19. Solomon SS, Mehta SH, Srikrishnan AK, Solomon S, McFall AM, Laeyendecker O, et al. Burden of hepatitis C virus disease and access to hepatitis C virus services in people who inject drugs in India: a cross-sectional study. Lancet Infect Dis. 2015;15:36–45.
20. Mathers BM, Degenhardt L, Phillips B, Wiessing L, Hickman M, Strathdee SA, et al. Global epidemiology of injecting drug use and HIV among people who inject drugs: a systematic review. Lancet. 2008;372:1733–45.
21. Gnatienko N, Han SC, Krupitsky E, Blokhina E, Bridden C, Chaisson CE, et al. Linking Infectious and Narcology Care (LINC) in Russia: design, intervention and implementation protocol. Addict Sci Clin Pract. 2016;11:10.
22. So-Armah KA, Edelman EJ, Cheng DM, Doyle MF, Patts GJ, Gnatienko N, et al. Effects of heavy drinking on T-cell phenotypes consistent with immunosenescence in untreated HIV infection. Alcohol Clin Exp Res. 2016; 40:1737–43.
23. National Institute on Drug Abuse: Seek, Test, Treat and Retain Initiative. HIV/HCV/STI testing status and organizational testing practices questionnaire. 2013. Available at: http://www.drugabuse.gov/researchers/research-resources/data-harmonization-projects/seek-test-treat-retain/addressing-hiv-among-vulnerable-populations (accessed 06 Oct 2015).
24. Needle R, Fisher DG, Weatherby N, Chitwood D, Brown B, Cesari H, et al. Reliability of self-reported HIV risk behaviors of drug users. Psychol Addict Behav. 1995;9:242–50.
25. Sheehan DV, Lecrubier Y, Sheehan KH, Amorim P, Janavs J, Weiller E, et al. The Mini-International Neuropsychiatric Interview (M.I.N.I.): the development and validation of a structured diagnostic psychiatric interview for DSM-IV and ICD-10. J Clin Psychiatry. 1998;59 Suppl 20:22–33.
26. Weatherby N, Needle R, Cesar H, Booth R, McCoy C, Watters J, et al. Validity of self-reported drug use among injection drug users and crack smokers recruited through street outreach. Eval Program Plann. 1994;17:347–55.
27. McLellan AT, Luborsky L, Cacciola J, Griffith J, Evans F, Barr HL, et al. New data from the Addiction Severity Index. Reliability and validity in three centers. J Nerv Ment Dis. 1985;173:412–23.
28. Broome K, Knight K, Joe G, Simpson D. Evaluating the drug-abusing probationer: clinical interview versus self-administered assessment. Crim Justice Behav. 1996;23:593–606.
29. Knight K, Simpson D, Morey J. Evaluation of the TCU Drug Screen. National Criminal Justice Reference Service. 2002. Report No.: 196682.
30. European Association for Study of Liver. EASL recommendations on treatment of hepatitis C 2015. J Hepatol. 2015;63:199–236.
31. Grebely J, Robaeys G, Bruggmann P, Aghemo A, Backmund M, Bruneau J, et al. Recommendations for the management of hepatitis C virus infection among people who inject drugs. Int J Drug Policy. 2015;26:1028–38.
32. Platt L, Easterbrook P, Gower E, McDonald B, Sabin K, McGowan C, et al. Prevalence and burden of HCV co-infection in people living with HIV: a global systematic review and meta-analysis. Lancet Infect Dis. 2016;16:797–808.
33. Thomas DL, Leoutsakas D, Zabransky T, Kumar MS. Hepatitis C in HIV-infected individuals: cure and control, right now. J Int AIDS Soc. 2011;14:22.
34. Vickerman P, Hickman M, May M, Kretzschmar M, Wiessing L. Can hepatitis C virus prevalence be used as a measure of injection-related human immunodeficiency virus risk in populations of injecting drug users? An ecological analysis. Addiction. 2010;105:311–8.
35. Ocheret D, Bikmukhametov D, Sultangaziev A, Matuizaite E. Current situation regarding access to hepatitis C treatment in Eastern Europe and Central Asia. Eurasian Harm Reduction Network (EHRN). 2013. Available at: https://www.harm-reduction.org/library/current-situation-regarding-access-hepatitis-c-treatment-eastern-europe-and-central-asia-0. Archived by WebCite® at http://www.webcitation.org/6c5CV08LL. (Accessed 6 Oct 2015).
36. Denniston MM, Jiles RB, Drobeniuc J, Klevens RM, Ward JW, McQuillan GM, et al. Chronic hepatitis C virus infection in the United States, National Health and Nutrition Examination Survey 2003 to 2010. Ann Intern Med. 2014;160:293–300.
37. Denniston MM, Klevens RM, McQuillan GM, Jiles RB. Awareness of infection, knowledge of hepatitis C, and medical follow-up among individuals testing positive for hepatitis C: National Health and Nutrition Examination Survey 2001-2008. Hepatology. 2012;55:1652–61.
38. Kwiatkowski CF, Fortuin CK, Booth RE. The association between knowledge of hepatitis C virus status and risk behaviors in injection drug users. Addiction. 2002;97:1289–94.
39. Bouscaillou J, Champagnat J, Luhmann N, Avril E, Inaridze I, Miollany V, et al. Hepatitis C among people who inject drugs in Tbilisi, Georgia: an urgent need for prevention and treatment. Int J Drug Policy. 2014;25:871–8.
40. Bowring AL, Luhmann N, Pont S, Debaulieu C, Derozier S, Asouab F, et al. An urgent need to scale-up injecting drug harm reduction services in Tanzania: prevalence of blood-borne viruses among drug users in Temeke District, Dar-es-Salaam, 2011. Int J Drug Policy. 2013;24:78–81.
41. Cachay ER, Hill L, Wyles D, Colwell B, Ballard C, Torriani F, et al. The hepatitis C cascade of care among HIV infected patients: a call to address ongoing barriers to care. PLoS One. 2014;9:e102883.
42. Tsui JI, Saitz R, Cheng DM, Nunes D, Libman H, Alperen JK, et al. Awareness of hepatitis C diagnosis is associated with less alcohol use among persons co-infected with HIV. J Gen Intern Med. 2007;22:822–5.
43. Tsui JI, Vittinghoff E, Hahn JA, Evans JL, Davidson PJ, Page K. Risk behaviors after hepatitis C virus seroconversion in young injection drug users in San Francisco. Drug Alcohol Depend. 2009;105:160–3.
44. World Health Organization. Draft global health sector strategies: viral hepatitis, 2016–2021. 2016. Report No.: A69/32.
45. Kirk GD, Mehta SH, Astemborski J, Galai N, Washington J, Higgins Y, et al. HIV, age, and the severity of hepatitis C virus-related liver disease: a cohort study. Ann Intern Med. 2013;158:658–66.
46. Weber R, Sabin CA, Friis-Moller N, Reiss P, El-Sadr WM, Kirk O, et al. Liver-related deaths in persons infected with the human immunodeficiency virus: the D:A:D study. Arch Intern Med. 2006;166:1632–41.
47. de Ledinghen V, Barreiro P, Foucher J, Labarga P, Castera L, Vispo ME, et al. Liver fibrosis on account of chronic hepatitis C is more severe in HIV-positive than HIV-negative patients despite antiretroviral therapy. J Viral Hepat. 2008;15:427–33.
48. Martin NK, Vickerman P, Grebely J, Hellard M, Hutchinson SJ, Lima VD, et al. Hepatitis C virus treatment for prevention among people who inject drugs: modeling treatment scale-up in the age of direct-acting antivirals. Hepatology. 2013;58:1598–609.
49. Grebely J, Matthews GV, Lloyd AR, Dore GJ. Elimination of hepatitis C virus infection among people who inject drugs through treatment as prevention: feasibility and future requirements. Clin Infect Dis. 2013;57:1014–20.

10

Strengthening hepatitis B and C surveillance in Europe: results from the two global hepatitis policy surveys (2013 and 2014)

Jeffrey V. Lazarus[1*], Antons Mozalevskis[2], Kelly Safreed-Harmon[1] and Irina Eramova[2]

Abstract

Background: Hepatitis B and C are major public health threats in the World Health Organization (WHO) European Region. Viral hepatitis surveillance shortcomings have resulted in many WHO Member States having insufficient data available to guide decision-making. This study describes surveillance in the region based on a quantitative sub-analysis of findings from the 2013 WHO viral hepatitis policy report and a qualitative analysis of civil society survey responses associated with these findings.

Methods: Descriptive statistics were created from information that national government focal points for viral hepatitis in 44 countries had previously reported in response to the WHO survey. Bivariate analysis was performed to compare data from within and outside of the European Union/European Economic Area (EU/EEA). Survey responses from civil society organizations in the countries of the WHO European Region were collated, and a descriptive analysis of the comments on surveillance-related questions was performed to identify key themes.

Results: The response rate for the survey of governments was 83 % among both EU/EEA countries (25/30) and non-EU/EEA countries (19/23). More than 90 % of governments reported having national surveillance systems for the acute forms of hepatitis B and hepatitis C, but less than two-thirds reported surveillance for the chronic forms of both diseases. High proportions of governments reported having central registries for the reporting of deaths (96 %) and liver cancer cases (80 %), while less than half reported regularly conducting viral hepatitis sero-surveys. All responding Member States reported having adequate laboratory capacity nationally to support hepatitis outbreak investigations and other surveillance activities. Target populations for sero-surveys most commonly included people who inject drugs (27 %), the general population (25 %), men who have sex with men (20 %) and pregnant women (20 %). Few statistically significant differences were found between EU/EEA and non-EU/EEA countries.

Conclusions: Study findings indicated a capacity for robust viral hepatitis surveillance across the WHO European Region, with most countries having important surveillance components in place, but notable weaknesses were also identified. There is an urgent need for countries throughout the region to strengthen their surveillance programs in order to maximize the population-level impact of advances in HBV and HCV prevention and treatment.

Keywords: Hepatitis, Surveillance, Survey, Europe

* Correspondence: Jeffrey.Lazarus@regionh.dk
[1]CHIP, Centre for Health and Infectious Disease Research and WHO Collaborating Centre on HIV and Viral Hepatitis, Rigshospitalet, University of Copenhagen, Copenhagen, Denmark
Full list of author information is available at the end of the article

Background

Hepatitis B virus (HBV) and hepatitis C virus (HCV) are increasingly recognized as major public health threats worldwide. These two viruses are estimated to cause approximately 1.4 million deaths annually [1]. An estimated 57 % of liver cirrhosis cases and 78 % of primary liver cancer cases are attributable to HBV and HCV infections [2]. In the World Health Organization (WHO) European Region, more than 18 million adults are estimated to be carrying the hepatitis B surface antigen (HBsAg) [3], which is a marker of chronic HBV infection. An estimated 15 million adults in this region have HCV-RNA [3], which is a marker of HCV infection. Two-thirds of HBsAg-positive people and HCV-RNA-positive people live in the countries outside of the European Union (EU) and European Free Trade Association (EFTA), even though those countries account for only 42 % of the WHO European Region's adult population [3]. Throughout the Region, high levels of HCV transmission, and to a lesser extent, HBV transmission, are known to occur through injecting drug use [4]. Eighty percent of new HCV infections with a known transmission route in EU and European Economic Association (EEA) countries are attributable to injecting drug use [5]. Regarding HBV, additional transmission pathways of note in the region are heterosexual sex and sex between men. In some European countries, nosocomial transmission of HBV also contributes to the disease burden. Available epidemiological evidence on HBV and HCV among migrants suggests that many migrant groups are also disproportionately affected in several European countries [3, 6, 7].

Major advances in the prevention and treatment of chronic HBV and HCV infections are influencing the course of both epidemics. An effective hepatitis B vaccine became available in 1982, and the mass immunization campaigns that followed led to a sharp decline in new infections. For example, a recent study in Tajikistan demonstrated seven-fold lower prevalence of HBsAg among the vaccinated birth cohorts compared with the baseline among unvaccinated cohorts [8]. The strategy of providing the first dose of HBV vaccine within 24 h of birth is effective for preventing mother-to-child HBV transmission and may ultimately help to bring about the eradication of the virus [9]. In the last decade, treatment options for chronic HBV and HCV infection have dramatically improved, resulting in better short-term and long-term survival as well as better quality of life for people with these diseases. Effective antiviral agents can supress replication of the hepatitis B virus in most infected people [10], and recent HCV treatment breakthroughs have made it possible to cure chronic HCV infection in more than 90 % of patients [11]. Consequently, people with access to HBV and HCV treatment can greatly reduce their risk of developing cirrhosis, liver cancer and liver failure [10, 12]. In light of the potential impact of these developments, combined with other essential prevention interventions, WHO has made the elimination of viral hepatitis as a public health threat by 2030 the overarching goal of its ambitious first-ever global health sector strategy on viral hepatitis [13].

In order to take full advantage of advances in viral hepatitis prevention, treatment and care, decision-makers need to work from a strong evidence base that includes accurate surveillance data [14, 15]. Case reporting, based on regular notification by clinicians and laboratories, has traditionally been the foundation of viral hepatitis surveillance. At the same time, other information sources aimed at assessing disease burden and outcomes, such as serological surveys and cancer and death registries, are important for measuring the impact of hepatitis infections and evaluating the efficacy of interventions [14]. The importance of reliable information gathered through epidemiological surveillance was recognized by the World Health Assembly in its 2010 resolution on viral hepatitis [16]. Four years later, in a second viral hepatitis resolution, the World Health Assembly noted that "most Member States lack adequate surveillance systems for viral hepatitis to enable them to take evidence-based policy decisions" and repeated its 2010 call for Member States (MS) to remedy this situation [17]. The new resolution also called on MS to develop and implement national viral hepatitis strategies "based on the local epidemiological context," further calling attention to the need for robust surveillance. WHO has provided technical support to MS by publishing in February 2016 its first comprehensive viral hepatitis surveillance guidance [18] and in April 2016, a monitoring and evaluation framework for the global health sector strategy on viral hepatitis [19].

In recent years, the European Centre for Disease Prevention and Control (ECDC) has led efforts to improve and harmonize viral hepatitis surveillance in the 28 EU MS, along with three EEA countries (Iceland, Liechtenstein and Norway). A key ECDC accomplishment has been the introduction of an enhanced hepatitis B and C surveillance program, which calls for EU/EEA countries to provide case-based data using standardized case definitions to the European Surveillance System (TESSy), a web-based data management platform [20]. Two 2015 publications indicated that, while the program has brought about considerable improvements to the quality of the data collected, some aspects of viral hepatitis surveillance, such as the completeness of the data and the task of classifying cases as acute or chronic, remain challenging. Furthermore, the current EU case definitions have yet to be adopted in all countries, which makes it difficult to compare data among countries [21, 22].

No comparable supra-national initiative has been undertaken in the non-EU/EEA countries. Publications documenting viral hepatitis surveillance practices in non-EU/EEA countries are scarce. The purpose of this study is to describe HBV and HCV surveillance policies and practices across the entire WHO European region based on a sub-analysis of surveillance-related findings from the WHO global viral hepatitis policy survey [23] and to present complementary qualitative findings from a civil society survey [24].

Methods

We carried out the following study using two existing datasets.

WHO global viral hepatitis policy survey

WHO, in collaboration with the World Hepatitis Alliance and the University of Copenhagen, conducted a survey of national policy responses to viral hepatitis among its 194 MS between 2012 and 2013. Findings were published in July 2013 in the *Global Policy Report on the Prevention and Control of Viral Hepatitis in WHO Member States* [23]. The quantitative data analyzed in this article are drawn from this survey. The data collection process for the survey is described in detail in Annex D of the report. In brief, a survey tool (Additional file 1) was developed for the purpose of collecting information about how national governments are addressing various aspects of viral hepatitis, including surveillance. After being piloted in 13 MS, it was distributed to all MS worldwide. In each MS, the national government focal point for viral hepatitis was asked to complete the survey. Data collection took place between July 2012 and February 2013. A total of 126 MS responded to the survey (65 %).

This article analyzes the data collected from the WHO European Region MS that participated in the survey. Responses were extracted for 18 questions pertaining to viral hepatitis surveillance; collection and use of other strategic information such as registries for death, liver cancer and HIV/hepatitis co-infection; viral hepatitis serosurveys; and screening of blood donors and pregnant women. We performed a descriptive analysis of all responses in accordance with the WHO European Region's geographical divisions for its 53 MS (West, Centre and East), as well as a comparison between EU/EEA countries and non-EU/EEA countries.

EU/EEA membership was determined in accordance with member status at the end of 2013. Thirty MS were defined as EU/EEA countries, including Croatia, which was in the process of joining the EU at that time. Lichtenstein was excluded since it is not a WHO MS. Twenty-three WHO MS were non-EU/EEA countries.

Basic statistical analysis of the data was undertaken and differences between the EU/EEA and non-EU/EEA regions were analyzed using the Chi-squared test. Bivariate analyses were two-tailed with a significance level of 0.05. All analyses were carried out using IBM SPSS version 20.0 software (Armonk, NY, USA).

Community hepatitis policy survey

In 2014, the World Hepatitis Alliance followed up the WHO policy survey with a global community hepatitis policy survey designed to give stakeholders outside of government the opportunity to share their perspectives. This survey, which was carried out by the University of Copenhagen, asked civil society organizations and community-based organizations, including patient groups, to assess the accuracy of their governments' responses to the earlier WHO survey (Additional file 2). Respondents were also invited to comment further on hepatitis policy issues in their countries. Findings were published in July 2014 in the *Global Community Hepatitis Policy Report* [24].

This survey was written in English, and responses were sought from World Hepatitis Alliance members (patient groups) as well as other non-governmental organizations (NGOs), academic institutions and medical associations. The survey was distributed via e-mail to approximately 800 organizations worldwide identified by the World Hepatitis Alliance and the University of Copenhagen, including 253 organizations in the WHO European Region. Data collection took place between February 1, 2014 and June 15, 2014.

The first part of the survey requested information about the responding organization. The second part asked each respondent to review 25 items of information provided by the respondent's country to the WHO survey, and to indicate whether he or she considered this information to be accurate. Respondents could also provide comments about each item. In the third part of the survey, respondents were invited to write statements about key national hepatitis policy issues of their choosing. Civil society stakeholders in countries where governments had not provided information to WHO were invited to complete a different survey that asked them to write statements about key national hepatitis policy issues of their choosing.

Responses from civil society organizations in the countries of the WHO European Region were collated for this study, and a descriptive analysis of the comments on surveillance-related questions was performed to identify key themes.

Results

WHO hepatitis policy survey

Respondents

Forty-four (83 %) of the 53 MS in the WHO European Region replied to the survey and were included in the analysis. Across the three sub-regions, 18 of the 23 MS in the West responded (78 %), as did 13 of the 15 MS in the Centre (87 %) and 13 of the 15 MS in the East (87 %). The response rate was 83 % among both EU/EEA countries (25/30) and non-EU/EEA countries (19/23) (Fig. 1).

Descriptive findings

National coordination and routine surveillance Thirteen responding MS (30 %) reported having a written national prevention and control strategy or plan for viral hepatitis: 5 (28 %) in the West, 3 (23 %) in the Centre and 5 (39 %) in the East. Twelve of those 13 MS (92 %) indicated that this strategy included a surveillance component (Table 1; Additional file 3). Ninety-eight percent of responding MS reported having national surveillance systems for acute hepatitis B, and 93 % for acute hepatitis C. Sixty-five percent of MS reported having a surveillance system for chronic hepatitis B, and 61 % for chronic hepatitis C. Ninety-six percent of MS reported having standard case definitions for viral hepatitis infections. Twenty-three percent responded that no viral hepatitis infections were reported to the national surveillance system as "undifferentiated" or "unclassified." All responding MS reported having adequate laboratory capacity nationally to support hepatitis outbreak investigations and other surveillance activities for HBV and HBC. Finally, 89 % of responding MS reported that viral hepatitis disease reports were published at least once a year (Table 2; Additional file 4).

Other sources of strategic information and capacities for disease burden estimation Ninety-six percent of MS responding to the survey reported having central registries for the reporting of deaths, including deaths related to viral hepatitis, and 80 % for the reporting of liver cancer cases. Sixty-six percent reported having national HIV/viral hepatitis co-infection registries. A total of 20 MS (46 %) reported undertaking viral hepatitis sero-surveys regularly. Target populations for sero-surveys most commonly included people who inject drugs (27 %), the general population (25 %), men who have sex with men (20 %) and pregnant women (20 %). Universal HBV screening for pregnant women was reported to take place in 77 % of responding MS. All countries with blood transfusion services reported screening all donated blood

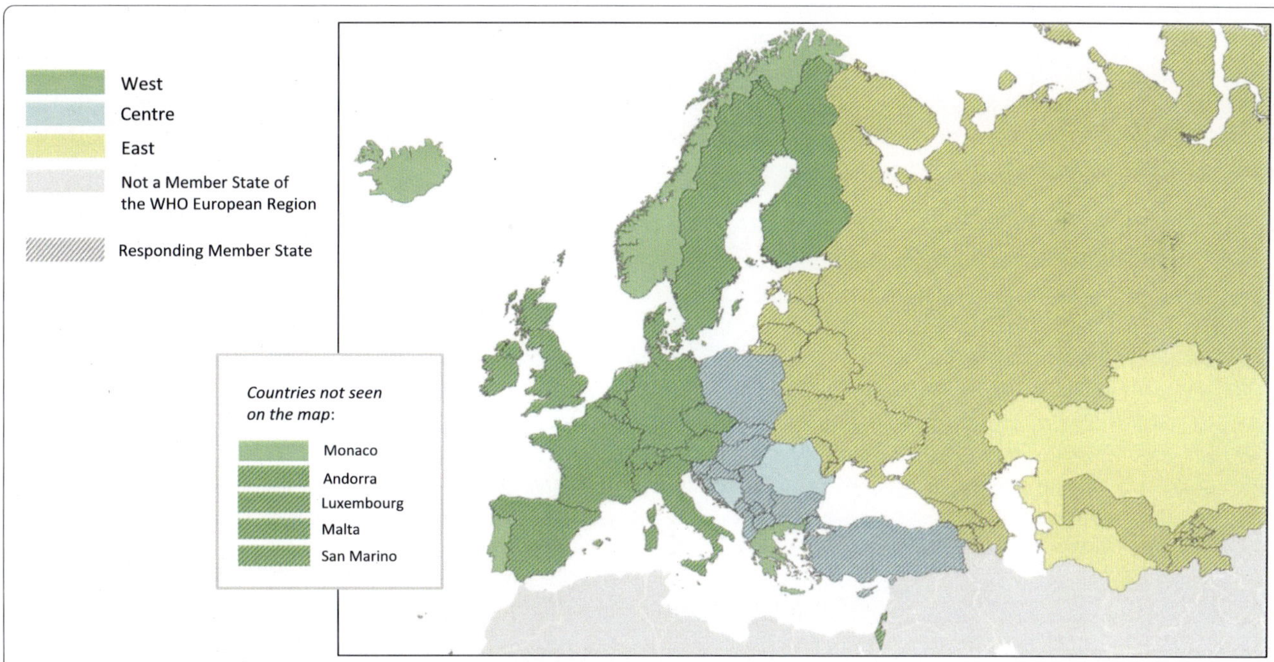

The Member States of the WHO European Region are grouped as follows:

- West, 23 countries: **Andorra**, **Austria***, **Belgium***, **Denmark***, **Finland***, **France***, **Germany***, Greece*, Iceland*, **Ireland***, **Israel**, **Italy***, **Luxembourg***, **Malta***, Monaco, **Netherlands***, Norway*, Portugal*, **San Marino**, **Spain***, **Sweden***, **Switzerland**, **United Kingdom***
- Centre, 15 countries: **Albania**, Bosnia and Herzegovina, **Bulgaria***, **Croatia***, **Cyprus***, **Czech Republic***, **Hungary***, **the former Yugoslav Republic of Macedonia**, **Montenegro**, **Poland***, Romania*, **Serbia**, **Slovakia***, **Slovenia***, **Turkey**
- East, 15 countries: **Armenia**, **Azerbaijan**, **Belarus**, **Estonia***, **Georgia**, Kazakhstan, **Kyrgyzstan**, **Latvia***, **Lithuania***, **Republic of Moldova**, **Russian Federation**, **Tajikistan**, Turkmenistan, **Ukraine**, **Uzbekistan**

* Countries which constitute the EU/EEA as of 1 of July 2013
(**Responding Member States**)

Fig. 1 Geographical/epidemiological divisions of the WHO European Region

Table 1 Reporting by Member States on the existence of a written national viral hepatitis strategy or plan

	World Health Organization European sub-region			Total
	West	Centre	East	
	N = 18 (%)	N = 13 (%)	N = 13 (%)	N = 44 (%)
Existence of a written national strategy or plan that focuses exclusively or primarily on the prevention and control of viral hepatitis:				
yes	5 (27.8)	3 (23.1)	5 (38.5)	13 (29.6)
no	13 (78.2)	10 (76.9)	8 (61.5)	31 (70.5)
If there is a strategy or plan, does it include a surveillance component?				
	N = 5 (%)	N = 3 (%)	N = 5 (%)	N = 13 (%)
yes	5 (100)	3 (100)	4 (80.0)	12 (92.3)
no	0 (0)	0 (0)	1 (20.0)	1 (7.7)
If there is a strategy or plan, is it exclusive for viral hepatitis or does it also address other diseases?				
	N = 5 (%)	N = 3 (%)	N = 5 (%)	N = 13 (%)
exclusive for viral hepatitis	1 (20.0)	1 (33.3)	2 (40.0)	4 (30.8)
only for HBV	0 (0)	1 (33.3)	0 (0)	1 (7.7)
only for HCV	1 (20.0)	0 (0)	0 (0)	1 (7.7)
integrated with other diseases	3 (60.0)	1 (33.3)	3 (60.0)	7 (53.8)

units for HCV infection, and all but Kyrgyzstan reported screening for HBV infection (Table 3; Additional file 5).

Areas in which Member States might want assistance from WHO Seventeen responding MS (39 %) indicated that they might want assistance from WHO in developing national viral hepatitis prevention and control plans, with the majority ($n = 10$; 77 %) of those MS located in the East. Ten countries (23 %) expressed interest in receiving WHO assistance with viral hepatitis surveillance, and 15 countries (34 %) did likewise for estimating the national burden of viral hepatitis. Again, much of the interest in receiving assistance came from the East, with eight MS (62 %) providing this response to both survey items (Table 4; Additional file 6).

Differences in survey findings between EU/EEA and non-EU/EEA member states

With regard to routine surveillance, slightly more countries in the EU/EEA than in non-EU/EEA MS reported conducting surveillance for chronic hepatitis, and all EU/EEA countries had standard case definitions, but these differences were not statistically significant. There were also non-significant differences regarding liver cancer registries and central death registries, with slightly more EU/EEA MS reporting that both were in place in their countries. Statistically significant differences occurred for only two survey items. More non-EU/EEA countries expressed interest in two forms of assistance from WHO: assistance developing national plans for viral hepatitis prevention and control (58 % versus 24 %, $p = 0.024$); and assistance with surveillance (42 % versus 8 %, $p = 0.010$) (Table 5).

Global community hepatitis policy survey

Forty organizations from 27 countries in the WHO European Region responded to the World Hepatitis Alliance's global community policy survey. Fifteen organizations (38 %) identified themselves as hepatitis patient groups and another seven (18 %) identified themselves as NGO direct service providers. Other types of organizations included other types of NGOs as well as medical societies and private foundations. Twenty-three of these countries (12 from the countries outside of the EU/EEA) had responded to the 2013 WHO global policy survey, and thus, the 35 respondents based in those countries were able to comment on the accuracy of their governments' responses.

In their comments, a number of respondents disputed or questioned the information that their governments had reported to WHO about surveillance policies and practices. Areas of disagreement related to the existence of routine viral hepatitis surveillance, the registration of liver cancer cases and cases of HIV/hepatitis co-infection, and the publication of hepatitis disease reports.

> *There is definitely no national registry for hepatocellular cancer. The information provided [for the WHO survey] is a misunderstanding, because it looks like the government representative who completed the survey confused the voluntary reporting system that exists in Poland with a register which contains all crucial data about particular patients. Of course data on hepatocellular carcinoma and hepatitis patients are collected by the National Health Fund but they are not analyzed and not provided upon the request of medical societies or even pharmaco-economic agencies.* –
> Polish Association for the Study of the Liver (Poland)

Table 2 Reporting by Member States on routine surveillance of viral hepatitis B and C

	World Health Organization European sub-region			Total
	West	Centre	East	
	N = 18 (%)	*N* = 13 (%)	*N* = 13 (%)	*N* = 44 (%)
National surveillance system for acute HBV:				
yes	17 (94.4)	13 (100)	13 (100)	43 (97.3)
no	1 (5.6)	0 (0)	0 (0)	1 (2.3)
National surveillance system for acute HCV:				
yes	15 (83.3)	13 (100)	13 (100)	41 (93.2)
no	3 (16.7)	0 (0)	0 (0)	3 (6.8)
National surveillance system for chronic HBV:				
yes	11 (61.1)	7 (53.8)	10 (76.9)	28 (63.6)
no	7 (38.9)	6 (46.2)	3 (23.1)	16 (36.4)
National surveillance system for chronic HCV:				
yes	10 (55.6)	7 (53.8)	10 (76.9)	27 (61.4)
no	8 (44.4)	6 (46.2)	3 (23.1)	17 (38.6)
Standard case definitions for viral hepatitis infections:				
yes	17 (94.4)	13 (100)	12 (92.3)	42 (95.5)
no	1 (5.6)	0 (0)	1 (7.7)	2 (4.5)
% of hepatitis cases reported as "undifferentiated" or "unclassified":				
zero	6 (33.3)	2 (15.4)	2 (15.4)	10 (22.7)
less than 5 %	2 (11.1)	4 (30.8)	3 (23.1)	9 (20.5)
5–15 %	0 (0)	2 (15.4)	3 (23.1)	5 (11.4)
more than 15 %	1 (5.6)	2 (15.4)	1 (7.1)	4 (9.1)
no response	9 (50.0)	3 (23.1)	4 (30.8)	16 (36.4)
Adequate laboratory capacity nationally to support hepatitis outbreak investigations and other surveillance activities for HBV and HBC:				
yes	18 (100)	13 (100)	13 (100)	44 (100)
Hepatitis outbreaks required to be reported to the government and further investigated:				
yes	17 (94.4)	13 (100)	12 (92.3)	42 (95.5)
no	1 (5.6)	0 (0)	1 (7.7)	2 (4.5)
Hepatitis disease reports published regularly (at least once per year):				
yes	15 (83.3)	13 (100)	11 (84.6)	39 (88.6)
no	3 (16.7)	0 (0)	2 (15.4)	5 (11.4)

> *I have never seen a hepatitis disease report from government. Very curious to [know what the survey submitted to WHO] means regarding a "hepatitis disease report."* – Associazione EpaC (Italy)

Additionally, some respondents indicated that, although their governments had reported having surveillance systems in place, the systems did not function adequately with regard to distinguishing between acute and chronic viral hepatitis or capturing other important information.

> *There is an inefficient [surveillance] system, which has been improved recently by shifting the reporting from the physicians to the virology laboratories. However, there is no information available on the clinical scenario, and no distinction is possible between acute and chronic hepatitis. Also, this is not routine surveillance in a strict sense but just opportunistic surveillance, finding cases by chance if the treating physician decides to order a test.* – Österreichische Gesellschaft für Gastroenterologie und Hepatologie (Austria)

> *This is a misunderstanding. Government recognizes as a "surveillance system" the voluntary reporting of hepatitis cases by physicians. So this is a passive*

Table 3 Reporting by Member States on other sources of strategic information and capacities for disease burden estimation

	World Health Organization European sub-region			Total
	West	Centre	East	
	N = 18 (%)	*N* = 13 (%)	*N* = 13 (%)	*N* = 44 (%)
Deaths, including from hepatitis, reported to a central registry:				
yes	17 (94.4)	13 (100)	12 (92.3)	42 (95.5)
no	1 (5.6)	0 (0)	0 (0)	1 (2.3)
no response	0 (0)	0 (0)	1 (7.7)	1 (2.3)
Liver cancer cases registered nationally:				
yes	15 (83.3)	11 (84.6)	9 (69.2)	35 (79.5)
no	3 (16.7)	2 (15.4)	3 (23.1)	8 (18.2)
do not know	0 (0)	0 (0)	1 (7.7)	1 (2.3)
Cases of HIV/hepatitis co-infection registered nationally:				
yes	10 (55.6)	10 (76.9)	9 (69.2)	29 (65.9)
no	8 (44.4)	3 (23.1)	4 (30.8)	15 (34.1)
Viral hepatitis serosurveys conducted regularly:				
yes	8 (44.4)	5 (38.5)	7 (53.8)	20 (45.5)
no	10 (55.6)	6 (46.2)	6 (46.2)	22 (50.0)
do not know	0 (0)	2 (15.4)	0 (0)	2 (4.5)
Target populations for serosurveys (respondents were given the options of "children", "general population", "people who inject drugs", "men who have sex with men", and "other groups", with space for identifying other groups):				
children	2 (11.1)	1 (7.7)	2 (15.4)	5 (11.4)
general population	4 (22.2)	5 (38.5)	2 (15.4)	11 (25.0)
people who inject drugs	4 (22.2)	3 (23.1)	5 (38.5)	12 (27.3)
men who have sex with men	2 (11.1)	4 (30.8)	3 (23.1)	9 (20.5)
pregnant women	2 (11.1)	2 (15.4)	5 (38.5)	9 (20.5)
prisoners	2 (11.1)	2 (15.4)	2 (15.4)	6 (13.6)
health care workers	0 (0)	2 (15.4)	4 (30.8)	6 (13.6)
sex workers	1 (5.6)	2 (15.4)	2 (15.4)	5 (11.4)
people living with HIV	0 (0)	1 (7.7)	2 (15.4)	3 (6.8)
blood donors	0 (0)	1 (7.7)	3 (23.1)	4 (9.1)
military	0 (0)	0 (0)	2 (15.4)	2 (4.5)
Roma youth	0 (0)	1 (7.7)	0 (0)	1 (2.3)
All pregnant women screened for HBV:				
yes	16 (88.9)	9 (69.2)	9 (69.2)	34 (77.3)
no	2 (11.1)	4 (30.8)	4 (30.8)	10 (22.7)
All donated blood (including family donations) screened for HBV:				
Yes	17 (94.4)	13 (100)	12 (100)	42 (95.5)
no	0 (0)	0 (0)	1 (7.7)	1 (2.3)
N/A (no blood centres)	1 (5.6)	0 (0)	0 (0)	1 (2.3)
All donated blood (including family donations) screened for HCV:				
yes	17 (94.4)	13 (100)	13 (100)	43 (97.7)
N/A (no blood centres)	1 (5.6)	0 (0)	0 (0)	1 (2.3)

system. There is no active surveillance program based on the screening of high-risk populations. ... The data collected by the National Institute of Health – recognized as a surveillance system – provides just a reporting rate and not a prevalence rate. – Polish Association for the Study of the Liver (Poland)

Table 4 Reporting by Member States regarding areas in which they might want assistance from WHO

	World Health Organization European sub-region			Total
	West	Centre	East	
	N = 18 (%)	*N* = 13 (%)	*N* = 13 (%)	*N* = 44 (%)
Areas in which government might want WHO assistance:				
national plan	2 (11.1)	5 (38.5)	10 (76.9)	17 (38.6)
surveillance	1 (5.6)	1 (7.7)	8 (61.5)	10 (22.7)
burden estimation	1 (5.6)	6 (46.2)	8 (61.5)	15 (34.1)

Table 5 Member States of the WHO European region reporting on surveillance-related activities by EU/EEA membership

	EU/EEA		non-EU/EEA		
	N = 25	%	*N* = 19	%	p-value
National coordination					
Existence of a written national strategy or plan that focuses exclusively or primarily on the prevention and control of viral hepatitis and includes a surveillance component	6	24.0	6	31.6	0.412
Routine surveillance of viral hepatitis B and C					
National surveillance system for acute HBV	25	100	18	94.7	0.432
National surveillance system for acute HCV	23	92.0	18	94.7	0.604
National surveillance system for chronic HBV	18	72.0	10	52.6	0.157
National surveillance system for chronic HCV	17	68.0	10	52.6	0.234
Standard case definitions for viral hepatitis infections	25	100	17	89.5	0.181
Regular hepatitis disease reports published	22	88.0	17	89.5	0.632
Hepatitis outbreaks required to be reported to the government and further investigated	23	92.0	19	100	0.317
Adequate laboratory capacity nationally to support hepatitis outbreak investigations and other surveillance activities for HBV and HBC	25	100	19	100	-
Other sources of strategic information and capacities for disease burden estimation					
Deaths, including from hepatitis, reported to a central registry	25	100	17	89.5	0.181
Liver cancer cases registered nationally	22	88.0	13	68.4	0.122
Cases of HIV/hepatitis co-infection registered nationally	16	64.0	13	68.4	0.508
Viral hepatitis serosurveys conducted regularly	10	40.0	10	52.6	0.299
If yes, please specify the target populations:					
- children	3	12.0	2	10.5	0.632
- general population	8	32.0	3	15.8	0.191
- people who inject drugs	6	24.0	6	31.6	0.412
- men who have sex with men	3	12.0	6	31.6	0.112
- other groups	7	28.0	10	52.6	0.089
All pregnant women screened for HBV	21	84.0	13	68.3	0.195
All donated blood (including family donations) screened for HBV	25	100	17[a]	94.4	0.419
All donated blood (including family donations) screened for HCV	25	100	18[a]	100	0.432
Areas in which Member States might want assistance from WHO					
National plan	6	24.0	11	57.9	0.024
Surveillance	2	8.0	8	42.1	0.010
Burden estimation	6	24.0	9	47.4	0.097

[a]Andorra is not included in this calculation because Andorra does not have blood donation centres

In a case when someone died from cirrhosis, the autopsy says "death from cirrhosis" but it is never specified whether it was caused by hepatitis and what kind. – National Association for Fighting Hepatitis – Hepasist (Bulgaria)

Some respondents expressed concern about surveillance systems not gathering information on treatment uptake or treatment coverage.

In England noone knows how many people are treated each year for HCV or HBV or what the outcomes are, an extraordinary situation given the cost. – The Hepatitis C Trust (United Kingdom)

The governmental structures receive partial information on acute hepatitis, and the information is spread by word-of-mouth. There are no follow-up data on what happens to those diagnosed with acute hepatitis and whether they receive treatment. – National Association for Fighting Hepatitis – Hepasist (Bulgaria)

Discussion

This sub-analysis of surveillance-related data from the WHO *Global Policy Report on the Prevention and Control of Viral Hepatitis in WHO Member States* demonstrates that key surveillance components are in place in most MS, suggesting that there is considerable potential to acquire better data for decision-making. However, substantial systemic shortcomings in hepatitis B and C surveillance were reported throughout the WHO European Region. Survey findings for EU/EEA and non-EU/EEA MS did not differ significantly for the most part, suggesting that attention should be given to strengthening surveillance and strategic information systems across the entire region.

While more than 90 % of MS reported conducting surveillance for acute HBV and HCV infections, the surveillance of chronic HBV and HCV infections was less common. One reason for this may be that viral hepatitis surveillance systems historically have focused on collecting data on acute infections, primarily for the purpose of identifying outbreaks. When WHO last published recommendations on viral hepatitis surveillance in 2003, the recommendations addressed surveillance of only acute infection [25]. Another influential source of technical guidance for the EU/EEA countries, ECDC, has only distinguished chronic infection with a revision of the EU case definitions for hepatitis B and C surveillance in conjunction with the recent implementation of its enhanced surveillance program. Data collected by the ECDC from the 31 countries it serves indicated that in 2013, only 17 countries were able to provide data on chronic HBV infection [26], and 12 on chronic HCV infection [5]. The ECDC experience, coupled with our own findings, suggests that surveillance systems may not be evolving rapidly enough to keep pace with recent developments in viral hepatitis prevention and treatment. A greater orientation toward chronic disease surveillance would contribute to efforts to understand the hepatitis disease burden, assess the impact of prevention and treatment efforts, and maximize the impact of resources [27].

The classification of viral hepatitis infection as acute versus chronic is a widely recognized challenge, especially for hepatitis C [28]. Data from our study indicate that only 10 MS (23 %) have no hepatitis cases reported as "undifferentiated" or "unclassified." Some community survey respondents' comments provided further evidence that distinguishing between acute and chronic hepatitis might not be possible in their countries. While most countries have case definitions, these vary across countries, making it difficult to compare data between countries. Progress has been made in the EU/EEA with the 2012 adoption of the revised EU case definitions [29], but further work is needed in this area, including the development of more accurate serological tests to better distinguish between acute and chronic HCV infection, and, to a lesser extent, for HBV infection as well.

All responding countries stated that they have adequate laboratory capacity nationally for outbreak investigations and other surveillance activities related to HBV and HCV, an indication that there might be considerable potential to improve and enhance viral hepatitis surveillance, including electronic-based reporting from laboratories. The survey information, however, should be regarded cautiously, as laboratory capacity at the central level might differ substantially from laboratory capacity at the regional and local levels.

The viral hepatitis disease burden can be assessed more accurately when data from case reporting are considered in conjunction with data from other sources such as death registries and disease registries. Almost all responding MS in our study reported having central death registries. Although these can potentially be used to assess the proportions of deaths attributable to HBV and HCV, the contribution of viral hepatitis to chronic liver disease-related mortality may be underestimated if death records are the only source of information [30, 31]. Since most deaths from HBV and HCV are due to complications of liver disease rather than being directly attributable to the viral infection, viral hepatitis may not be specified on the death certificate. Nonetheless, the usefulness of death registries in assessing the HBV and HCV disease burden and evaluating the population-level impact of treatment could be improved by linking such registries to viral hepatitis diagnosis databases [32]. Disease registries are another potentially valuable source of hepatitis information. In Europe, up to 15 % of primary liver cancer cases are caused by HBV, and up to 70 % by HCV [33]. The majority of European countries responding to the WHO survey reported the existence of national liver cancer registries, but the use of these data might be problematic, as noted by a community survey respondent from Poland. The feasibility of using liver cancer incidence indicators associated with cancer registries for evaluating the burden of chronic viral hepatitis infection has been demonstrated [34], but the accurate contribution of HBV and HCV infection to worldwide cancer trends is not well defined [35].

Two-thirds (66 %) of responding MS reported having national registries for HIV/viral hepatitis co-infection. Such databases can be used as additional data sources for chronic hepatitis surveillance and for identifying high-prevalence groups that should be targeted for screening [36]. In most jurisdictions globally, comprehensive HIV/AIDS surveillance has been in place for many years. The ECDC and the WHO Regional Office for Europe have effectively collaborated to jointly coordinate HIV/AIDS surveillance since 2008 for all 53 countries in the WHO European Region, although data on HIV/viral hepatitis co-infection are not currently being reported at the regional level [37]. The example of the joint ECDC/WHO surveillance for HIV/AIDS may serve as a useful model for strengthening viral hepatitis surveillance at the regional level in the future.

Data from sero-surveys can make a unique contribution to assessments of the burden of HBV and HCV disease because sero-surveys identify the many asymptomatic undiagnosed infections. Systematically repeated sero-surveys can be considered a form of surveillance, while single surveys provide a baseline measure of disease prevalence. In addition, the results can be compared and integrated with simultaneously collected epidemiologic information or case reporting data [38]. Only 20 of 44 (45 %) responding study countries reported conducting viral hepatitis sero-surveys regularly, and three other countries (Croatia, Czech Republic and Latvia) reported that they had conducted sero-surveys at least occasionally. It is likely that the complexity and expense of conducting sero-surveys are both factors limiting their role in HBV and HCV surveillance in the WHO European Region.

Many national surveillance programs may be able to make good use of HBV and HCV seroprevalence data that are already being recorded for two populations: blood donors and pregnant women. Both populations are subject to routine testing in accordance with health care standards in many countries. In our study, almost all responding MS reported having routine blood donor screening for both HBV and HCV. In most cases, data on the prevalence of HBV and HCV among blood donors is readily available, thus providing a basis for estimating seroprevalence within the general population. However, this is not a good proxy in most countries due to pre-screening selection of donors. HBV and HCV seroprevalence data for pregnant women may be more informative, but these data are not always as readily available as data from blood transfusion services because of less strictly regulated reporting from maternity services to public health officials. Furthermore, far fewer countries screen pregnant women for HCV than HBV [6]. In our study, 77 % of responding MS reported having routine HBV screening for pregnant women for HBV.

The lack of statistically significant differences between EU/EEA countries and non-EU/EEA countries in regard to the existence of chronic hepatitis surveillance and national death and liver cancer registries was somewhat surprising considering that EU/EEA countries generally have higher income levels and greater health spending. Twenty-two responding EU/EEA MS (88 %) were high-income countries, while 15 non-EU/EEA respondents (79 %) were low/middle income countries ($p < 0.001$), as determined by World Bank 2012 country income classifications. Also, EU/EEA countries might be expected to benefit from the ECDC's ongoing work to harmonize and improve viral hepatitis surveillance in the region that it serves. The finding that non-EU/EEA countries were interested in potential assistance from WHO on national planning and surveillance-related activities could be partly explained by the fact that countries in Eastern Europe and Central Asia traditionally have received technical assistance from WHO, and thus may be more likely to request it in the future. At the same time, the finding indirectly suggests that their surveillance systems may need greater attention than those in EU/EEA countries.

Responses from the global community hepatitis policy survey raise the following issues. First, some disagreements with government information regarding national surveillance policies and practices may indicate areas in which governments misreported facts for the WHO global policy survey. It is also possible that civil society respondents may have questioned the accuracy of some government information that was actually correct but was not sufficiently communicated to all relevant stakeholders. For example, civil society stakeholders in two countries made statements questioning their governments' assertions that hepatitis disease reports are published. One explanation may be that government agencies are compiling and disseminating reports internally but not making people outside of those agencies aware of their existence. Beyond civil society respondents' concerns about the accuracy of what their governments reported, some of their statements appear to offer informed opinions about surveillance issues. While public health surveillance by its nature is largely, or entirely, carried out by governments, findings from this study suggest that civil society stakeholders in some settings may be able to make important contributions to strengthening viral hepatitis surveillance. Governments should consider this point as they take action on the World Health Assembly's 2014 viral hepatitis resolution, which, among other points, urges MS "to promote the involvement of civil society in all aspects of preventing, diagnosing and treating viral hepatitis" [17].

In sum, virtually all responding countries in the WHO European Region reported having viral hepatitis surveillance systems in place, and there seem to be similar challenges and opportunities for improvement across the Region. However, it should be emphasized that the WHO survey collected information about the existence of policies and practices from national focal points but did not assess the extent or quality of implementation. Thus, it would be premature to draw conclusions about the overall effectiveness or ineffectiveness of national viral hepatitis surveillance systems based on the findings of this study. Furthermore, before such systems can be rigorously assessed, clarity is needed regarding the aims, outcomes and capacities of surveillance. It may be that many countries are achieving their stated viral hepatitis surveillance aims even if they do not have all of the components of what might be considered an ideal surveillance system. It would be beneficial for the WHO European Region as a whole to have a shared understanding of the specific ways in which surveillance is intended to support effective responses to HBV and HCV. This approach might entail recognizing, for example, the importance of surveillance data for developing estimates of adverse outcomes of HBV and HCV, such as those presented in the Global Burden of Disease study [39], even while the surveillance data are understood to provide an incomplete picture. It also might entail adopting common definitions in order to avoid confusion about issues such as those brought to light by the Polish civil society respondent who asserted that, what the government considers to be a surveillance system, is merely a record of physicians' voluntary reporting of hepatitis cases. The prospect of large numbers of people with chronic HCV gaining access to new treatments with high cure rates in the coming years further underscores the need for clarification about what national surveillance systems can contribute to tracking the changing epidemiology of this disease.

Limitations

Our study suffers from a number of limitations in addition to those already identified. First, although the European Region had the second-highest response rate to the WHO global policy survey among the six WHO regions, the absence of information from nine European MS (13 %) limits the generalizability of study findings. Other limitations relate to language and terminology. Survey respondents were restricted to using five languages (English, French, Spanish, Portuguese and Russian), and this may have resulted in some respondents not fully comprehending all of the survey questions. Furthermore, some questions in the survey might have been understood differently by respondents in different settings. Finally, the data in the WHO *Global Policy Report* were submitted by the identified focal points from MS, and researchers did not verify the accuracy of the data prior to publication of the report.

To some extent, the World Hepatitis Alliance's civil society survey provides useful complementary information, although that survey was not designed to verify governments' responses to individual survey items. Also, many respondents may not be fully qualified to have a complete overview of the national surveillance system and to assess whether responses to the WHO survey were indeed correct. The civil society survey has additional limitations as a robust source of data. Survey responses were received from only about half of all European countries, and some countries were represented by a single civil society respondent while others were represented by multiple civil society respondents. Furthermore, organizations that disagreed with the data provided by governments may have been more likely to respond to the survey than organizations that agreed. These factors limit the extent to which generalizations can be made on the basis of specific civil society survey findings.

Conclusions

To conclude, our study indicates that there is high overall capacity for robust HBV and HCV surveillance throughout the WHO European Region, but that existing surveillance systems have substantial weaknesses. Many governments have surveillance systems in place, along with laboratory capacity, and many governments are producing surveillance reports on at least an occasional basis. However, findings from the WHO policy survey and the follow-up civil society survey point to shortcomings, such as a lack of surveillance for chronic HBV and HCV disease, a lack of serosurveillance and an absence of mechanisms for tracking treatment outcomes in many MS. International organizations such as WHO and ECDC have the potential to play an important role in supporting country-level efforts to improve viral hepatitis surveillance and developing a comprehensive framework for the collection, analysis and use of strategic information. There is an urgent need for European countries to strengthen their surveillance programs to be able to monitor national progress toward achieving ambitious global targets relating to the elimination of viral hepatitis and to maximize the population-level impact of advances in HBV and HCV prevention and treatment.

Additional files

Additional file 1: Annex E: Responding to viral hepatitis: the World Health Organization/World Hepatitis Alliance 2012 survey of national governments. (PDF 85 kb)

Additional file 2: Annex B: World Hepatitis Alliance 2014 Survey of Civil Society Stakeholders. (PDF 114 kb)

Additional file 3: Reporting by Member States on the existence of a written national viral hepatitis strategy or plan. (DOCX 30 kb)

Additional file 4: Reporting by Member States on routine surveillance of viral hepatitis B and C. (DOCX 36 kb)

Additional file 5: Reporting by Member States on other sources of strategic information and capacities for disease burden estimation. (DOCX 39 kb)

Additional file 6: Reporting by Member States regarding areas in which they might want assistance from WHO. (DOCX 25 kb)

Abbreviations

ECDC, European Centre for Disease Prevention and Control; EEA, European Economic Area; EFTA, European Free Trade Association; EU, European Union; HBsAg, hepatitis B surface antigen; HBV, hepatitis B virus; HCV, hepatitis C virus; MS, Member States; NGOs, non-governmental organizations; WHO, World Health Organization

Acknowledgments

We would like to thank everyone who responded to the WHO global viral hepatitis policy survey and the community hepatitis policy survey. We also are grateful to Ida Sperle, who was a co-author of both global hepatitis policy reports, and to Erika Duffel of the European Centre for Disease Prevention and Control for providing very helpful comments on an earlier draft of this paper. We further extend our thanks to Tim Nguyen, Hande Harmanci and Stefan Wiktor of the World Health Organization and to Charles Gore and Raquel Peck of the World Hepatitis Alliance.

Funding

The World Hepatitis Alliance provided funding for the surveys upon which this study was based.

Authors' contributions

JVL and KSH developed and administered the surveys that this article is based on. AM and IE contributed to the analysis. KSH, JVL and AM drafted the article. All authors read and approved the final manuscript.

Authors information

No additional information.

Competing interests

The authors declare that they have no competing interests.

Author details

[1]CHIP, Centre for Health and Infectious Disease Research and WHO Collaborating Centre on HIV and Viral Hepatitis, Rigshospitalet, University of Copenhagen, Copenhagen, Denmark. [2]World Health Organization (WHO) Regional Office for Europe, Copenhagen, Denmark.

References

1. GBD 2013 Mortality and Causes of Death Collaborators. Lancet. 2015; 385(9963):117–71.
2. Perz JF, Armstrong GL, Farrington LA, Hutin YJF, Bell BP. The contributions of hepatitis B virus and hepatitis C virus infections to cirrhosis and primary liver cancer worldwide. J Hepatol. 2006;45(4):529–38.
3. Hope VD, Eramova I, Capurro D, Donoghoe MC. Prevalence and estimation of hepatitis B and C infections in the WHO European Region: a review of data focusing on the countries outside the European Union and the European Free Trade Association. Epidemiol Infect. 2014;142(2):270–86.
4. Nelson P, Mathers B, Cowie B, Hagan H, Jarlais DD, Horyniak D, et al. The epidemiology of viral hepatitis among people who inject drugs: Results of global systematic reviews. Lancet. 2011;378(9791):571–83.
5. European Centre for Disease Prevention and Control. Hepatitis C surveillance in Europe – 2013 [Internet]. Stockholm; 2015. Available from: http://ecdc.europa.eu/en/publications/Publications/hepatitis-c-surveillance-in-europe-2013.pdf.
6. European Centre for Disease Prevention and Control. Hepatitis B and C in the EU neighbourhood: prevalence, burden of disease and screening policies [Internet]. Stockholm; 2010. Available from: http://ecdc.europa.eu/en/publications/Publications/TER_100914_Hep_B_C%20_EU_neighbourhood.pdf.
7. Schweitzer A, Horn J, Mikolajczyk RT, Krause G, Ott JJ. Estimations of worldwide prevalence of chronic hepatitis B virus infection: a systematic review of data published between 1965 and 2013. Lancet. 2015. doi:10.1016/S0140-6736(15)61412-X [Epub ahead of print].
8. Khetsuriani N, Tishkova F, Jabirov S, Wannemuehler K, Kamili S, Pirova Z, et al. Substantial decline in hepatitis B virus infections following vaccine introduction in Tajikistan. Vaccine. 2015;33(32):4019–24.
9. Chen D-S. Hepatitis B vaccination: the key towards elimination and eradication of hepatitis B. J Hepatol. 2009;50(4):805–16.
10. World Health Organization. Guidelines for the prevention, care and treatment of persons with chronic hepatitis B infection [Internet]. Geneva; 2015 [cited 2015 Jul 24]. Available from: http://apps.who.int/iris/bitstream/10665/154590/1/9789241549059_eng.pdf?ua=1&ua=1
11. Pawlotsky J-M, Feld JJ, Zeuzem S, Hoofnagle JH. From non-A, non-B hepatitis to hepatitis C virus cure. J Hepatol. 2015;62(1 Suppl):S87–99.
12. World Health Organization. Guidelines for the screening, care and treatment of persons with hepatitis C infection [Internet]. Geneva; 2014 [cited 2015 Jan 28]. Available from: http://apps.who.int/iris/bitstream/10665/111747/1/9789241548755_eng.pdf?ua=1&ua=1.
13. World Health Organization. Draft global health sector strategy on viral hepatitis, 2016–2021: the first of its kind (draft: 13.11.2015) [Internet]. Available from: http://www.who.int/hepatitis/strategy2016-2021/Draft_global_health_sector_strategy_viral_hepatitis_13nov.pdf?ua=1.
14. Wiktor SZ. Where next for hepatitis B and C surveillance? J Viral Hepat. 2015;22(7):571–3.
15. World Health Organization. Prevention and control of viral hepatitis infection: framework for global action. 2012. Available from: http://apps.who.int/iris/bitstream/10665/130012/1/WHO_HSE_PED_HIP_GHP_2012.1_eng.pdf?ua=1&ua=1.
16. Sixty-third World Health Assembly. WHA63.18 Hepatitis. [Internet]. 2010. Available from: http://apps.who.int/gb/ebwha/pdf_files/WHA63-REC1/WHA63_REC1-en.pdf.
17. Sixty-seventh World Health Assembly. WHA67.6 Hepatitis [Internet]. 2014. Available from: http://apps.who.int/gb/ebwha/pdf_files/WHA67/A67_R6-en.pdf.
18. World Health Organization. Technical considerations and case definitions to improve surveillance for viral hepatitis: technical report [Internet]. 2016 [cited 2016 May 5]. Available from: http://apps.who.int/iris/bitstream/10665/204501/1/9789241549547_eng.pdf?ua=1
19. World Health Organization. Monitoring and evaluation for viral hepatitis B and C: recommended indicators and framework [Internet]. 2016. Available from: http://apps.who.int/iris/bitstream/10665/204790/1/9789241510288_eng.pdf.
20. European Centre for Disease Prevention and Control. Hepatitis B and C surveillance in Europe 2012 [Internet]. Stockholm; 2014. Available from: http://ecdc.europa.eu/en/publications/Publications/hepatitis-b-c-surveillance-europe-2012-july-2014.pdf.
21. Duffell EF, van de Laar MJW, Amato-Gauci AJ. Enhanced surveillance of hepatitis B in the EU, 2006–2012. J Viral Hepat. 2015;22(7):581–9. doi:10.1111/jvh.12364. Epub 2014 Nov 24.

22. Duffell EF, van de Laar MJW, Amato-Gauci AJ. Enhanced surveillance of hepatitis C in the EU, 2006–2012. J Viral Hepat. 2015;22(7):590–5. doi:10.1111/jvh.12367. Epub 2014 Nov 25.
23. World Health Organization. Global policy report on the prevention and control of viral hepatitis in WHO Member States. 2013.
24. World Hepatitis Alliance. Global Community Hepatitis Policy Report [Internet]. London; 2014. Available from: http://www.worldhepatitisalliance.org/sites/default/files/resources/documents/Community%20policy%20report.pdf.
25. World Health Organization. WHO-recommended standards for surveillance of selected vaccine-preventable diseases. 2003.
26. European Centre for Disease Prevention and Control. Hepatitis B surveillance in Europe – 2013 [Internet]. Stockholm; 2015. Available from: http://ecdc.europa.eu/en/publications/Publications/hepatitis-b-surveillance-in-europe-2013.pdf.
27. Committee on the Prevention and Control of Viral Hepatitis Infections; Institute of Medicine. Hepatitis and liver cancer: a national strategy for prevention and control of hepatitis B and C. [Internet]. 2010. Available from: http://www.nap.edu/catalog/12793.html.
28. Irving WL, Brown RJP. Acute hepatitis C virus infection: a dynamic-and challenging-concept. J Infect Dis. 2010;202(12):1765–7.
29. 2012/506/EU: Commission Implementing Decision of 8 August 2012 amending Decision 2002/253/EC laying down case definitions for reporting communicable diseases to the Community network under Decision No 2119/98/EC of the European Parliament and of the Council [Internet]. 2012. Available from: http://eur-lex.europa.eu/LexUriServ/LexUriServ.do?uri=OJ:L:2012:262:0001:0057:EN:PDF.
30. Manos MM, Leyden WA, Murphy RC, Terrault NA, Bell BP. Limitations of conventionally derived chronic liver disease mortality rates: Results of a comprehensive assessment. Hepatol. 2008;47(4):1150–7.
31. Asrani SK, Larson JJ, Yawn B, Therneau TM, Kim WR. Underestimation of liver-related mortality in the United States. Gastroenterology. 2013; 145(2):375–382-2.
32. Aspinall EJ, Hutchinson SJ, Janjua NZ, Grebely J, Yu A, Alavi M, et al. Trends in mortality after diagnosis of hepatitis C virus infection: an international comparison and implications for monitoring the population impact of treatment. J Hepatol. 2015;62(2):269–77.
33. Hatzakis A, Wait S, Bruix J, Buti M, Carballo M, Cavaleri M, et al. The state of hepatitis B and C in Europe: report from the hepatitis B and C summit conference*: The state of hepatitis B and C in Europe. J Viral Hepat. 2011;18:1–16.
34. Kanwal F, Hoang T, Kramer JR, Asch SM, Goetz MB, Zeringue A, et al. Increasing prevalence of HCC and cirrhosis in patients with chronic hepatitis C virus infection. Gastroenterology. 2011;140(4):1182–1188.e1.
35. Center MM, Jemal A. International trends in liver cancer incidence rates. Cancer Epidemiol Biomark Prev Publ Am Assoc Cancer Res Cosponsored Am Soc Prev Oncol. 2011;20(11):2362–8.
36. Brogueira P, Costa A, Miranda A, Peres S, Baptista T, Aldir I, et al. Improve screening of HCV infection by targeting high prevalence aged groups: analysis of a cohort of HCV and HIV co-infected patients. J Int AIDS Soc. 2014;17(4 Suppl 3):19601.
37. European Network for HIV/AIDS Surveillance [website] [Internet]. [cited 2016 Feb 9]. Available from: http://ecdc.europa.eu/en/healthtopics/aids/hiv-network/Pages/index.aspx.
38. Giesecke J. Modern infectious disease epidemiology. 3rd ed. London: Arnold; 2002.
39. Lozano R, Naghavi M, Foreman K, Lim S, Shibuya K, Aboyans V, et al. Global and regional mortality from 235 causes of death for 20 age groups in 1990 and 2010: a systematic analysis for the Global Burden of Disease Study 2010. The Lancet. 2013;380(9859):2095–128.

11

State of viral hepatitis knowledge and testing uptake in Brazil: Findings from the National Survey of Knowledge, Attitudes and Practices (PCAP-2013)

Silvano Barbosa de Oliveira[1], Meritxell Sabidó[2*], Ana Roberta Pati Pascom[1], Juliana Machado Gisiviez[1], Adele Schwartz Benzaken[1,2] and Fábio Mesquita[1]

Abstract

Background: Data were obtained from the third National Survey of Knowledge, Attitudes and Practices of HIV and other Sexually Transmitted Infections (STI) (PCAP-2013) and used to describe the current state of viral hepatitis (VH) knowledge and screening as well as the prevalence of viral hepatitis B (HBV) vaccination in Brazil and to assess the factors associated with testing uptake.

Methods: A probability sample survey of 12,000 individuals (50 % men) aged between 15 and 64 years was conducted between October and December of 2013. The participants completed the survey in their own homes through computer-assisted face-to-face interviews and self-interviews. We analysed data related to self-reported knowledge of VH routes and screening uptake after weighting the variables to account for unequal selection probabilities and correct for differences in sex, age and region according to 2010 census figures.

Results: The levels of correct knowledge regarding HBV and HCV transmission through unprotected sex were 33.1 and 34.3 %, respectively. The levels of correct knowledge regarding HBV and HCV transmission through tattooing/piercing were 26.4 and 24.5 %, respectively. Overall, 29 % of the respondents reported having underwent VH screening and 73.9 % reported prior HBV vaccination. VH screening was associated with the following factors: age between 25 and 49 years (adjusted male odds ratio (OR): 2.29, [95 % confidence interval (CI): 1.83–2.87]; female OR: 1.36, [95 % CI: 1.10-1.67]); age between 50 and 64 years (male OR: 1.52, [CI: 1.13–2.03]; female OR: 1.29, [CI: 1.02–1.63]); initial sexual intercourse before the age of 15 years in men (OR: 1.32, [CI: 1.10–1.57]); higher socioeconomic statuses of group A (male OR: 2.38, [CI: 1.81–3.13]; female OR: 2.10, [CI: 1.66–2.68]) and B (female OR: 1.56, [CI: 1.27–1.93]); and having ever been tested for HIV (male OR: 7.50, [CI: 5.82–8.53]; female OR: 7.13, [CI: 5.97–8.54]).

Conclusions: This study revealed low levels of knowledge regarding VH transmission and screening practices in the general Brazilian population, especially among younger individuals and those with lower socioeconomic status. Efforts to enhance awareness campaigns and expand testing sites are needed to remove barriers to testing.

Keywords: Hepatitis, Viral, Knowledge, Testing, Brazil

* Correspondence: xellsabido@gmail.com
[2]Fundação de Medicina Tropical Doutor Heitor Vieira Dourado (FMT-HVD), Avenida Pedro Teixeira 25, CEP: 69040-000 Manaus, AM, Brazil
Full list of author information is available at the end of the article

Background

Globally, viral hepatitis (VH) affects approximately 500 million people and is responsible for 1.4 million deaths every year [1]. An estimated 57 % of cirrhosis and 78 % of hepatocellular carcinoma cases can be attributed to chronic hepatitis B or C infections [1]. In Brazil, a population-based survey conducted from 2005 to 2009 [2] revealed that 39.5 % of individuals aged between 5 and 19 years had been exposed to hepatitis A virus (HAV). The prevalence of individuals exposed to hepatitis B virus (HBV) (based on serological evidence of antibodies to hepatitis B core antigen [anti-HBc]) was 7.4 %, and the prevalence of those exposed to hepatitis C virus (HCV) was 1.4 %, although variation across regions was observed [3, 4]. The burden of chronic HBV has been estimated at 0.65 %, with 1 in 275,813 individuals being positive for hepatitis B surface antigen (HBsAg) [5]. Studies have also shown that the prevalence of exposure to hepatitis E virus (HEV) in adults is approximately 3 % [6], although little is known regarding the presence of HEV in the Brazilian population. Hepatitis D virus (HDV) infections in HBV cases have been observed in Amazonas [7]. In Brazil, the number of newly reported cases per 100,000 people in 2010 was 3.6 for HAV, 6.9 for HBV and 5.4 for HCV [8], and the annual number of deaths per 100,000 people was estimated at 0.03 for HAV, 0.3 for HBV and 1 for HCV [8]. Overall, 10 % of all deaths in Latin America (2008–2010) have been attributed to causes related to VH [9]. In Brazil, cirrhosis of the liver was ranked as the tenth leading cause of death in 2012 [10]. In Brazil, HCV infection is a major cause of cirrhosis, hepatocellular carcinoma (8040 new cases per year), and liver transplantation (30 % of transplants in 2011) [11].

In Brazil, VH response is integrated within the national HIV programme. The country has taken a leading role in raising awareness of VH at the intergovernmental level [12]. Policy regarding VH, as well as procurement of and payment for vaccination, falls under the responsibility of the Ministry of Health, and vaccination administration is free in Brazil's municipalities. Domestic production of a HAV vaccine by public institutions has been planned [9]. Brazil has also introduced new efforts to expand the diagnosis and treatment of VH, and the country incorporated the use of rapid tests to improve early detection in 2011 [8]. Universal access to hepatitis treatment has been adopted, and clinical guidelines for HBV and HCV have been updated [13]. Several public media hepatitis campaigns have been undertaken, and since 2010 Brazil has commemorated World Hepatitis Day [13]. Despite these efforts, further improvements are still required. Knowledge and awareness of VH among the general population are limited, which might affect the adoption of preventative actions, such as testing uptake [14]. Indeed, most individuals with chronic hepatitis B or C infections are unaware of their status and remain untreated.

Over the past two decades, detailed information regarding the Brazilian population's awareness of sexual health, HIV status and knowledge of other sexually transmitted infections (STIs) has been obtained through the National Survey of Knowledge, Attitudes and Practices (PCAP) [15, 16]. However, this large probability sample survey only included questions on VH in its third PCAP round (PCAP-2013). In the present study, we assessed the state of knowledge related to VH and prior testing for HBV and HCV and the factors associated with testing uptake in a general population sample from Brazil to provide actionable information for clinicians and policy makers.

Methods

The PCAP-2013 survey interviewed a representative sample of 12,000 Brazilian men and women aged between 15 and 64 years between October and December of 2013. Brazil, one of the five largest countries in the world, has over 200 million inhabitants and a land area of more than 8,500,000 km^2 [17].

Sample design

The PCAP is a multistage, clustered and stratified probability sample survey. Census tracts with more than 60 permanent households were selected as primary sampling units (PSUs). Special sectors, such as military bases, boats, prisons, hospitals and convents, were excluded. Addresses within the census tracts were selected in the second stage, and only one eligible person per household was selected in the final stage. Prior to selection, the PSUs were stratified by region, main city, population density and rural versus urban contexts based on data from the 2010 census. The census tracts were selected systematically, and each sector was given a probability of selection that was proportional to its total number of households, with heads of households being stratified according to literacy level and education level of the sector being used as a proxy. Within each census tract, 16 households were systematically selected, and within each household, one person was selected based on sex, age group and cohabitation status [18].

The sample size of the PCAP study conducted in 2013 was calculated to provide robust estimates of the major parameters (e.g., consistent condom use with any type of partner, which was approximately 20 %) and a bilateral error of 2.5 %. Accounting for the complex sample design, the target sample size was set to 12,000 individuals. The sample was distributed by region, such that 1600 participants were from the north and central west, 2400 were from the south, and 3200 were from the northeast and southeast. Additionally, the sample contained equal numbers of men and women to provide sufficient statistical power to estimate the proportion of intravenous drug users, which was approximately 0.5 % with a bilateral error of 0.18 %.

Data collection

Professional interviewers visited each address, established whether any of the residents were eligible, and selected one individual per household. Computer-assisted personal interviews were performed in the households. The more sensitive questions were previously validated through focus group discussions, and these were self-completed. The participants were asked questions related to the following factors: 1) sociodemographic status, including sex, age, education level and household assets; 2) sexual behaviours, including age at initial sexual intercourse, sexual encounters with members of the same sex, number of casual partners during the last year, and condom use during recent sexual intercourse; 3) drug use, including intravenous drug use; 4) VH transmission route knowledge; and, 5) self-reported hepatitis screening, including VH type, self-reported screening during the last 12 months, screening with the rapid test, screening sites, reasons for screening, knowledge of the test results, and self-reported vaccination history against HBV. Data were stored in a secured, password-protected location and they were encrypted before being sent online to the coordination centre.

Study measures

To measure each participant's socioeconomic status, a combination of educational level (completed/did not complete high school) and number of household assets (e.g., television, video player/recorder, radio, refrigerator, freezer, washing machine, dish-washing machine, fixed telephone, cellular phone, automobile, etc.) was used. Three socioeconomic status categories were established according to the Brazilian Association of Research Companies (ABEP) [19]. Group A/B individuals had six or more household assets and completed high school, group D/E individuals had fewer than six household assets and did not complete high school, and group C individuals were all remaining participants.

As knowledge indicators, we considered the percentages of individuals who correctly reported whether HBV or HCV can be transmitted via unprotected sexual intercourse (only HBV), needles, manicure/pedicure equipment, dental treatments, dialysis, endoscopy and tattooing or piercing. As a denominator, we used those who spontaneously reported that each route could transmit VH. We defined having ever been screened for VH as being previously tested, regardless of the VH type tested. We defined a participant as being "vaccinated" if he or she reported at least one (lifetime) previous dose of HBV vaccine and as "fully vaccinated" if he or she completed all three doses.

Statistical analysis

All analyses were undertaken using the complex survey functions included in Stata 11 (StataCorp LP, College Station, TX, USA), which can incorporate weighting, clustering and stratification of data. Regarding the knowledge indicators, we reported proportions using 95 % confidence intervals (CIs) for male and female participants, who were further divided according to age group and socioeconomic status. We explored the prevalence rates of the knowledge indicators, screening and hepatitis B vaccination practices within the PCAP according to age group and socioeconomic status, which were further stratified by sex.

To identify the factors associated with having ever reported VH, weighted bivariable and multivariable logistic regression models were used. Variables with unadjusted odds ratios (ORs) of < 0.25 were included in the initial multivariable model. A backward fitting procedure was used, and variables were retained in the model when the *P*-value of the likelihood ratio test was less than 0.05. The magnitudes of the associations were estimated with weighted OR and 95 % CIs.

Ethics

The PCAP study was granted ethical approval from the National Research Ethics Committee (reference: 64485/12). The interviewers explained the survey contents to the participants, and each of the participants was asked to sign a consent form.

Results

In total, 6000 men and 6000 women were interviewed. The estimated response rate for the PCAP 2013 was 91.7 %. In each geographic region, the age and sex distributions of the sample were compared with the 2010 Demographic Census population distribution, and small differences (less than 1 %) were identified.

Knowledge of VH transmission

Table 1 illustrates the weighted age-specific knowledge of the enrolled men and women. Regarding knowledge indicators related to transmission, the proportion of individuals who correctly identified all transmission routes of both HBV and HCV was much lower than those who correctly identified the transmission routes of each individual infection. A higher proportion of women than men correctly identified that HBV and HBV/HCV can be transmitted through dental treatments, dialysis and endoscopy (29.9 % vs. 25.5 % for women, respectively, $p = 0.007$; 11.6 % vs. 9.5 % for men, respectively, $p = 0.01$). Among the women, a higher proportion of those aged between 25 and 49 years correctly identified that HCV can be transmitted through unprotected sexual intercourse, sharing needles and tattooing or piercing.

Table 1 Correct knowledge related to viral hepatitis transmission among individuals aged between 15 and 64 years according to sex and age in Brazil as measured by the PCAP-2013

		Men					Women				
	Total	15–24 years	25–49 years	50–64 years	All age groups	*p*-value	15–24 years	25–49 years	50–64 years	All age groups	*p*-value
Unprotected sexual intercourse											
HBV	33.1 (30.3–35.9)	41.6 (33.8–49.9)	37.3 (32.5–42.4)	32.7 (26.0–40.2)	37.5 (33.0–42.3)	0.17	27.9 (22.1–34.5)	30.1 (26.0–34.7)	23.9 (18.6–30.1)	28.6 (25.4–32.0)	0.27
HCV	34.3 (31.6–37.0)	33.1 (26.4–40.6)	36.8 (32.2–41.8)	30.6 (24.1–37.9)	34.9 (31.1–38.9)	0.29	27.5 (21.5–34.4)	38.2 (33.5–43.2)	25.6 (19.9–32.1)	33.7 (30.3–37.3)	0.002
HBV/HCV	17.1 (14.8–19.5)	17.2 (12.1–23.7)	19.3 (15.6–23.7)	18 (13.0–24.3)	18.6 (15.3–22.4)	0.72	12.8 (8.7–18.4)	17.7 (14.3–21.8)	11.6 (7.9–16.6)	15.6 (13.0–18.6)	0.06
Sharing needles											
HBV	30.0 (27.5–32.6)	25.8 (20.4–32.1)	32 (27.7–36.8)	29.7 (23.5–36.7)	30.1 (65.8–34.2)	0.13	29.4 (23.9–35.6)	29.9 (26.2–33.9)	30.8 (24.7–37.7)	29.9 (26.8–33.2)	0.95
HCV	27.0 (24.7–29.3)	25.8 (20.3–32.2)	28.5 (24.4–32.9)	25.2 (19.7–31.7)	27.3 (23.9–30.8)	0.57	21.5 (16.8–27.2)	30.1 (26.5–34.0)	21.0 (16.3–26.6)	26.6 (23.9–29.5)	0.004
HBV/HCV	12.0 (10.3–13.8)	10.4 (6.8–15.4)	13.5 (10.9–16.7)	12.6 (8.4–18.6)	12.6 (10.3–15.4)	0.43	10.3 (6.9–15.2)	12.3 (9.9–15.1)	9.6 (6.6–13.9)	11.4 (9.5–13.7)	0.45
Sharing manicure/pedicure equipment											
HBV	30.4 (28.2–32.6)	30 (23.8–37.0)	30 (25.8–34.5)	31.4 (25.6–37.9)	30.2 (26.6–34.1)	0.90	31.5 (27.1–36.2)	31.7 (28.5–35.0)	25.2 (20.9–30.0)	30.6 (28.0–33.3)	0.06
HCV	27.2 (25.0–29.4)	31.1 (24.9–38.0)	28.8 (25.1–32.8)	23.4 (18.5–29.0)	28.4 (25.2–31.8)	0.15	24.2 (20.0–28.9)	28.0 (24.8–31.4)	23.2 (19.2–27.8)	26.3 (23.8–29.0)	0.12
HBV/HCV	9.7 (8.2–11.2)	11.3 (7.1–17.6)	10.5 (8.1–13.6)	11.8 (8.4–16.3)	10.9 (8.7–13.6)	0.85	7.7 (5.5–10.9)	9.4 (7.4–11.7)	8.2 (5.9–11.2)	8.8 (7.3–10.6)	0.52
Dental treatment, dialysis or endoscopy											
HBV	28.0 (25.6–30.4)	24.7 (19.0–31.5)	25.4 (21.7–29.5)	28.9 (22.7–35.9)	25.9 (22.6–29.5)	0.56	29.0 (23.3–35.4)	30.1 (26.4–34.2)	30.2 (24.4–36.6)	29.9 (26.7–33.3)	0.93
HCV	27.4 (25.1–30.0)	27 (21.0–33.9)	30.3 (26.2–34.8)	22.7 (17.6–28.8)	28.2 (24.8–31.2)	0.10	24.6 (19.5–30.6)	27.9 (24.1–32.1)	24.5 (19.5–30.3)	26.6 (23.6–29.9)	0.42
HBV/HCV	10.6 (9.0–12.2)	8.6 (5.3–13.6)	9.1 (7.0–11.9)	11.6 (7.8–16.9)	9.5 (7.6–11.8)	0.53	9.5 (6.4–13.9)	12.5 (9.9–15.7)	10.9 (7.6–15.5)	11.6 (9.5–14.1)	0.37
Tattooing or piercing											
HBV	26.4 (24.0–28.7)	22.5 (17.3–28.8)	26.4 (22.5–30.8)	27.0 (21.0–34.1)	25.6 (22.3–29.2)	0.43	23.5 (18.6–29.2)	29.3 (25.6–33.4)	23.6 (18.7–29.5)	27.1 (24.1–30.3)	0.07
HCV	24.5 (27.1–31.8)	30.3 (23.8–37.7)	28.9 (24.8–33.3)	28.3 (22.1–35.5)	29.1 (25.7–32.9)	0.89	23.6 (18.6–29.4)	33.4 (29.6–37.4)	25.1 (20.0–31.1)	29.8 (26.932.8)	0.003
HBV/HCV	11.3 (9.6–13.0)	7.9 (4.9–12.5)	10.3 (7.8–13.5)	11.8 (7.9–17.0)	10.0 (7.9–12.5)	0.37	9.0 (6.0–13.4)	15.1 (12.3–18.4)	7.9 (5.3–11.6)	12.5 (10.4–15.0)	0.001
Denominators											
Unweighted	12000	1503	3002	1495	6000		1499	3002	1499	6000	
Weighted	12000	1577	3208	1081	5867		1565	3362	1207	6133	

Percentages indicate those with correct knowledge related to viral hepatitis transmission. The data in parentheses are 95 % CIs

Among all of the socioeconomic status groups, the men with C-level socioeconomic status exhibited the highest level of knowledge that unprotected sex is a transmission route for HBV. For HCV, the proportions of men and women who correctly reported that unprotected sex and sharing needles are transmission routes for infection decreased as socioeconomic status decreased (Fig. 1).

Screening for VH and vaccination against HBV

Overall, 29.0 % of the individuals (23.7 % of the men and 34.0 % of the women) reported having been screened for VH (Table 2). Among these respondents, 44.6 % were screened for HBV, 32.0 % were screened for HCV, and 16.8 % were screened for HDV. The proportion of participants who reported VH screening within the previous 12 months was higher among the men than the women (39.1 % vs. 34.3 %, respectively, $p = 0.004$). Additionally, among the women, this proportion decreased significantly with age. Overall, 17.5 % of the participants had been screened with a rapid test. The proportion of women who reported having been screened for the virus using rapid testing significantly decreased with age. Overall, 89.9 % of the participants who had been screened were aware of the results of their last VH test and 38.7 % knew of a service that provided testing for HBV and HCV free of charge. This proportion was higher among the women than the men (45.1 % vs. 32.1 %, respectively) and varied with age in both genders. The majority of the respondents (73.9 %) declared that they had been vaccinated against HBV (irrespective of the number of vaccination doses administered), and 18.3 % declared that they had completed the three-dose regimen.

Figure 2 illustrates the distribution of testing sites for the most recently recorded VH tests and details the reasons for testing according to sex. The majority of the respondents were tested in public hospitals or via primary health services (60.0 %), while 22.9 % were tested in private health services, and 6.2 % were tested at voluntary counselling and testing (VCT) sites. When dividing the respondents by sex, greater proportions of men reported having been last tested at a VCT site (13.8 % vs. 4.4 %) or a blood bank (9.4 % vs. 2.7 %). The majority of patients were screened because of a medical indication (29.7 %). Regarding the reasons for screening, greater

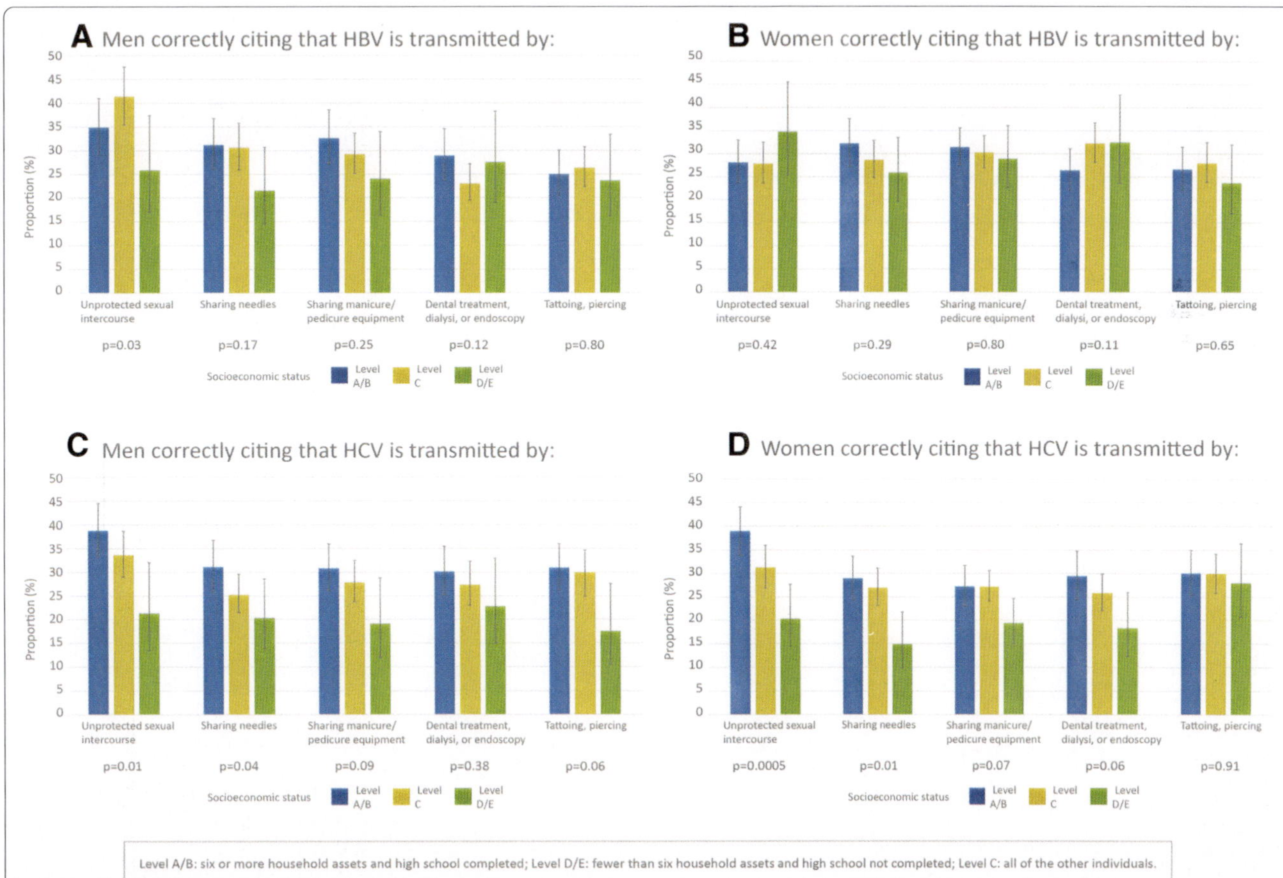

Fig. 1 Knowledge related to viral hepatitis transmission among individuals aged between 15 and 64 years according to socioeconomic status and social class in Brazil as measured by the PCAP-2013

Table 2 Screening for viral hepatitis and hepatitis B vaccinations among individuals aged between 15 and 64 years according to sex and age in Brazil as measured by the in the PCAP-2013

		Men					Women				
	Total	15–24	25–49	50–64	All age groups	*p*-value	15–24	25–49	50–64	All age groups	*p*-value
VH screening, ever	29 (27.6–30.4)	14.3 (11.9–17.1)	27.7 (25.6–29.9)	25.5 (22.3–28.9)	23.7 (22.1–25.3)	<0.001	24.5 (21.6–27.6)	41 (38.4–43.6)	26.6 (23.8–29.6)	34 (32–36)	<0.001
HBV	44.6 (42.2–47.2)	46.2 (37.2–55.5)	47.4 (42.9–52)	39.9 (33–47.3)	45.8 (42–49.6)	0.25	49.4 (42.9–55.9)	43.6 (39.8–47.5)	38.5 (32.5–44.8)	43.9 (40.1–47.2)	0.05
HCV	32 (29.7–34.5)	36.3 (27.6–46.1)	33.5 (29.2–38)	32.8 (26.4–40)	33.8 (30.3–37.6)	0.79	29.3 (23.2–36.4)	31.5 (27.9–35.4)	29.8 (24.1–36.2)	30.8 (27.7–34.1)	0.77
HDV	16.8 (13.7–19)	15.7 (10–23.8)	16.8 (13.8–20.3)	14.5 (10.3–20.1)	16.2 (16.7–19)	0.77	17.6 (12.4–24.3)	16.9 (14.1–20.1)	14.9 (10.8–20.2)	16.7 (14.2–19.6)	0.73
VH screening, last 12 months	36.2 (35.5–42.7)	38.5 (29.7–48)	40 (35.7–44.5)	36.3 (29.5–43.8)	39.1 (35.5–42.7)	0.70	45 (38.4–51.7)	33.2 (29.5–37.1)	26.3 (21–32.3)	34.3 (31.4–37.2)	0.0003
VH screening using rapid testing, ever	17.5 (15.6–19.6)	16.2 (10.1–25.1)	21 (17.3–25.2)	16.3 (11.8–22.2)	19.3 (16.5–22.4)	0.31	24 (18.2–31.1)	14.7 (12.1–17.8)	14.1 (10.1–19.3)	16.3 (13.8–19.2)	0.002
Knowledge of last VH test results	89.9 (88.3–91.3)	84.2 (75.2–90.4)	88.7 (84.7–91.8)	89.9 (84.3–93.7)	88.3 (85.2–90.7)	0.36	89.8 (85.5–93)	91.4 (89–93.3)	90.2 (86.6–93)	90.9 (89–92.5)	0.61
Knowledge of any health service that offers free screening for VH	38.7 (37–40.5)	26 (23–29.2)	34.6 (32.1–37.3)	33.3 (29.9–36.9)	32.1 (30–34.2)	<0.001	36 (32.8–40)	50.4 (47.6–53.3)	42.3 (38.9–46)	45.1 (42.7–47.5)	<0.001
HBV vaccination (1 dose)	73.9 (72.4–75.4)	68.8 (65.3–72)	71.3 (68.6–73.8)	72.2 (68.8–75.4)	70.8 (68.5–73)	0.19	76.8 (73.9–79.5)	76.4 (74–78.6)	78.6 (75.8–81.2)	76.9 (75–78.8)	0.38
HBV vaccination (3 doses)	18.3 (17.0–19.6)	10.3 (8.4–12.5)	14.3 (12.6–16.3)	12.8 (10.6–15.3)	13.0 (11.6–14.5)	0.01	24.7 (22.0–27.6)	24.6 (22.2–27.2)	17.9 (15.5–20.5)	23.3 (21.3–25.5)	<0.001
Denominators											
Unweighted	12000	1503	3002	1495	6000	...	1499	3002	1499	6000	...
Weighted	12000	1577	3208	1081	5867	...	1565	3362	1207	6133	...

... not statistically significant

proportions of men than women reported work-related reasons (17.1 % vs. 2.9 %, respectively) and blood donation (4.7 % vs. 1.6 %, respectively).

Table 3 illustrates the results for the variables associated with having been screened for VH. The proportion of men who reported undergoing screening for VH was greatest among those aged between 50 and 64 years; among the women, this proportion was greatest among those aged between 25 and 49 years. Among the men, screening increased significantly with age, whereas among

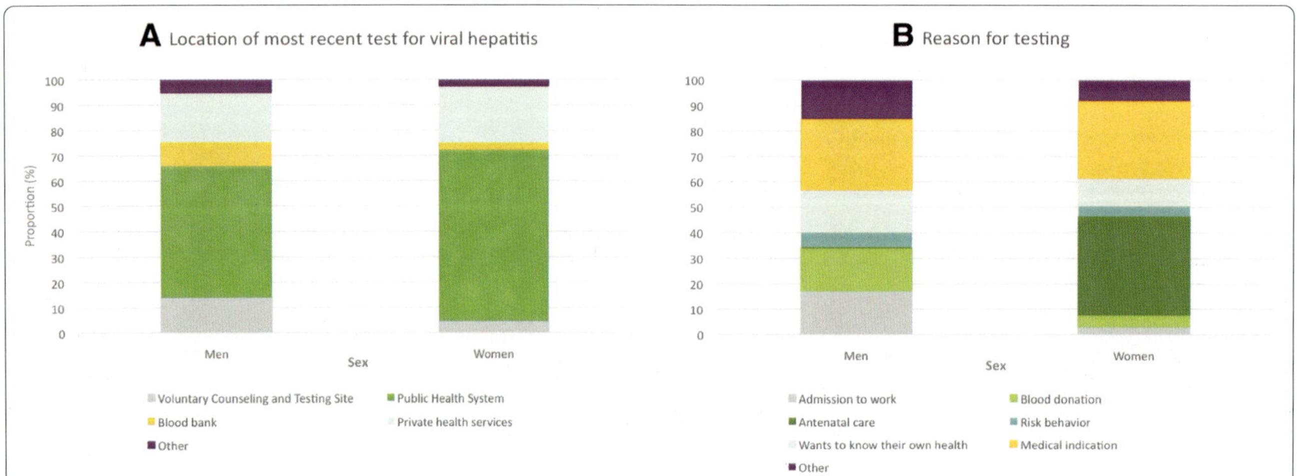

Fig. 2 Location of most recent test for viral hepatitis and reasons for testing according to sex

Table 3 Reporting of hepatitis screening in relation to demographic status, behavioural variables and HIV testing history according to sex

	Men			Women		
	Percentage reporting hepatitis screening	Crude OR	Adjusted OR	Percentage reporting hepatitis screening	Crude OR	Adjusted OR
All	23.7 (22.1–25.3)			34 (32–36)		
Demographic characteristics						
Age groups						
15 – 24 years	14.3 (11.9 – 17.1)	1	1	24.5 (21.6 – 27.6)	1	1
25 – 49 years	27.7 (25.6 – 29.9)	2.29 (1.83 – 2.87)	1.33 (1.03 – 1.71)	41 (38.4 – 43.6)	2.14 (1.79 – 2.56)	1.36 (1.10 – 1.67)
50 – 64 years	25.5 (22.3 – 28.9)	2.05 (1.59 – 2.64)	1.52 (1.13 – 2.03)	26.6 (23.8 – 29.6)	1.12 (0.90 – 1.38)	1.29 (1.02 – 1.63)
Socioeconomic status						
A/B	30.6 (27.4 – 34)	2.38 (1.81 – 3.13)	1.78 (1.34 – 2.37)	40.6 (36.9 – 44.5)	2.35 (1.89 – 2.94)	2.10 (1.66 – 2.68)
C	22 (20 – 24.1)	1.52 (1.18 – 1.94)	1.14 (0.88 – 1.47)	34.4 (32 – 36.9)	1.80 (1.49 – 2.18)	1.56 (1.27 – 1.93)
D/E	15.7 (12.9 – 18.9)	1	1	22.5 (19.8 – 25.5)	1	1
Sexual behaviour						
Age at initial intercourse						
< 15 years	28.1 (25.4 – 30.9)	1.32 (1.23 – 1.60)	1.32 (1.10 – 1.57)	33 (29.2 – 37.1)	0.83 (0.68 – 1.00)	
≥ 15 years	22.8 (20.9 – 24.8)	1	1	37.4 (35.1 – 39.7)	1	...
Sex with same sex, ever						
No	24.4 (22.6 – 26.1)	1		36.6 (34.5 – 38.9)	1	
Yes	30 (24.5 – 36.1)	1.33 (1.00 – 1.77)		38.6 (31.1 – 46.6)	1.08 (0.78 – 1.51)	...
Condom use at last sexual intercourse						
Yes	24.6 (22.2 – 27.3)	1		38.2 (34.7 – 41.9)	1	
No	26.7 (24.3 – 29.2)	1.11 (0.93 – 1.35)	...	39.1 (36.4 – 41.7)	1.03 (0.87 – 1.23)	...
Number sexual partners over the lifetime						
≤ 10	21.7 (19.2 – 24.3)	1		42.1 (39.2 – 45)	1	
> 10	27.9 (25.4 – 30.6)	1.40 (1.16 – 1.69)	...	38.7 (33.8 – 43.9)	0.87 (0.70 – 1.09)	...
Having casual partner, last 12 months						
No	27 (24.9 – 29.2)	1		39.7 (37.3 – 42.1)	1	
Yes	23.6 (21 – 26.4)	0.84 (0.70 – 0.99)	...	33.6 (28.8 – 38.7)	0.76 (0.61 – 0.96)	...
Intravenous drugs, ever						
No	23.8 (22.2 – 25.5)	1		34 (32 – 36)	1	
Yes	19.9 (10.1 – 35.4)	0.80 (0.36 – 1.76)	...	29.7 (18 – 44.8)	0.82 (0.43 – 1.58)	...
Tested for HIV, ever						
No/don't know	13 (11.6 – 15.6)	1	1	16.5 (14.8 – 18.4)	1	1
Yes	53.8 (50.4 – 57.1)	7.79 (6.46 – 9.39)	7.05 (5.82 – 8.53)	60.1 (57.1 – 63)	7.62 (6.44 – 9.00)	7.13 (5.97 – 8.54)

The data in parentheses are 95 % CIs
COR crude odds ratio, *AOR* adjusted odds ratio
... not statistically significant

the women the adjusted OR was highest for the 25- to 49-year-old group (AOR: 1.36, [95 % confidence interval: 1.10–1.67]) and decreased thereafter. Among the men, initial sexual intercourse before 15 years of age was significantly associated with VH screening. For both the men and the women, reported screenings decreased significantly with decreasing socioeconomic status. Overall, the proportions of men and women who reported undergoing VH screening were higher among those who had been tested for HIV, and this association remained after adjustment of variables.

Discussion

This study is the first to report the low level of knowledge related to HBV and HCV transmission in Brazil and the low screening rates for VH within the general population. The strengths of this study are the high response rate and large probability sample, which reflected a broad Brazilian population in terms of demographic characteristics.

For all of the assessed knowledge indicators, fewer than 35 % of the participants correctly identified the transmission routes for both HBV and HCV. Although the major HBV transmission route in Brazil is sexual intercourse [13], only 33.1 % of the respondents correctly identified this transmission route. This percentage is lower than the percentages observed in other population-based studies; for example, 44 % of a sample from Hong Kong correctly identified this transmission route [20], while approximately 60 % of a sample in Germany [21, 22], 70 % of a sample in France [23], and 77.6 % of a sample in the Netherlands [21] provided correct identification.

In Brazil, donated blood is routinely screened for HCV, and measures are in place to facilitate infection control and safe-injection practices; thus, HCV is now transmitted primarily through injected drug use. The prevalence of markers of hepatitis B and C among intravenous drug users are high at 63.9 and 55.8 %, respectively [24]; however, knowledge related to the transmission of HCV through shared needles was low. A similar result was observed for HBV. These results are inconsistent with those reported by other studies. For example, 44 % of respondents in Hong Kong [20] and 95 % in Germany [22] correctly identified that HBV can be transmitted by sharing needles. A similar result was obtained for knowledge related to HBV transmission through tattooing and piercing, with much lower levels of knowledge reported in Brazil than in Hong Kong (37 %) [20] and Germany (73 %) [22].

Furthermore, the proportion of respondents who correctly identified the transmission routes of both HBV and HCV substantially dropped relative to the proportions of individuals who identified the transmission routes of the individual virus types. This confusion within the general population regarding the specificities associated with each hepatitis type has also been observed in previous studies [4, 20–22].

The commemoration of World Hepatitis Day (named in the 2010 resolution WHA63.18) [25] is helping to raise awareness and mobilize governments and resources to aid in the fight against VH in Latin America [14]. In Brazil, although World Hepatitis Day campaigns have been conducted since 2010, knowledge related to VH remains low. Because increasing the knowledge of HBV and HCV is an effective means of preventing or reducing the spread of infection [26–28], additional efforts are needed to improve public education regarding the transmission routes and specificities of HBV and HCV.

Our results revealed that there is an urgent need to improve overall testing uptake for VH. Such screening is a necessary first step toward providing access to prevention, care and treatment services. Only one third of the participants in this study had ever been screened for VH; this proportion was higher for HBV (44.6 %) than for HCV (32 %). Early diagnosis of VH is among the main priorities of the Department of STIs, AIDS and VH of the Brazilian Ministry of Health [29]. Since 2004, free testing for VH has been offered at VCT sites located in clinics and specialized centres [30], although only a small proportion of our participants (6.2 %) reported having been screened for VH at such sites. Members of the general population may be reluctant to undergo testing at these sites because the sites are designed to offer VH and HIV testing specifically for populations who are at a greater risk of exposure to HIV and other STIs, such as men who have sex with men, sex workers and intravenous drug users. Moreover, studies have shown that VCT sites exhibit low levels of performance with regards to installed capacity and present significant limitations in terms of the quality of diagnostic services and the promotion of prevention measures [31]. As a strategy to improve access to diagnosis, Brazil implemented rapid testing in 2011 within the public health system [30]. However, our results indicated that only 17.5 % of the respondents had been screened with such tests, which suggests that rapid testing has not been widely implemented. Only a small proportion of participants reported engagement in high-risk behaviours as a reason for testing, suggesting that testing was performed for reasons other than individual perceptions of risk, which is a factor that has been associated with not being tested in other studies.

Among the enrolled women, VH screening coverage was also low, which is surprising because such screening is offered during pregnancy: 96 % of pregnant women in Brazil receive antenatal care [32], and 83.5 % of pregnant women are tested for HIV [33]. Although this result is subject to respondent recall bias, this low reported coverage among women might be explained by a possible lack of information provided by health professionals to pregnant women with regard to VH screening. Providers might not always communicate VH screening results to women if they do not pose a threat to the patient or baby, such as when results are negative or indicate past infection. Another possible explanation is that many women might not be aware that they are being screened for VH during pregnancy. The provision of appropriate pre- and post-test counselling for VH during antenatal care should be improved by providing appropriate training to doctors and mid-wives [14].

In our multivariate analysis, the participants who reported having undergone VH screening were seven times more likely to have been tested for HIV compared with those who had never been tested for VH. One potential explanation for this finding is that the same services offer testing for both infections, which are a part of the screening package used to evaluate pregnant women and high-risk groups, such as sex workers and men who have sex with men [29]. The HIV testing rate (54 % in men and 60 % in women) was higher than the VH testing rate; however, despite this difference, the HIV testing rate was strikingly low considering that HIV prevention has been the subject of broad testing provisions, effective testing promotion at all levels of health services, testing campaigns and widespread community advocacy and awareness campaigns [34]. This result indicates that difficulties remain in overcoming the general population's reluctance to seek testing, although it can be used as a lesson for VH advocacy.

The enrolled men who were aged between 50 and 64 years old were significantly more likely to have been screened. Several studies have identified an association between increased age [35, 36] and testing status, whereas other studies have not found this association [28]. Socioeconomic differences were observed in various aspects of this study. Multivariable analysis identified associations between lower socioeconomic status and a lack of screening in both men and women. Moreover, the participants of lower socioeconomic status exhibited generally poorer knowledge of VH transmission, a finding that has been corroborated by several authors [20, 21]. This lack of knowledge is particularly important because the prevalence of VH is higher in individuals in economically and socially vulnerable situations [3, 23].

We found that 73.9 % of the respondents had received hepatitis B vaccines. This proportion is higher than those reported in previous population-based studies conducted in other countries [20, 22, 23]. However, the proportion of respondents who had completed all three doses of the vaccine was considerably lower at 18.3 %. In this study, no vaccination cards were verified or cross-referenced and therefore this result is subject to respondent recall bias. Importantly, 30 % of the men and 23 % of the women under 24 years of age had not been vaccinated against HBV, and sexual transmission of HBV remains a concern among unvaccinated adolescents in Brazil. Nevertheless, vaccination against HBV was extended to young individuals (aged 20–24 years) in 2011 to increase the coverage rate.

The current study has several limitations. The PCAP-2013 relied on self-reported data, which are subject to recall and desirability biases. These biases might have influenced the high rate of HBV vaccine coverage, which was not cross-checked against vaccination records. Additionally, questions related to certain behaviours were sensitive and might have been under-reported. We sought to minimize this bias by using a self-interview technique for the survey sections regarding sexual practices and drug use. Several studies have demonstrated that it is difficult for the general population to differentiate between various types of VH [4, 20, 22]. Consequently, interpretations of specific knowledge indicator values should be assessed with caution [20]. However, our findings are valuable as baseline information and can be assessed in future rounds of the PCAP, which should take into account changes in census tracts when establishing a longitudinal comparison.

Conclusions

The PCAP-2013 provides a novel assessment of VH in Brazil. In measuring the extent of knowledge related to VH across a large representative sample, we found that our study participants possessed low levels of knowledge related to hepatitis B and C. This study also underscores the need to improve screening practices used in the general population and to specifically target younger and lower socioeconomic status populations. Based on these findings, current preventive measures must be reinforced. Efforts to enhance education through awareness campaigns, increased testing resources and expanded testing sites are needed to remove barriers to testing and improve access to treatment.

Abbreviations

ABEP: Association of Research Companies; AOR: adjusted odds ratio; CIs: confidence intervals; FMT-HVD: Fundação de Medicina Tropical Doutor Heitor Vieira Dourado; HAV: hepatitis A virus; HBV: viral hepatitis B; HCV: hepatitis C virus; HDV: hepatitis D virus; HEV: hepatitis E virus; OR: odds ratio; PCAP: Survey of Knowledge, Attitudes and Practices of HIV and Other Sexually Transmitted Infections; PCAP-2013: Third round of the Survey of Knowledge, Attitudes and Practices of HIV and Other Sexually Transmitted Infections; PSUs: primary sampling units; STIs: sexually transmitted infections; VCT: voluntary counselling and testing; VH: viral hepatitis.

Competing interests
The authors declare that they have no competing interests.

Authors' contributions
FM and ASB provided institutional support and coordinated the study. SBO, ARP and JMG designed the study and supervised field work. MS analyzed data and wrote the manuscript. All of the authors interpreted data, critically revised the manuscript for important intellectual content and gave final approval for this version to be published.

Acknowledgements
We thank the government officials and experts in the study areas. This study was funded by the Department of STI, AIDS and Viral Hepatitis of the Brazilian Ministry of Health.

Author details
[1]Department of STI, AIDS, and Viral Hepatitis, Brazil Ministry of Health, Brasília, DF, Brazil. [2]Fundação de Medicina Tropical Doutor Heitor Vieira Dourado (FMT-HVD), Avenida Pedro Teixeira 25, CEP: 69040-000 Manaus, AM, Brazil.

References

1. World Health Organization. A63/15 viral hepatitis: report by the secretariat. 2010. http://apps.who.int/gb/ebwha/pdf_files/WHA63/A63_15-en.pdf. Accessed 23 Jan 2016.
2. Ximenes RA, Pereira LM, Martelli CM, Merchan-Hamann E, Stein AT, Figueiredo GM, et al. Methodology of a nationwide cross-sectional survey of prevalence and epidemiological patterns of hepatitis A, B and C infection in Brazil. Cad Saude Publica. 2010;26:1693–704.
3. Pereira LM, Martelli CM, Moreira RC, Merchan-Hamman E, Stein AT, Cardoso MR, et al. Prevalence and risk factors of Hepatitis C virus infection in Brazil, 2005 through 2009: a cross-sectional study. BMC Infect Dis. 2013;13:60.
4. Universidade de Pernambuco. Estudo de prevalência de base populacional das infecções pelos vírus das Hepatitis A, B, e C nas capitais do Brasil. Brasil: Universidade de Pernambuco, Núcleo de Pós-Graduação; 2010.
5. Schweitzer A, Horn J, Mikolajczyk RT, Krause G, Ott JJ. Estimations of worldwide prevalence of chronic hepatitis B virus infection: a systematic review of data published between 1965 and 2013. Lancet. 2015;386:1546–55.
6. World Health Organization. The global prevalence of hepatitis E virus infection and susceptibility: a systematic review. WHO/IVB/10.14. Geneva: World Health Organization; 2010.
7. Pascarella S, Negro F. Hepatitis D virus: an update. Liver Int. 2011;31:7–21.
8. Brazil Ministry of Health. 2012 epidemiological bulletin on viral hepatitis. Brasília: Ministry of Health, Health Surveillance Secretariat, Department of STI, AIDS and Viral Hepatitis; 2012. http://www.aids.gov.br/sites/default/files/anexos/publicacao/2012/51820/boletim_epidemiol_gico_hepatites_virais_2012_ve_12026.pdf. Accessed 23 Jan 2016.
9. Gomez B. The Latin American Response Viral Hepatitis. Session: The Impact & Response to Viral Hepatitis in Different Scenarios. X Congress on HIV/AIDS, III Congress on Viral Hepatitis; Nov 2015. João Pessoa: 2015. http://www.aidshvbrasil2015.aids.gov.br/pt-br/latin-american-response-viral-hepatitis-session-impact-response-viral-hepatitis-different-scenarios. Accessed 23 Jan 2016.
10. World Health Organization. WHO: Country statistics and global health estimates. Brazil: WHO statistical profile; 2015.
11. Ferreira PR, Brandão-Mello CE, Estes C, Gonçales Júnior FL, Coelho HS, Razavi H, et al. Disease burden of chronic hepatitis C in Brazil. Braz J Infect Dis. 2015;19:363–8.
12. Mesquita F. Response to Viral Hepatitis in Brazil. X Congress on HIV/AIDS III Congress on Viral Hepatitis; 17–20 November. João Pessoa: 2015. http://aidshvbrasil2015.aids.gov.br/pt-br/resposta-hepatites-virais-no-brasil Accessed 23 Jan 2016.
13. Brazil Ministry of Health. Viral hepatitis in Brazil: situation, actions, and agenda. Brasília: Ministry of Health, Health Surveillance Secretariat, Department of STD, AIDS and Viral Hepatitis; 2011. http://www.aids.gov.br/sites/default/files/anexos/publicacao/2011/50069/agendahepatites_2011_pdf_19532.pdf. Accessed 23 Jan 2016.
14. Díez-Padrisa N, Castellanos LG. PAHO viral hepatitis group. Viral hepatitis in Latin America and the Caribbean: a public health challenge. Rev Panam Salud Publica. 2013;34:275–81.
15. Brazil Ministry of Health. Study about knowledge, attitudes and practices among Brazilian population aged 15 to 24 years - PCAP 2004. Brasília: Ministry of Health, Health Surveillance Secretariat, National Program of STD and AIDS; 2005.
16. Brazil Ministry of Health. Study about knowledge, attitudes and practices among Brazilian population aged 15 to 64 years - PCAP 2008. Brasília: Ministry of Health, Health Surveillance Secretariat, Department of DST, AIDS, and Viral Hepatitis; 2011. http://www.aids.gov.br/sites/default/files/anexos/publicacao/2009/40352/pcap_2008_f_pdf_13227.pdf. Accessed 23 Jan 2016.
17. Instituto Brasileiro de Geografia e Estadística (IBGE). Sinopse do Censo Demográfico 2010. Tabela 1.4 - População nos Censos Demográficos, segundo as Grandes Regiões e as Unidades da Federação - 1872/2010. Rio de Janeiro: Directoria Geral de Estatística; 2010. http://www.ibge.gov.br/home/estatistica/populacao/censo2010/tabelas_pdf/Brasil_tab_1_4.pdf. Accessed 16 May 2013.
18. Kish L. Survey sampling. Hoboken: Wiley; 1965.
19. Associação Brasileira de Empresas de Pesquisa (ABEP). Critério de classificação econômica. Brasil: 2008. [cited 2015 4 Oct]. http://www.abep.org. Accessed 23 Jan 2016.
20. Leung CM, Wong WH, Chan KH, Lai LS, Luk YW, Lai JY, et al. Public awareness of hepatitis B infection: a population-based telephone survey in Hong Kong. Hong Kong Med J. 2010;16:463–9.
21. Crutzen R, Goritz AS. Public awareness and practical knowledge regarding Hepatitis A, B, and C: a two-country survey. J Infect Public Health. 2012;5:195–8.
22. Schenkel K, Radun D, Bremer V, Bocter N, Hamouda O. Viral hepatitis in Germany: poor vaccination coverage and little knowledge about transmission in target groups. BMC Public Health. 2008;8:132.
23. Brouard C, Gautier A, Saboni L, Jestin C, Semaille C, Beltzer N, et al. Hepatitis B knowledge, perceptions and practices in the French general population: the room for improvement. BMC Public Health. 2013;13:576.
24. Nelson PK, Mathers BM, Cowie B, Hagan H, Des Jarlais D, Horyniak D, et al. Global epidemiology of hepatitis B and hepatitis C in people who inject drugs: results of systematic reviews. Lancet. 2011;378:571–83.
25. World Health Organisation. Sixty-third World Health Assembly resolution WHA63.18: viral hepatitis. 2010. [cited 2012 4 Jan]. http://apps.who.int/gb/ebwha/pdf_files/WHA63/A63_R18-en.pdf. Accessed 23 Jan 2016.
26. Chao J, Chang ET, So SK. Hepatitis B and liver cancer knowledge and practices among healthcare and public health professionals in China: a cross-sectional study. BMC Public Health. 2010;10:98.
27. Munoz Sastre MT, Bacq Y, Mullet E, Sorum PC. Misconceptions regarding hepatitis C in the French public. Prev Med. 2002;34:596–9.
28. van der Veen YJ, Voeten HA, de Zwart O, Richardus JH. Awareness, knowledge and self-reported test rates regarding Hepatitis B in Turkish-Dutch: a survey. BMC Public Health. 2010;10:512.
29. Brazil Ministry of Health. Departament: the role of the department. Brasília: Ministry of Health, Health Surveillance Secretariat, Department of STD, AIDS and Viral Hepatitis; 2013. http://www.aids.gov.br/en/pagina/departament. Accessed 23 Jan 2016.
30. Brazil Ministry of Health. Viral hepatitis: evolution of actions. Brasília: Ministry of Health; 2012. http://www.aids.gov.br/pagina/2013/54919. Accessed 23 Jan 2016.
31. Grangeiro A, Escuder MM, Wolffenbüttel K, Pupo LR, Nemes MIB, Monteiro PHN. Avaliação do perfil tecnológico dos centros de testagem e aconselhamento para HIV no Brasil. Rev Saude Publica. 2009;43:427–36.
32. Pan American Health Organization. 2014 update: elimination of mother-to-child transmission of HIV and syphilis in the Americas. Washington: PAHO; 2014.
33. Brazilian Ministry of Health. Vertical transmission of HIV and sífilis: strategies for reduction and elimination. Brasília: Brazilian Ministry of Health; 2014. [cited 2014 30 Dec]. http://www.aids.gov.br/publicacao/2014/transmissao-vertical-do-hiv-e-sifilis-estrategias-para-reducao-e-eliminacao. Accessed 23 Jan 2016.
34. Brazil Ministry of Health. Global AIDS response. Progress reporting, 2014. Narrative reporting. Brasília: Brazilian Ministry of Health; 2015. http://www.unaids.org/sites/default/files/country/documents//file%2C94421%2Ces..pdf. Accessed 23 Jan 2016.
35. Cheung J, Lee TK, Teh CZ, Wang CY, Kwan WC, Yoshida EM. Cross-sectional study of hepatitis B awareness among Chinese and Southeast Asian Canadians in the Vancouver-Richmond community. Can J Gastroenterol. 2005;19:245–9.
36. Choe JH, Taylor VM, Yasui Y, Burke N, Nguyen T, Acorda E, et al. Health care access and sociodemographic factors associated with hepatitis B testing in Vietnamese American men. J Immigr Minor Health. 2006;8:193–201.

12

Incidence of hepatitis C among people who inject drugs

Anne Marie Carew[1], Niamh Murphy[2], Jean Long[1], Kate Hunter[2], Suzi Lyons[1], Cathal Walsh[3,4] and Lelia Thornton[2*]

Abstract

Background: Comprehensive information on the incidence and duration of hepatitis C virus (HCV) infection for people who inject drugs (PWID) in Ireland is not available. We created an incidence curve of injecting drug use in Ireland and subsequently estimated incidence of hepatitis C virus (HCV) infection.

Methods: Anonymised data from the National Drug Treatment Reporting System (NDTRS) were used to identify all people who inject drugs (PWIDs) and who entered drug treatment for the first time between 1991 and 2014. A curve, estimating the incidence of injecting, was created to plot PWIDs by year of commencing injecting. The curve was adjusted for missing data on PWIDs in treatment and for PWIDs who were never treated. An adjustment was made to account for injectors who had never shared injecting equipment. The incidence of HCV infection and chronic infection in PWIDs was estimated by applying published rates.

Results: Between 1991 and 2014, 14,320 injectors were registered on NDTRS. The majority were young (median age 25 years), male (74%), lived in Dublin (73%) and injected an opiate (e.g. heroin) (94%). The estimated total number of injectors up to the end of 2014 was 16,382. An estimated 12,423 (95% CI 10,799-13,161) were infected with HCV, and 9,317 (95% CI 8,022-9,996) became chronically infected. The estimated annual number of new HCV infections among PWIDs increased steeply from the late 1970s and peaked in 1998. By 2014, almost 30% of injectors were estimated to have been infected for over 20 years.

Conclusions: This is the first comprehensive national estimate of the incidence of HCV in PWIDs in Ireland and will inform planning and developing appropriate health care services.

Keywords: Hepatitis C, Ireland, Injecting drug use, PWID, Incidence

Background

Hepatitis C (HCV) was first identified in 1989. The acute phase of infection is usually asymptomatic, but approximately 75% of those who are infected develop chronic infection, which can cause liver cirrhosis, hepatocellular carcinoma (HCC) and liver failure [1, 2]. The risk of developing cirrhosis or HCC is higher in males, those who consume excess alcohol, those with hepatitis B or HIV co-infection [1] and those who were infected at older ages [2]. Between 5 and 20% of those who are chronically infected will develop cirrhosis after approximately 20 years of infection. Of those with cirrhosis, approximately 4% progress to decompensated liver disease each year and 1.6% develop HCC annually [2].

* Correspondence: lelia.thornton@hse.ie
[2]HSE Health Protection Surveillance Centre, 25-27 Middle Gardiner Street, Dublin 1, Ireland
Full list of author information is available at the end of the article

The main modes of transmission of HCV infection in Ireland are injecting drug use and the receipt of contaminated blood or blood products before the introduction of routine screening for HCV in the early 1990s. Information on the epidemiology of HCV in Ireland is mostly available from National Virus Reference Laboratory (NVRL) data since 1989, routine surveillance data based on statutory laboratory and clinical notifications to the Health Protection Surveillance Centre (HPSC) since 2004, and special studies in high prevalence groups such as people who inject drugs (PWIDs) and prisoners.

A study using NVRL diagnostic data and HPSC notification data estimated that approximately 10,000 individuals had been diagnosed with HCV and were living with chronic infection in Ireland by the end of 2009 [3]. The extent of underdiagnosis in Ireland is not known, but assuming levels of between 50 and 67% would increase this estimate to between 20,000 and 30,000 individuals [4]. Drug use was the most likely risk factor in 80% of the cases of HCV diagnosed by the NVRL between 1989 and 2004, of which 53% were genotype 1 and 42% genotype 3 [3]. A further 4,813 cases of HCV were notified to HPSC between 2010 and 2014 and, where risk factor data were available, approximately 80% were PWIDs [5].

The most recent capture-recapture study found that there were approximately 12,000 known opiate users (ever-injectors and non-injectors) in Ireland in 2006 and estimated the total number of known and 'hidden' opiate users to be 20,790 (95% CI 18,136-23,576) [6, 7]. Testing for blood-borne viral infections is offered to PWIDs in Ireland when they first attend opiate substitution services (clinics, prisons, and general practice) and is repeated at regular intervals. An Irish opiate treatment outcomes study commissioned in 2002 showed that HCV testing was carried out for 82% of attendees entering treatment services in rural, urban and inner-city areas [8]. However, addiction treatment services were not widely available outside of Dublin until more recent years and the proportion of PWIDs with undiagnosed HCV infection is likely to be higher outside of Dublin. Studies of PWIDs in prisons, opiate substitution services and general practice in Ireland, between 1992 and 2006, estimated the HCV antibody prevalence in this population to be between 52 and 84% [9–17]. Using a weighted average of the estimates from these studies (based on sample size), the national prevalence of HCV in PWIDs was calculated to be approximately 70% [16]. More recently, a cross-sectional study in 2011 reported lower levels of HCV antibody positivity in the prison population, with 41.5% of those with a self-reported history of ever injecting drugs testing positive for anti-HCV [18]. Of note, the prevalence of HCV infection differed depending on the type of drug injected; for example, 54% (80/149) of heroin injectors, 66% (66/100) of cocaine injectors and 62% (42/68) of benzodiazepine injectors tested HCV antibody positive, whereas only 21% (14/66) of steroid injectors tested positive [19].

The incidence and duration of HCV infection in Ireland have never been comprehensively described. The aim of this study was to estimate the incidence of HCV infection among PWIDs in Ireland. The objectives were: (1) to create an incidence curve of injecting drug use, (2) to estimate the annual incidence of HCV in PWIDs and (3) to estimate the number of PWIDs who developed chronic HCV infection.

Methods

Anonymised individualised data from the National Drug Treatment Reporting System (NDTRS) formed the basis of this study. The NDTRS records information on treated problem drug use in Ireland using an agreed Europe-wide protocol (http://www.emcdda.europa.eu/publications/manuals/tdi-protocol-3.0) and covers 76% of drug and alcohol treatment services in Ireland. It was established in the Greater Dublin Area in 1990 by the Health Research Board and was extended in 1995 to cover all areas of the country [20]. Treatment data for problem drug use in Ireland are provided to the NDTRS by statutory and non-statutory services, including outpatient services, residential centres and general practices. Clients who attend needle-exchange services are not included in this reporting system. The database records client information on the date of treatment, whether a client has ever previously received drug treatment (incident case identifier), ever injected drugs, age when they first injected, and recent injection behaviour, in addition to detailed demographic, drug use and treatment data. The NDTRS does not contain information on HCV status.

Injecting and HCV infection curves were created using a four-stage process.

1. **Original injector data and imputed missing values**
   In 2016, all ever-injector individuals, whether current or former injectors, entering drug treatment for the first time between 1991 and 2014 were identified and extracted from the NDTRS. The length of time an individual injected before coming to their first treatment as an injector was ascertained and an injecting curve was created for the number of cases starting to inject each year. The year of commencing injecting was missing for a proportion of cases. Factors associated with missing values were investigated and discovered not to be completely random. Therefore, in order to account for this, missing data were generated using Expectation-Maximization (EM) methods. The original and imputed data were combined to create an epidemic curve based on the year of commencing injecting for all PWIDs registered on the NDTRS up to the end of 2014.
2. **Estimating injectors not in treatment**
   Treated PWIDs represent a proportion of the injecting drug population. Estimates for the proportion of PWIDs not in treatment were used to adjust the epidemic curve for all PWIDs. In the absence of Irish data for this proportion, Scottish rates were applied to each yearly estimate of injectors residing in Dublin (6% of injectors never attended treatment in Glasgow between 2008 and 2010) [21]). Scottish data were considered the most appropriate as the drug situation in Dublin has been likened to that in Glasgow [22]. For injectors living outside Dublin, a worst case scenario estimate of 50% non-attendance was used based on the 2006 capture-recapture estimate [7], as appropriate harm

reduction and treatment services were not historically available to a large proportion of these. No adjustment was made to take account of PWIDs who died prior to the commencement of the NDTRS in 1991. Using a Mann–Whitney *U* test, the estimated number of injectors was validated by comparing it with published data available for four time points, from capture recapture studies estimating the number of opiate users in Ireland [6, 7]. The number of opiate users who were injectors was derived using the known percentage of opiate injectors in the NDTRS.

3. **Estimating HCV infections**
In order to adjust for injectors who were not at risk of infection a conservative 21% deduction was made from the total estimate of injectors to allow for those who had never shared injecting equipment. The 21% was based on the lowest annual proportion of cases (worst case scenario) who reported through the NDTRS that they had never shared and had been in treatment for drug use two or more times during the 23 year time period [unpublished NDTRS data]. In order to estimate the incidence of HCV infection among PWIDs, published HCV incidence rates in PWID populations for different time periods in Ireland were applied to the injecting curve. Incidence data were available for two time periods. Smyth et al. found a HCV incidence rate of 66 per 100 person years (95% CI 51–84) in a study carried out between 1992 and 1998 [23]. This rate and its 95% confidence intervals (CI) were used for those who commenced injecting between 1992 and 1998. In a study carried out in 2001, Grogan et al. [13] estimated that the infection rate for clients in opiate substitution services in the parts of Dublin and surrounding areas was 24 per 100 person years (95% CI 12.2–43.8) but included both injectors and non-injectors in their denominator. We adjusted this rate and its 95% confidence intervals using the proportion of opiate users entering treatment in the area in 2001 who were recorded in the NDTRS as having reported injecting (70%) and thus estimated the infection rate in PWIDs to be 35 per 100 person years (95% CI 17.4–62.6). This rate and its 95% confidence intervals were applied to 2001 and continued for the period 2001 to 2014 as these were the most recent estimates. As no published data were available for the period 1953 to 1991, the mid-point between the highest and lowest incidence and its confidence intervals for the two periods with known incidence rates were applied; these were a rate of 50.7 per 100 person years and 95% CI of 17.4–84. For 1999 and 2000 the mid-points of the rate and the upper and lower confidence intervals for the two periods with known incidence rates on either side of the timeline were applied (50 per 100 person years, and 95% CI 34.6–73.4).
4. **Estimating chronic HCV**
In order to obtain an estimate of chronic HCV infections, an internationally accepted 75% conversion from acute to chronic HCV was applied to the HCV infections curve [2].

Results

Original injector data and imputed missing values

During the 23-year study period (1991–2014), 14,320 ever-injectors entered addiction treatment and were registered on the NDTRS. The majority were male (74.3%) and lived in Dublin (73.0%). The median age for injectors entering treatment was 25 years (90% central range 18–40 years) while the median age at commencing injecting was 20 years (90% central range 15–31 years). Half of all PWIDs had injected for 3 years or more before entering addiction treatment (90% central range 0–18 years). Opiates were the main problem drug reported by 94.1% of PWIDs. Seventy one per cent reported problem use of more than one drug and 14.7% had been in treatment as a smoker and later returned to treatment as an injector. Problem alcohol use was reported by 9.1% of injectors on entering treatment. Data necessary to calculate the year of first injecting were available for 86.4% ($n = 12{,}375$) and missing for 13.6% ($n = 1{,}945$). The most common missing information was age first injected ($n = 1{,}929$, 13.5%). Using logistic regression, year of treatment and main problem drug were found to be significantly associated with the probability of a patient's record not having data on age first injected. An imputed year of first injecting was assigned to individuals with missing data using the pattern of observed data for similar injectors (Fig. 1).

The resulting injecting curve shows few new PWIDs in Ireland prior to 1970 ($n = 36$, 1957 to 1969); the estimated number of new PWIDs increased steadily in the late 1970s and then continued to increase at a lower rate into the 1980s (Fig. 1). Incidence of injecting increased again in the late 1980s and early 1990s, peaking in 1998. Data from 2011 to 2014 are likely to be incomplete due to the lag time between injecting and first attending treatment.

Estimating injectors not in treatment

Adjusting for PWIDs who had never attended drug treatment services and therefore who were not registered on the NDTRS, added a further 2,062 injectors to the curve. The total estimated number of PWIDs up to the end of 2014 is 16,382 (Fig. 1).

Estimates from the injecting curve were validated against the number of opiate injectors estimated using opiate user data from Irish capture recapture studies

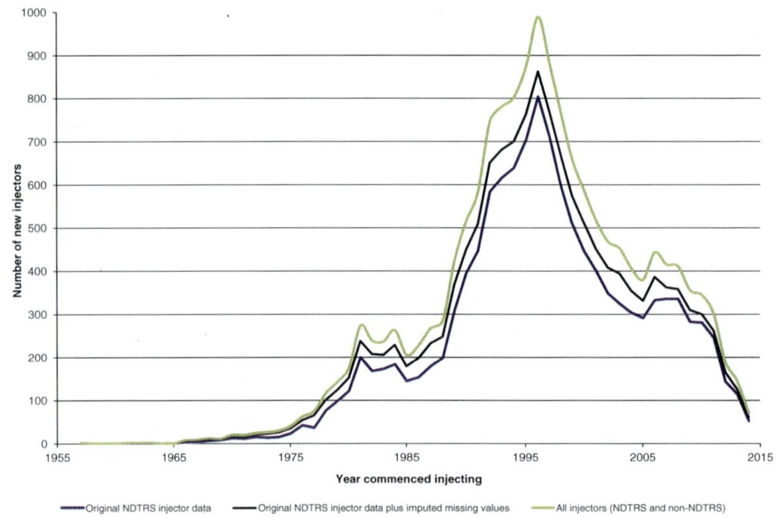

Fig. 1 New injectors by year of commencing injecting

over four different years [6, 7] and data on the percentage of opiate users who were injecting in those years from the NDTRS (Table 1). Overall the estimates were not statistically significantly different ($U = 5.00$, $p = 0.49$).

Estimated HCV infections

After adjusting for injectors who had never shared injecting equipment, it is estimated that 12,423 (95% CI 10,799-13,161) PWIDs were infected with HCV over the entire period (Fig. 2) and that 9,317 (95% CI 8,022-9,996) became chronically infected (Fig. 3). The estimated number of new infections peaked in 1997. By 2014, more than one quarter (27.0%) of PWIDs with chronic HCV infection were estimated to have been infected for 0–10 years, 43.4% for 11–20 years, 22.8% for 21–30 years and 6.7% for over 30 years.

Discussion

This study is the first comprehensive national estimate of the incidence of injecting drug use in Ireland along with the incidence and extent of the hepatitis C epidemic in this population. Results show an estimated 16,400 PWIDs in Ireland during the 24 year study period (1991–2014). The majority of injectors were young, male, lived in Dublin and injected heroin. Over 12,000 PWIDs were estimated to have been infected with HCV by 2014, with over 9,000 likely to have become chronically infected. More than 40% of injectors were estimated to have been infected for 11–20 years by 2014 and almost 30% were estimated to have been infected for over 20 years. However, some of these injectors will have since died or may have been successfully treated for HCV infection and the cumulative incidence numbers presented in this paper do not take account of these events. In relation to deaths, the National Drug-Related Death Index reported that 937 PWID who were hepatitis C-infected died between the years 1998 and 2014 (Personal communication: Dr Suzi Lyons, Senior Researcher, National Health Information Systems, Health Research Board. 8 November 2016). In relation to treatment for hepatitis C, a national programme set up at the end of 2014 offering direct acting antivirals to individuals testing positive for hepatitis C and meeting pre-defined clinical criteria reported that 138 PWID were successfully

Table 1 Comparison of estimates from the injecting curve with published data from a capture recapture study

Year	Opiate users in capture recapture[a]	95% CI	% opiate injectors in NDTRS	Estimated opiate injectors in capture recapture	Opiate injectors calculated from injecting curve	% difference between capture recapture and injecting curve
1996	13461	12037–15306	65%	8750	8469	−3.2
2000	14158	12884-15883	83%	11751	11362	−3.3
2001	14452	13405–15819	78%	11273	11879	+5.4
2006	20790	18136–23576	65%	13513	14024	+3.8

[a][6, 7]

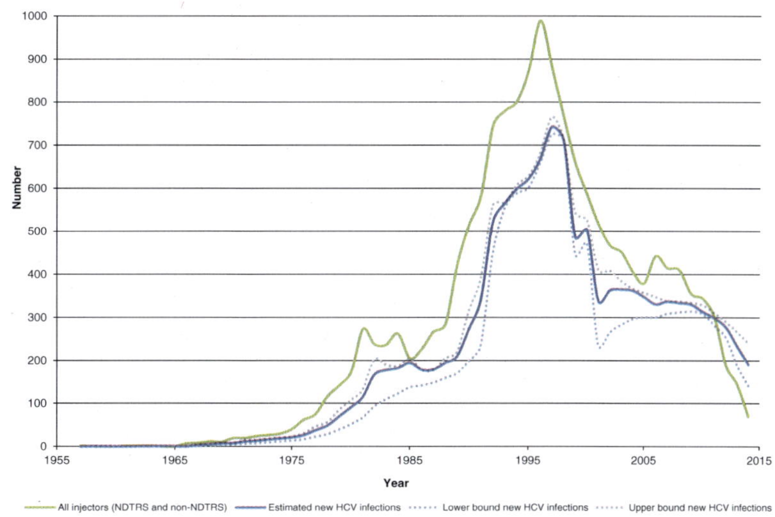

Fig. 2 Estimates of new injectors by year commenced injecting and new HCV infections by year infected

treated (measured by a sustained virological response) between December 2014 and August 2016 (Personal communication: Michele Tait, Programme Manager, HSE Hepatitis C Treatment Programme. 3 November 2016). Prior to this, research published in 2007 indicated that few PWID were suitable for (13%) or commenced (3%) antiviral treatment [15]. Thus the overall numbers successfully treated or who died are likely to be small and do not change the overall estimate of the extent of the hepatitis C epidemic.

The overall size and pattern of the estimated hepatitis C incidence curve is similar to a hepatitis C infection curve based on the date of laboratory diagnoses, despite a different study approach [3]. Both studies found that hepatitis C incidence is now decreasing in Ireland. This is supported by routine surveillance data which show that statutory notifications have declined significantly since 2012 [5]. Given this fall in the number of newly diagnosed cases and the fact that the most recent incidence study dates to 2001, the authors acknowledge that there may be a corresponding overestimate in later years. As PWIDs make up the majority of known hepatitis C infected people in Ireland, the results from this study are of benefit in estimating the extent of the overall HCV epidemic in Ireland. The other known large cohort is people infected through blood and blood products in the past in Ireland. This is a historical cohort of over 1,700 people, approximately 390 of whom remained alive and chronically infected at the end of 2013 [24]. Undiagnosed infection in this population would be expected to be rare due to extensive national screening programmes. There may, however, be a significant

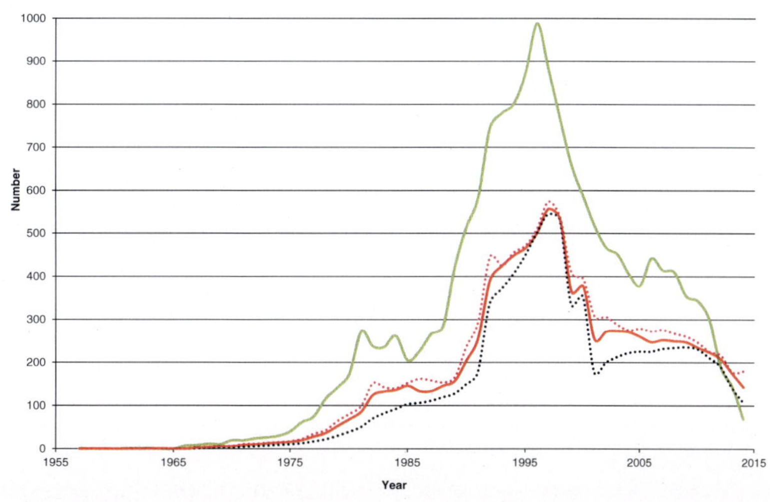

Fig. 3 Estimates of new injectors by year commenced and chronic HCV infections by year infected

number of undiagnosed cases of HCV in the recent migrant population in Ireland. Although asylum seekers are routinely offered infectious disease screening, there is no systematic testing for other migrants. At the time of the 2011 census, there were 766,770 non-Irish nationals living in Ireland. Based on census data on the number of people living in Ireland by country of birth (CSO unpublished data, Olive Pluck, CSO) and published data on the prevalence of anti-HCV by country of birth [25, 26], over 10,000 of these are likely to be chronically infected with HCV. This assumes that the prevalence of HCV in the migrant population in Ireland is similar to published data for the general population in their country of birth.

There are a number of limitations to the methods used in this study. The number of PWIDs who never accessed drug treatment was unknown and was estimated. However, the estimates of PWIDs were validated against capture recapture studies [6, 7] and were not statistically different. The hepatitis C infection rates that were applied were based on incidence studies during two specific time periods and varied considerably from 66 to 35%. This is not surprising as HCV incidence rates for Glasgow show similar variations although their injecting curve is approximately 10 years ahead of the Irish curve; for example, model-based rates estimated for Glasgow were 6–40, 78–89 and 18–30 per 100 injector-years during the periods 1960–1976, 1977–1986 and 1990–2000 respectively [27]. The decrease in the incidence of HCV infection in opiate users in Ireland may be due to the provision of opiate detoxification and substitution in prisons and the increased provision of such programmes in the community, in particular outside Dublin [28]. Another limitation was that we did not have data on whether individuals ceased to inject. Therefore HCV infection rates were applied to each individual each year. However, a proportion of individuals may have ceased injecting prior to becoming HCV infected and no longer have been at risk of infection. A proportion of individuals may also have died, and this is not reflected in the estimates described here. Our interval estimates in Figs. 2 and 3 account for known uncertainties in the inputs, but do not account for other uncertainties and modelling assumptions the impact of which is not explicitly known. Despite these limitations, as already stated, modelled curves are broadly in line with those described by laboratory diagnoses and by surveillance data [3, 5].

Modelling the progression of disease for the population is of interest from a public health perspective, especially in the context of emerging treatments for HCV. This work is ongoing by one of the authors (CW), involving the calibration of disease models, and evidence syntheses for treatments that are available, and is due for publication in the near future. The additive effect of alcohol use on progression of HCV-related cirrhosis [1] will be an important factor to take into account, as PWIDs in Ireland have been shown to have a high prevalence of problem alcohol consumption. Only 9% reported problem alcohol use on first entry to treatment; however, data on previously treated opiate users indicate that 21% reported problem alcohol use [18] and 35% of opiate users receiving methadone in general practice in Dublin were harmful alcohol users [29]. Recent drug treatment data show that the number of injectors entering drug treatment for the first time in Ireland has dropped slightly in recent years [30]. However, injecting drug use remains a significant issue. The European Monitoring Centre for Drugs and Drug Addiction (EMCDDA) recommends the collection of accurate data on the incidence of injectors entering treatment as this is an indicator of problem drug use [31]. Therefore, this analysis demonstrates the wider usefulness of routine drug treatment data collected by the NDTRS. It is important that harm reduction strategies continue to be implemented and evaluated in order to achieve reductions in injecting risk behaviours and HCV transmission. Although the incidence of injecting and the incidence of HCV have declined in recent years, unless substantial numbers receive treatment for their HCV infection the burden of HCV-related liver complications will be high over the next few decades. The information from this study will be of benefit in planning cost-effective approaches to the use of the highly effective but expensive direct acting antiviral treatments now available.

Conclusions

This paper is the first comprehensive national estimate of the incidence of injecting drug use in Ireland, along with the incidence and extent of the hepatitis C epidemic in this population. The findings will inform those responsible for planning and developing health care services and will be of benefit in planning cost-effective approaches to the use of the highly effective but expensive new treatments for hepatitis C that have recently become available.

Abbreviations

EMCDDA: European Monitoring Centre for Drugs and Drug Addiction; HCC: Hepatocellular carcinoma; HCV: Hepatitis C virus; HPSC: Health Protection Surveillance Centre; NDTRS: National Drug Treatment Reporting System; NVRL: National Virus Reference Laboratory; PWID: People who inject drugs

Acknowledgements
NDTRS team, Aline Brennan, Mary O'Meara, Joe Barry, Seamus Dooley, Bobby Smyth, Melissa Canny, Jennifer Kieran, Susi Schmitz and Michele Tait.

Funding
We received no specific funding for this study.

Authors' contributions
JL, LT, and KH initiated and designed the study. AMC, JL and KH performed the data extraction and prepared the dataset for analysis. AMC, NM, JL, SL, CW and LT analysed and interpreted the data. AMC, NM, JL, SL and LT wrote a first draft of the paper. All authors read, commented on and approved the final manuscript.

Competing interests
The authors declare that they have no competing interests.

Author details
[1]Health Research Board, Grattan House, 67-72 Lower Mount Street, Dublin 2, Ireland. [2]HSE Health Protection Surveillance Centre, 25-27 Middle Gardiner Street, Dublin 1, Ireland. [3]Department of Statistics, Trinity College Dublin, Dublin, Ireland. [4]Health Research Institute (HRI) and MACSI, University of Limerick, Limerick, Ireland.

References

1. World Health Organization. Guidelines for the screening, care and treatment of persons with Hepatitis C infection. Geneva: World Health Organization; 2014.
2. Global Burden Of Hepatitis C Working Group. Global burden of disease (GBD) for hepatitis C. J Clin Pharmacol. 2004;44:20–9.
3. Thornton L, Murphy N, Jones L, Connell J, Dooley S, Gavin S, Hunter K, Brennan A. Determination of the burden of hepatitis C virus infection in Ireland. Epidemiol Infect. 2012;140:1461–8.
4. Hepatitis C in the UK: 2013 report. (http://www.gov.uk/government/uploads/system/uploads/attachment_data/file/364074/Hepatitis_C_in_the_UK_2013.pdf). Accessed 26 June 2014. [Available at: https://www.gov.uk/government/uploads/system/uploads/attachment_data/file/364074/Hepatitis_C_in_the_UK_2013.pdf]
5. Health Protection Surveillance Centre. Hepatitis C annual reports 2010–2014. Accessed 1 Nov 2016. [Available at: http://www.hpsc.ie/A-Z/Hepatitis/HepatitisC/HepatitisCreports/HepatitisAnnualReports/]
6. Kelly A, Carvalho M, Teljeur C: A 3-source capture recapture study of the prevalence of opiate use in Ireland 2000 to 2001: key findings summary tables.: Department of Community Health & General Practice, Trinity College Dublin; 2003.
7. Kelly A, Teljeur C, Carvalho M. Prevalence of opiate use in Ireland 2006: a 3-Source capture recapture study. Dublin: National Advisory Committee on Drugs; 2009.
8. Comiskey C, Cox G, Sheehy L, Kelly PA, Leckey Y, O'Duill B. ROSIE baseline data.: National Advisory Committee on Drugs. 2007.
9. Smyth R, Keenan E, Dorman A, O'Connor J. Hepatitis C infection among injecting drug users attending the National Drug Treatment Centre. Ir J Med Sci. 1995;164:267–8.
10. Smyth BP, Keenan E, O'Connor JJ. Bloodborne viral infection in Irish injecting drug users. Addiction. 1998;93:1649–56.
11. Smyth BP, Keenan E, O'Connor JJ. Evaluation of the impact of Dublin's expanded harm reduction programme on prevalence of hepatitis C among short-term injecting drug users. J Epidemiol Community Health. 1999;53:434–5.
12. Cullen W, Bury G, Barry J, O'Kelly F. Drug users attending general practice in Eastern Regional Health Authority (ERHA) area. Ir Med J. 2000;93:214–7.
13. Grogan L, Tiernan M, Geogeghan N, Smyth B, Keenan E. Bloodborne virus infections among drug users in Ireland: a retrospective cross-sectional survey of screening, prevalence, incidence and hepatitis B immunisation uptake. Ir J Med Sci. 2005;174:14–20.
14. Cullen W, Bury G, Barry J, O'Kelly FD. Hepatitis C infection among drug users attending general practice. Ir J Med Sci. 2003;172:123–7.
15. Cullen W, Stanley J, Langton D, Kelly Y, Bury G. Management of hepatitis C among drug users attending general practice in Ireland: baseline data from the Dublin area hepatitis C in general practice initiative. Eur J Gen Pract. 2007;13:5–12.
16. Long J. Blood-borne viral infections among injecting drug users in Ireland, 1995 to 2005. Overview 4. Dublin: Health Research Board; 2006.
17. Allwright S, Bradley F, Long J, Barry J, Thornton L, Parry JV. Prevalence of antibodies to hepatitis B, hepatitis C, and HIV and risk factors in Irish prisoners: results of a national cross sectional survey. BMJ. 2000;321:78–82.
18. Drummond A, Codd M, Donnelly N, McCausland D, Mehegan J, Daly L, Kelleher C. Study on the prevalence of drug use,including intravenous drug use, and blood-borne viruses among the Irish prisoner population: National Advisory Committee on Drugs and Alcohol. 2014.
19. Garavan C, Long J, Lyons S. Prevalence of drug use and blood-borne viruses in Irish prisons, 2011. Drugnet Ireland. 2014;Issue 50(Summer 2014):7–11.
20. Carew AM, Bellerose D, Lyons S, Long J. Trends in treated problem opiate use in Ireland, 2002 to 2007. In: HRB Trends Series 7. Dublin: Health Research Board; 2009.
21. University of the West of Scotland HPS, University of Strathclyde and the West of Scotland Specialist Virology Centre. The Needle Exchange Surveillance Initiative (NESI): Prevalence of HCV and injecting risk behaviours among people who inject drugs attending injecting equipment provision services in Scotland, 2008/2009 & 2010. Paisley: University of the West of Scotland; 2012.
22. Hay G, Gannon M, Casey J, McKeganey N. Estimating the National and Local Prevalence of Problem Drug Misuse in Scotland. Glasgow: University of Glasgow; 2009. http://www.scotpho.org.uk/downloads/drugs/Prevalence_Report_%202006.pdf.
23. Smyth BP, O'Connor JJ, Barry J, Keenan E. Retrospective cohort study examining incidence of HIV and hepatitis C infection among injecting drug users in Dublin. J Epidemiol Commun Health S2- Br J Prev Soc Med. 2003;57:310–1.
24. Health Protection Surveillance Centre: National Hepatitis C Database. 2015 Report. Dublin: Health Service Executive; 2015. (http://www.hpsc.ie/A-Z/Hepatitis/HepatitisC/HepatitisCDatabase/BaselineandFollow-upReports/File,15238,en.pdf
25. Mohd Hanafiah K, Groeger J, Flaxman AD, Wiersma ST. Global epidemiology of hepatitis C virus infection: new estimates of age-specific antibody to HCV seroprevalence. Hepatology. 2013;57:1333–42.
26. Lavanchy D. Evolving epidemiology of hepatitis C virus. Clin Microbiol Infect. 2011;17:107–15.
27. Hutchinson S. Modelling the hepatitis C virus disease burden among injecting drug users in Scotland (dissertation). Glasgow: University of Glasgow, 2004. https://core.ac.uk/download/pdf/9654527.pdf.
28. Health Research Board. Drugs Misuse Research Division: 2004 National Report to the EMCDDA by the Reitox National Focal Point. Ireland. New developments, trends and in-depth information on selected issues. Dublin: Health Research Board; 2004.
29. Ryder N, Cullen W, Barry J, Bury G, Keenan E, Smyth BP. Prevalence of problem alcohol use among patients attending primary care for methadone treatment. BMC Fam Pract. 2009;10:42.
30. Statistical bulletin. Treatment demand indicator (TDI). Available at http://www.emcdda.europa.eu/stats/archive. Accessed 11 June 2014.
31. European Monitoring Centre for Drugs and Drug Addiction: PDU (Problem drug use) revision summary. European Monitoring Centre for Drugs and Drug Addiction. 2013.

13

Predisposing, enabling, and need factors associated with utilization of HCV testing services among PWID in two settings

Ruchi Sogarwal*, Varada Madge, Pratyush Bishi, Apam Woleng and Rishi Garg

Abstract

Background: The Hepatitis C virus (HCV) is very common among people who inject drugs (PWID), yet PWID in India have suboptimal access to HCV testing and treatment. This study sought to identify HCV risk factors among male PWID who utilized a free needle and syringe exchange program and to examine the predisposing, enabling, and need factors associated with utilization of HCV testing services by those PWID reporting that they had been tested.

Methods: A cross-sectional study was conducted in Imphal, Manipur and Amritsar, Punjab. These two settings have high HCV prevalence and large numbers of PWID. A team of 18 field investigators obtained data through face-to-face interviews using a structured multiple-choice questionnaire. The questionnaire was administered to 1241 of 2644 male PWID aged 15 years and above enrolled in the needle and syringe program of India's AIDS Control Program, with study participants selected through consecutive sampling. Statistical analyses included descriptive statistics and multivariate regression.

Results: Twenty-four percent of PWID in our study sample reported having been tested for HCV. Unlike PWID in Imphal, more than half of PWID in Amritsar reported unprotected sex and use of alcohol or non-injecting drugs as being among their HCV risk factors (67.1 and 77.8 %, respectively). However, opioid substitution therapy non-adherence was reported more often in Imphal than in Amritsar. Education, marital status, place of residence and duration of injecting drug use were found to significantly enable access to HCV testing while alcohol use, frequent mobility and unprotected sex were found to significantly inhibit access to HCV testing for PWID after controlling for other explanatory variables.

Conclusions: Predisposing and enabling determinants provide an area for developing effective interventions to improve HCV testing practices among PWID. HCV prevention programs that address safe injecting and sexual practices, OST adherence and frequent mobility customized for PWID by age are strongly recommended.

Keywords: Hepatitis C virus, People who inject drugs, India

* Correspondence: ruchi.dr@gmail.com; ruchis@mamtahimc.org
MAMTA Health Institute for Mother and Child, New Delhi, India

Background

Hepatitis C virus (HCV) is a global public health problem, with around 150 million people chronically infected [1]. Approximately 2.7 % of all deaths annually are thought to be attributable to HCV [2]. This translates into one million deaths, most resulting from HCV-associated cirrhosis or HCV-associated liver cancer [3–5]. People who inject drugs (PWID) have disproportionately high HCV prevalence worldwide (50–90 %) in comparison to the general population [6]. Indian studies have reported HCV sero-positivity in PWID to be between 20 and 90 %. Some Indian PWID populations have extremely high HCV seroprevalence, while others have HCV seroprevalence in the more moderate range of 30 to 50 % [7–10]. Despite the high burden of disease in Indian PWID, the problem has not been addressed in a systematic way. Recently, national initiatives to increase case finding have been proposed, including recommendations for improved laboratory-based surveillance [11]. These initiatives are timely since recent treatment advances have resulted in most cases of chronic HCV being curable with the use of direct-acting antiviral regimens [12–14]. The prospects of translating these advances into population-level declines in HCV disease are currently limited by the fact that 50 to 75 % of HCV-infected individuals are unaware of their sero-status. Those under age 30 are particularly likely to be undiagnosed or to have experienced a late diagnosis [15–17].

In light of overlapping risk factors for transmission of viral hepatitis and HIV infection, as well as limited public health resources in many settings, the World Health Organization along with other experts has recommended integrating HCV and HIV services [18, 19]. In 2014, with the support of the Bristol-Myers Squibb Foundation [20], MAMTA Health Institute for Mother and Child [21] launched an initiative to reduce transmission of HCV and to improve patient care by integrating viral hepatitis prevention into existing public health programs providing HIV-related services to PWID in two settings in India: Amritsar District, in the state of Punjab, and Imphal District, in the state of Manipur. Historically, injection drug use was concentrated in the northeastern part of India, including Manipur, but rapidly growing populations of injection drug users have been reported in Punjab [22, 23]. Estimated HCV prevalence among PWID is 64.9 % in Imphal and 48.7 % in Amritsar [7].

The MAMTA intervention sought to empower people to seek health services early in regard to HCV screening, diagnosis and treatment, as well as to build the capacity of frontline health workers. It used the existing HIV program as a pathway for the expansion of viral hepatitis services, including vaccination, screening, confirmatory testing, and referral to care and treatment. In the first phase of the intervention, testing PWID for HCV was regarded as a key strategy and also an opportunity to promote health services and risk reduction services. However, program planners were hampered by a lack of knowledge about the characteristics of the population being targeted.

This study addresses the need for information in two ways. First, it investigates HCV risk factors among PWID utilizing a free needle and syringe exchange program. Second, it investigates which predisposing, enabling, and need factors were associated with utilization of HCV testing services by PWID. The conceptual framework for the study is based on the Gelberg-Andersen Behavioral Model for Vulnerable Populations [24], which has been extensively applied to the study of HIV testing in high-risk individuals [25–28]. *Predisposing* factors are demographic and other personal characteristics that influence the likelihood of obtaining care. *Enabling* factors are personal, family and community resources that support or encourage efforts to access health services. *Need* factors arise from the real or perceived need for health services and provide motivation for individuals to seek those services. In the absence of any similar research on HCV testing, we utilised the HIV literature to develop the hypothesis that are tested in this study. The hypothesis is that the predisposing factors would be associated with lower odds of utilisation of HCV testing as compared to enabling and need factors.

By comparing risk factors and HCV testing behavior in two settings that vary in regard to the nature of their drug use epidemics and HCV epidemics, this study also presents an opportunity to investigate whether different areas of India may benefit from different HCV prevention and testing approaches.

Methods

Study setting and participants

We surveyed male PWID utilizing a free multi-site needle and syringe exchange program in the districts of Amritsar and Imphal. Needle and syringe exchange took place at the community organization facilities of the Indian government's State AIDS Control Program [29]. Facilities were selected to participate in the study if they met three criteria: willingness of facility managers; available financial resources; and more than 200 PWID enrolled for services. These criteria resulted in one out of nine facilities in Amritsar serving as a study site, along with five out of 23 facilities in Imphal. Consecutive individuals who were at least 15 years old and reported a history of injecting drug use were invited to participate in the study when they attended the needle and syringe exchange facilities at these six sites from April 2015 through July 2015.

Instrument and variables

The data were obtained through face-to-face interviews by a team of 18 field investigators using a structured multiple-choice questionnaire that addressed prominent risk factors for HCV infection. The questionnaire included five domains relating to socio-demographic characteristics of the respondents, injecting patterns and practices, sexual practices, and other risk behaviors related to HCV including information about spouses and parents. The questionnaire was developed in English then translated into Hindi and Manipuri. All study participants were interviewed in the primary local language (Hindi in Amritsar and Manipuri in Imphal).

The main variable of interest (dependent variable) was self-report of ever receiving HCV testing. For the analysis of this study, we categorized independent variables into predisposing, enabling, and need factors in accordance with the previously described Gelberg-Andersen Behavioral Model for Vulnerable Populations [24]. Predisposing factors included age, education level, marital status, and use of alcohol and/or non-injecting drugs in the previous 1 month. Variables categorized as enabling factors included income status, 'below-poverty-line' status, level of mobility, district of residence, tattoo/piercing, unprotected sex in last 1 month, and sex with female sex workers in the last 1 month. Study participants were classified as belonging to either below-poverty-line (BPL) households or non-BPL households as defined by the government of India on the basis of three categories of vulnerability: residential, occupational and social [30]. Study participants were considered to be highly mobile if they spent more than 10 days per month interacting with other PWID at locations outside of the community where they resided [31]. The variables included as need factors were HCV-positive status of spouse or either parent; ever had transfusion of blood or blood components; ever had medical/dental surgery or hemodialysis; ever had needle stick injury; and sexually transmitted infection symptoms or treatment reported in last 1 month. Since frequency of injecting drug use is associated with likelihood of HCV transmission [32, 33], we included variables measuring current injecting drug use, injecting in groups in last 1 month, sharing needles/syringes and other equipment in last 1 month, and duration of injecting drug use.

Statistical analysis

Descriptive analyses were used to assess the characteristics of study participants and the occurrence of HCV risk factors among younger PWID (aged 15–29) and older PWID (aged 30–44). In order to understand differentials in level of HCV risk factors by age and district of residence, ratios were computed. A ratio value of less than 1 would mean that the levels of risk factors were relatively higher for clients in the reference category compared to other clients, and a ratio value of more than 1 would mean the opposite, while a value of 1 would indicate no difference in the risk factors by age (reference category: <30 years) or district of residence (reference category: Amritsar). Bivariate analysis examined associations between the dependent variable and predisposing, enabling, and need factors. All variables that were significantly associated with the dependent variable were included in multivariate regression modeling. All p-values less than 0.05 were considered significant. Results are presented as odds ratios (ORs), with the relationship between exposure (independent variable) and an outcome (i.e. HCV testing) compared to no exposure. We reported higher odds (OR > 1) when this relationship is positive, and lower odds (OR < 1) when the relationship is negative. All statistical analyses were performed using SPSS 21.0 (IBM Corp, Armonk NY, 2012).

Results

Among 2644 needle and syringe exchange users invited to participate in the study, 1241 agreed (46.9 %). Two hundred and eighty eight of the 1241 study respondents were HIV positive. The overall mean age of study participants was 33.4 years. Imphal had a much larger proportion of study participants aged 30 and above (81.2 %) than did Amritsar (37.3 %) (Table 1). Less than 10 % of study participants had no formal education, and most reported completing either primary education (22.0 %) or secondary education (55.9 %). Just over half of study participants reported currently being married, while 42.3 % had never been married. More than four-fifths of people were employed, including those who reported part-time employment and self-employment. More than three-quarters had a monthly income of 6000 Indian Rupees (INR) or less (38.3 %, <3000 INR; 41.9 %, 3001–6000 INR), and approximately one-third met the criteria for below-poverty-line status. Study participants in Amritsar had engaged in injecting drug use for a median of 3.0 years, while those in Imphal had engaged in injecting drug use for a median of 8.6 years.

Self-reported HCV risk factors

Findings for self-reported HCV risk factors were disaggregated by both place of residence (Amritsar versus Imphal) and age (<30 years versus ≥30 years) (Table 2).

The Amritsar study cohort had more people under age 30 than age 30-plus who reported injecting daily in the last 1 month (11.6 versus 6.4 %; ratio: 0.6). The inverse relationship was seen in Imphal, where 28.7 % of people under age 30 and 34.4 % of people age 30-plus reported injecting daily in the last 1 month (ratio: 1.2). A similar pattern was seen for non-adherence to opioid substitution therapy. More Amritsar study participants under age 30 than age 30-plus reported non-adherence (22.5 versus 15.8 %; ratio: 0.7), while more Imphal study participants age 30-plus reported non-adherence (60.0 %)

Table 1 Sociodemographic characteristics of PWID in Amritsar and Imphal districts, India

Characteristics	Amritsar (*N* = 507) *N* (%)	Imphal (*N* = 734) *N* (%)	Total (*N* = 1241) *N* (%)
Age (years)			
15–19	15 (3.0)	11 (1.5)	26 (2.1)
20–29	303 (59.8)	127 (17.3)	430 (34.6)
≥ 30	189 (37.3)	596 (81.2)	785 (63.3)
Education			
No formal education	65 (12.8)	50 (6.8)	115 (9.3)
Primary (up to 5 years of schooling)	174 (34.3)	99 (13.5)	273 (22.0)
Secondary (up to 10 years of schooling)	249 (49.1)	445 (60.6)	694 (55.9)
Higher (up to 12 years of schooling or beyond)	19 (3.7)	140(19.1)	159 (12.8)
Marital status			
Currently married	232 (45.8)	404 (55.0)	636 (51.2)
Widowed, divorced or separated	19 (3.7)	61(8.3)	80 (6.4)
Never married	256 (50.5)	269 (36.6)	525 (42.3)
Employment status			
Employed (including part-time employment and self-employment)	393 (77.5)	625 (85.1)	1018 (82.0)
Not employed	114 (22.5)	109 (14.9)	223 (18.0)
Monthly income (Indian Rupees)			
≤ 3000	122 (24.1)	353 (48.1)	475 (38.3)
3001–6000	270 (53.3)	250 (34.1)	520 (41.9)
6001–10,000	75 (14.8)	55 (7.5)	130 (10.5)
> 10,001	40 (7.9)	76 (10.4)	116 (9.3)
Below-poverty-level (BPL) status[a]			
Not below poverty level	383 (75.5)	438 (59.7)	821 (66.2)
Below poverty level	124 (24.5)	296 (40.3)	420 (33.8)
Age at sexual debut (years)			
Mean ± SD	18.0 ± 2.8	23.7 ± 5.7	21.2 ± 5.5
Median (range)	18.0 (10–31)	24.0 (10–48)	20.0 (10–48)
Duration of injecting drug use (years)			
≤ 1	130 (25.6)	42 (5.7)	172 (13.9)
2–5	292 (57.6)	137 (18.7)	429 (34.6)
6–10	49 (9.7)	190 (25.9)	239 (19.3)
≥ 11	36 (7.1)	365 (49.7)	401 (32.3)
Mean ± SD	±4.4	13.3 ± 11.0	9.5 ± 8.5
Median (range)	3.0 (1–35)	8.6 (1–35)	7 (1–35)

[a]BPL status was determined in accordance with the definition used by the Indian government (Planning Commission, Government of India: Report of the expert group to review the methodology for measurement of poverty; June 2014; http://planningcommission.nic.in/reports/genrep/pov_rep0707.pdf)

in comparison to the under-30 Imphal cohort (53.8 %) (ratio: 1.1)

In both Amritsar and Imphal, there was more reported sharing of injecting equipment in the last 1 month among under-30 study participants than among those age 30-plus, although the difference was greater in Amritsar (24.6 versus 16.9 %; ratio: 0.7). Similarly, larger proportions of under-30 study participants in both locations reported "ever had tattoo or piercing" as a risk factor. Regarding a third HCV risk factor, unprotected sex in the last 1 month, both locations had larger proportions of older study participants than younger study participants reporting that they had engaged in this behavior (Amritsar: <30 years, 67.1 %; ≥30 years, 78.4 %; ratio: 1.2; Imphal: <30 years, 29.5 %; ≥30 years, 51.8 %; ratio: 1.8).

When study participants under age 30 in Imphal were compared to study participants under age 30 in Amritsar, various differences were observed. A much larger proportion of the Imphal cohort than the Amritsar cohort reported injecting daily in the last month (28.7 versus 11.6 %; ratio: 2.5). On the other hand, smaller proportions of younger study participants in Imphal than in Amritsar reported other risk factors such as sharing of injecting equipment in the last 1 month (13.4 versus 24.6 %; ratio: 0.5), unprotected sex in the last month (29.5 versus 67.1 %; ratio: 0.4), and ever had tattoo or piercing (26.7 versus 32.7 %; ratio: 0.8). Regarding OST non-adherence in the last 1 month, 22.5 % of study participants under age 30 in Amritsar reported non-adherence, while 53.8 % of those under age 30 in Imphal did so (ratio: 2.4).

The age 30-plus study cohort had a similar pattern in risk factors across the two locations. A much larger proportion of older Imphal study participants reported being daily injectors in the last month in comparison to their counterparts in Amritsar (34.4 versus 6.4 %; ratio: 5.4). A much smaller proportion of older Amritsar study participants reported OST non-adherence in the last 1 month in comparison to the older Imphal cohort (15.8 versus 60.0 %; ratio: 3.8). Several other risk factors were reported by larger proportions of age 30-plus Amritsar residents than age 30-plus Imphal residents, including sharing of injecting equipment in the last 1 month (16.9 versus 12.0 %; ratio: 0.7); unprotected sex in the last 1 month (78.4 versus 51.8 %; ratio: 0.7); and ever had tattoo or piercing (24.5 versus 12.4 %; ratio: 0.5).

Factors associated with utilization of HCV testing

Two hundred and ninety-eight of the 1241 study participants (24.0 %) reported that they had been tested for HCV.

Three of four predisposing factors were significantly associated with HCV testing (Table 3). Study participants with any formal education were more likely to

Table 2 HCV risk factors reported by younger (<30 years) and older (≥30 years) study participants, by place of residence ($N = 1241$)

Reported HCV risk	Amritsar ($N = 507$)		Imphal ($N = 734$)		Ratio (≥30 years/ <30 years)		Ratio (IMP/AMR)	
	<30 years ($n = 318$)	≥30 years ($n = 189$)	<30 years ($n = 138$)	≥30 years ($n = 596$)	AMR	IMP	<30 years	≥30 years
Daily injector in last 1 month	36/311 (11.6)	12/ 188 (6.4)	37/129 (28.7)	178/518 (34.4)	0.6	1.2	2.5	5.4
More than 30 injecting episodes per month in last consecutive 3 months	24/153 (15.7)	10/73 (13.7)	46/104 (44.2)	177/369 (47.9)	0.9	1.1	3.2	3.4
Injecting in a group in last 1 month	134/314 (42.7)	57/188 (30.3)	55/126 (43.7)	153/502 (30.5)	0.7	0.7	1.0	1.0
Sharing of needles/ syringes and other equipment in last 1 month	77/313 (24.6)	32/189 (16.9)	17/126 (13.4)	62/516 (12.0)	0.7	0.9	0.5	0.7
Unprotected sex in last 1 month	186/277 (67.1)	131/167 (78.4)	38/129 (29.5)	275/531 (51.8)	1.2	1.8	0.4	0.7
Sex with female sex worker in last 1 month	42/314 (13.4)	13/188 (6.9)	4/133 (3.0)	11/578 (1.9)	0.5	0.6	0.2	0.3
STI symptoms or STI treatment in last 1 month	10/315 (3.2)	3/189 (1.6)	1/132 (0.8)	4/571 (0.7)	0.5	0.8	0.2	0.4
Use of alcohol and/or other non-injecting drugs in last 1 month	245/315 (77.8)	177/189 (77.8)	77/133 (57.9)	284/579 (49.1)	1.0	0.8	0.7	0.6
Opioid substitution therapy non-adherence in last 1 month	71/315 (22.5)	30/189 (15.8)	71/132 (53.8)	348/580 (60.0)	0.7	1.1	2.4	3.8
High mobility in last 1 month[a]	26/307 (8.5)	10/187 (5.3)	28/132 (21.2)	110/577 (19.1)	0.6	0.9	2.5	3.6
Mother, father or spouse ever tested HCV-positive	1/314 (0.3)	0/189 (0)	3/131 (2.3)	18/572 (3.1)	0.0	1.3	7.7	-
Ever had tattoo or piercing	102/312 (32.7)	46/188 (24.5)	35/131 (26.7)	72/581 (12.4)	0.7	0.5	0.8	0.5
Ever had transfusion of blood or blood components	18/314 (5.7)	15/189 (7.9)	1/132 (0.8)	18/579 (3.1)	1.4	3.9	0.1	0.4
Ever had medical or dental surgery, or hemodialysis	13/315 (4.1)	25/189 (13.2)	1/131 (0.8)	16/582 (2.7)	3.2	3.4	0.2	0.2
Ever had needle stick injury	0/315	1/188 (0.5)	3/130 (2.3)	10/573 (1.7)	-	0.7	-	3.4

[a]High mobility for PWID is defined as spending more than 10 days per month interacting with other PWID at locations outside of the community where one resides

report testing than those with no formal education (adjusted odds ratio [aOR] 3.5, 95 % confidence interval [CI] 1.2–10.4, $p = 0.022$). Currently married study participants were more likely to report testing than those who were not (aOR 2.4, CI 1.3–4.5, $p = 0.004$). Study participants who reported using alcohol and/or other non-injecting drugs in the last 1 month were less likely than those who did not to report testing (aOR 0.6, CI 0.4–0.9, $p = 0.016$). As for the fourth predisposing factor, 9.7 % of study participants under age 30 and 32.2 % of study participants age 30-plus reported testing, but the older age group did not have significantly higher odds of testing (aOR 1.4, CI 0.8–2.3, $p = 0.208$).

Three of seven enabling factors were significantly associated with HCV testing. Residents of Imphal were much more likely than residents of Amritsar to report testing (aOR 4.9, CI 2.7–8.8, $p < 0.001$). Study participants who reported using condoms in the last 1 month were less likely to report testing than those who did not (aOR 0.5, CI 0.3–0.9, $p = 0.015$), as were those who reported high mobility in the last 1 month in comparison to those who did not (aOR 0.5, CI 0.3–0.8, $p = 0.005$).

Among five need factors, only one was significantly associated with HCV testing. Study participants who had been injecting drugs for 11 or more years were more likely to report testing than those who had been injecting for 1 year or less (aOR 2.1, CI 1.0–4.2, $p = 0.050$).

Discussion

This cross-sectional study investigated prevalence of HCV risk factors among 1241 male PWID utilizing a free needle and syringe exchange program in two distinct settings in India, as well as assessing which factors were associated with utilization of HCV testing services. Study participants in Imphal, which has had an injection drug epidemic for longer than Amritsar, reported a much longer median number of years of injection drug use than their Amritsar counterparts. When reported HCV risk factors were compared across the study sites with study participants disaggregated into two age groups, some risk factors appeared to be more prominent among Amritsar PWID and other risk factors appeared to be more prominent among Imphal PWID regardless of age. For example, higher proportions of

Table 3 Univariate and multivariate logistic regression analyses of factors associated with previous HCV testing among PWID ($N = 1241$ unless otherwise noted)

Factors	Tested for HCV (%)	Univariate		Multivariate	
		OR (95 % CI)	*P*-value	Adjusted OR (95 % CI)	*P*-value
Predisposing factor					
Age (years)					
< 30	45/456 (9.7)	1	<0.001	1	0.208
≥ 30	253/785 (32.2)	4.4 (3.1–6.2)		1.4 (0.8–2.3)	
Education					
No formal education	13/115 (11.3)	1	0.001	1	0.022
Formal education (any)	285/1126 (25.4)	2.7 (1.5–4.8)		3.5 (1.2–10.4)	
Marital Status					
Widowed, divorced, separated or never married	112/605 (18.5)	1	<0.001	1	0.004
Currently married	186/636 (29.2)	1.8 (1.4–2.4)		2.4 (1.3–4.5)	
Use of alcohol and/or other non-injecting drugs in last 1 month ($N = 1186$)					
No	162/433 (37.4)	1	<0.001	1	0.016
Yes	129/753 (17.1)	0.4 (0.3–0.5)		0.6 (0.4–0.9)	
Enabling factor					
District of residence					
Amritsar	28/507 (5.5)	1	<0.001	1	<0.001
Imphal	270/734 (36.8)	10.1 (6.7–15.2)		4.9 (2.7–8.8)	
Employment status					
Not employed	263/1018 (25.8)	1		1	0.802
Employed	35/223 (15.7)	0.5 (0.4–0.8)	0.002	1.1 (0.6–1.8)	
Below-poverty-level (BPL) status[a]					
Not below poverty level	157/821 (19.1)	1	<0.001	1	0.598
Below poverty level	141/420 (33.6)	2.1 (1.6–2.8)		1.1 (0.8–1.6)	
Unprotected sex in last 1 month ($N = 1104$)					
Always used condoms for sex	131/474 (27.6)	1	0.05	1	0.015
Did not always use condoms for sex	143/630 (22.7))	0.8 (0.6–1.0)		0.5 (0.3–0.9)	
High mobility in last 1 month[b] ($N = 1203$)					
No	253/1029 (24.5)	1	0.099	1	0.005
Yes	33/174 (18.9)	0.7 (0.5–1.0)		0.5 (0.3–0.8)	
Sex with female sex worker in last 1 month ($N = 1213$)					
No	59/1143 (5.2)	1	0.106	1	0.195
Yes	11/70 (15.71)	0.6 (0.3–1.1)		2.1 (0.7–6.8)	
Ever had tattoo or piercing ($N = 1212$)					
No	238/957 (24.8)	1	0.083	1	0.259
Yes	50/255 (19.6)	0.7 (0.5–1.0)		1.3 (0.8–2.2)	
Need factor					
STI symptoms or STI treatment in last 1 month ($N = 1207$)					
No	280/1189 (23.5)	1	0.345	1	0.170
Yes	6/18 (33.3)	1.6 (0.6–4.3)		3.9 (0.5–27.2)	
Current injecting drug user ($N = 1211$)					

Table 3 Univariate and multivariate logistic regression analyses of factors associated with previous HCV testing among PWID (*N* = 1241 unless otherwise noted) *(Continued)*

No, but formerly	131/512 (25.6)	1	0.163	1	0.525
Yes, currently (injected drugs in last 3 months)	155/699 (22.2)	0.7 (0.6–1.0)		0.9 (0.6–1.3)	
Injecting in a group in last 1 month (*N* = 1130)					
No	171/731 (23.4)	1	0.009	1	0.619
Yes	67/399 (16.8)	0.7 (0.5–1.1)		1.1 (0.7–1.8)	
Sharing of needles/syringes and other equipment in last 1 month (*N* = 1144)					
No	214/956 (22.4)	1		1	0.365
Yes	34/188 (18.1)	0.7 (0.5–1.1)	0.179	1.3 (0.7–2.1)	
Duration of injecting drug use (years)					
≤ 1	21/172 (12.2)	1		1	0.021
2–5	46/429 (10.7)	0.8 (0.5–1.5)	0.585	0.9 (0.5–1.9)	0.861
6–10	60/239 (25.1)	2.4 (1.4–4.1)	0.001	1.3 (0.6–2.7)	0.491
≥ 11	171/401 (42.6)	5.4 (3.3–8.9)	<0.001	2.1 (1.0–4.2)	0.050

[a]BPL status was determined in accordance with the definition used by the Indian government (Planning Commission, Government of India: Report of the expert group to review the methodology for measurement of poverty. June 2014; http://planningcommission.nic.in/reports/genrep/pov_rep0707.pdf)
[b]High mobility for PWID is defined as spending more than 10 days per month interacting with other PWID at locations outside of the community where one resides

Amristar PWID in both age groups reported sharing needles/syringes and other injecting equipment in the last month, while higher proportions of Imphal PWID in both age groups experiencing OST non-adherence in the last month. Some risk factors also followed a consistent pattern across the two cities in relation to age. For example, higher proportions of PWID under age 30 in both cities reported injecting in groups in the last 1 month. At the same time, the two age groups exhibited different patterns of risk in different locations in certain regards. For example, more Amritsar PWID under age 30 had non-adherence to OST in the last month in comparison to older PWID in the same location, while older Imphal PWID reported this risk factor more often than did younger Imphal PWID. Among the subgroup of 298 study participants who reported previous HCV testing, Imphal residents were far more likely to do so than Amritsar residents, while age on the other hand was determined to not be a significant predictor of previous testing.

This study, by separately examining the potential influence of age and place of residence on PWID in relation to HCV risk, has provided evidence that some HCV-related needs vary considerably across different Indian PWID subpopulations. One factor that may help to account for this variation is the longevity of the injecting drug use epidemic. Two HCV risk factors reported by higher proportions of Amritsar residents than Imphal residents were sharing injection equipment and having unprotected sex. We speculate that Amritsar with its newer injection drug epidemic may lag behind Imphal in regard to the provision of a range of services for PWID, including interventions to reduce the sharing of injection equipment and promote condom use. At the same time, PWID in a setting with a longtime drug use epidemic, such as Imphal, may also have specific unmet needs. In our study, both younger and older PWID in Imphal, unlike their counterparts in Amritsar, reported quite high levels of non-adherence to opioid substitution therapy. Since the provision of OST is regarded as a key component of a comprehensive approach to reducing HCV transmission and preventing HCV reinfection among PWID, our study finding points to a problem that should be addressed through geographically targeted interventions. Furthermore, the finding that OST non-adherence was somewhat higher among older Imphal PWID (60.0 %) compared to younger Imphal PWID (53.8 %) suggests that age-targeted interventions addressing this issue might be beneficial in Imphal as well. One of the examples of the age-targeted intervention is the UFO (U Find Out) model for HCV prevention, a youth centered, collaborative and harm reduction based intervention, in which young IDU centered referral services are provided for early screening of HCV [34].

One-fourth of the PWID in our study reported ever being tested for HCV. In multivariate analysis, Imphal residents were almost five times as likely as Amritsar residents to report previous HCV testing. Nonetheless, when HCV testing findings were disaggregated by place of residence, the reported HCV testing level among Imphal residents was still only 36.8 %. Numerous factors may account for this disparity, such as diversity in drug use, epidemic stage of HCV and socio-demographic and risk behaviours [7, 8]. Additionally, prevention services such as the needle and syringe exchange are more numerous and accessible to Imphal residents; and PWID in this area may therefore have greater knowledge of available resources. There may be unmet needs for outreach services and a paucity of trained health care providers for PWID in less epidemic area. These results illustrate the need for expanded access to primary health care and prevention services that could be an important strategy to address an unmet need for individuals at high risk for HCV or detecting previously undiagnosed cases of HCV. For PWID who are not routinely engaged in medical care, NSEP may also be utilized resource for HCV screening.

Guided by Gelberg-Andersen model [24], we categorized multi-level factors that may facilitate or hinder HCV testing behavior of PWIDs. Contrary to our hypothesis, we found that most predisposing factors were associated with higher odds of utilisation of HCV testing as compared to enabling and need factors. This indicates that access to comprehensive services by PWID relates to socio-demographic factors. In the final adjustment model, education, marital status, place of residence and duration of injecting drug use were found to significant enable uptake of HCV testing services while alcohol use, mobility and unprotected sex were found to significantly inhibit uptake to HCV testing services. This indicates that targeting and reaching PWID who may be in need of HCV testing is complex, and cannot be determined by one element of vulnerability. This finding, coupled with the finding about variation in HCV risk factors across different age groups and settings, raises concern about an important dimension of the response to HCV in large heterogeneous countries such as India. National policies in India are translated into strategies and action plans at the state level. In order to develop an effective overall response, it is important to know which factors should be the highest-priority targets for interventions at the state and local levels. Multiple domains of information, including epidemiology as well as knowledge of program, geographic, and community settings, may be essential to develop effective interventions.

This study has several limitations. First, this sample was drawn from a group of organizations involved in implementing a specific National AIDS Control Program activity, and results cannot be assumed to represent PWID who are not receiving the same services. Second, study participants were recruited from the client rosters of the needle and syringe exchange facilities, and the dearth of female clients is reflected in the all-male composition of the study cohort. Study results thus do not reflect the experience of an important but often hidden segment of India's injection drug-using population. Results are further limited by fact that study participants were from two districts in different Indian states. Whether findings can be generalized to PWID in other parts of those states or other parts of the country remains to be determined. Additionally, we could not verify the accuracy of self-reported data on HCV testing. Some study participants may have answered this question incorrectly due to recall bias, social desirability bias or some other reason. The data that were collected provided little insight into system-level factors that may affect HCV testing uptake, such as funding, regulation and service delivery infrastructure. Despite these limitations, the study findings may inform comprehensive interventions for systems delivering care to specific high-risk groups. Our findings are important because they suggest identifiable characteristics that can be targeted to reduce the risk and spread of HCV infection.

Conclusion

Our findings highlight important factors that may be useful to increase HCV testing rates among PWID, which may strengthen prevention and reduce transmission of the infection. This study concludes that predisposing and enabling determinants provide an area for developing effective interventions to improve HCV testing practices and risk reduction. Prevention programs that address safe injecting and sexual practices, adherence to OST and frequent mobility customized for PWID by 'age' is strongly recommended to prioritize HCV risk reduction strategies. The priority factors found in this study coincide with the HIV prevention program in the country; hence integration of HCV within the harm reduction program could be a possible solution to address the HCV burden among PWID.

Abbreviations

BPL, Below Poverty Line; HCV, Hepatitis C Virus; HIV, Human Immunodeficiency Virus; NGO, Non-government Organization; NSEP, Needle Syringe Exchange Program; OST, Opioid Substitution Therapy; PWID, People who Inject Drugs; STI, Sexually Transmitted Infection; TI, Targeted Intervention

Acknowledgements

The authors would like to acknowledge the Bristol-Myers Squibb Foundation, which provided funding for the intervention. We acknowledge the guidance and support provided by state government authorities. Thanks are also extended to all healthcare providers of Manipur and Punjab states, particularly Imphal and Amritsar districts. The authors thank our implementation partners, the Manipur Network of Positive People and Abhivyakti Foundation, Punjab. The study would have not been possible without the active participation of people who inject drugs in Amritsar and Imphal districts.

Funding

This work was a part of the project funded by the Bristol-Myers Squibb Foundation (grant #1410).

Authors' contributions

RS conceptualized, defined the research theme and drafted the manuscript. PB, AW and RG performed the data collection and management. RS and PB performed the statistical analyses and interpreted the data. All authors read and critically revised the subsequent drafts of the manuscript. All authors approved the final manuscript.

Authors' information

All authors belong to MAMTA Health Institute for Mother and Child, New Delhi, India.

Competing interest

All authors declared no financial and non-financial competing interests.

References

1. World Health Organization. Hepatitis C: fact sheet no. 164. Available from: http://www.who.int/mediacentre/factsheets/fs164/en/. Accessed 10 Aug 2015.
2. Caccamo G, Saffioti F, Raimondo G. Hepatitis B virus and hepatitis C virus dual infection. World J Gastroenterol. 2014;20(40):14559–67. doi:10.3748/wjg.v20.i40.14559. PMCID:PMC4209523.
3. World Health Organization Executive Board (2009). Viral hepatitis. Report by the Secretariat. EB126/15, 12 November, 2009. Available from: http://apps.who.int/gb/ebwha/pdf_files/EB126/B126_15-en.pdf. Accessed 10 Aug 2015.
4. World Health Organization. Prevention and control of viral hepatitis infection. Framework for global action. Available from: http://www.who.int/csr/disease/hepatitis/GHP_Framework_En.pdf. Accessed 12 July 2015.
5. Perz JF, Armstrong GL, Farrington LA, Hutin YJ, Bell BP. The contributions of hepatitis B virus and hepatitis C virus infections to cirrhosis and primary liver cancer worldwide. J Hepatol. 2006;45:529–38.
6. Aceijas C, Rhodes T. Global estimates of prevalence of HCV infection among injecting drug users. Int J Drug Policy. 2007;18:352–58.
7. Solomon SS, Mehta SH, Srikrishnan AK, Solomon S, McFall AM, Laeyendecker O, et al. Burden of hepatitis C virus disease and access to hepatitis C virus services in people who inject drugs in India: a cross-sectional study. The Lancet. 2015;15:36–45.
8. Panda S, Roy T, Pahari S, Mehraa J, Sharma N, Singh G, et al. Alarming epidemics of human immunodeficiency virus and hepatitis C virus among injection drug users in the northwestern bordering state of Punjab, India: prevalence and correlates. Int J STD AIDS 2013;12:2-11. http://std.sagepub.com/content/early/2013/12/16/0956462413515659. Accessed 22 June 2016.
9. Basu D. Overview of substance abuse and hepatitis C virus infection and co-infections in India. J Neuroimmune Pharmacol. 2010;5:496–506.
10. Basu D et al. Hepatitis C virus (HCV) infection & risk factors for HCV positivity in injecting & non-injecting drug users attending a de-addiction centre in northern India. Indian Journal of Medical Research. 2015;142:311–6.
11. Government of India. Quarterly Newsletter of the National Center for Disease Control. January to March 2014;Vol 3: Issue 1. p. 7. http://ncdc.gov.in/writereaddata/linkimages/NewsLtr0103_20146480274026.pdf.
12. Sulkowski MS, Gardiner DF, Rodriguez-Torres M, the AI444040 Study Group, et al. Daclatasvir plus sofosbuvir for previously treated or untreated chronic HCV infection. N Engl J Med. 2014;370:211–21.
13. Afdhal N, Zeuzem S, Kwo P, the ION-1 Investigators, et al. Ledipasvir and sofosbuvir for untreated HCV genotype 1 infection. N Engl J Med. 2014;370:1889–98.
14. World Health Organisation, Hepatitis C treatment Guidelines, http://www.who.int/mediacentre/news/releases/2014/hepatitis-guidelines/en/. Accessed 12 Aug 2015.
15. World Health Organization. Key global facts and figures in 2011, Fact Sheet no 279. 2011.
16. Davis KL, Mitra D, Medjedovic J, Beam C, Rustgi V. Direct economic burden of chronic hepatitis C virus in a United States managed care population. J Clin Gastroenterol. 2011;45(2):e17–24.
17. Islam MM, Topp L, Day CA, Dawson A, Conigrave KM. The accessibility, acceptability, health impact and cost implications of primary healthcare outlets that target injecting drug users: a narrative synthesis of literature. Int J Drug Policy. 2012;23(2):94–102.
18. Joanna Buffington and T. Stephen Jones, M. Integrating Viral Hepatitis Prevention into Public Health Programs Serving People at High Risk for Infection: Good Public Health. Public Health Reports. 2007;Suppl 2:122. http://www.publichealthreports.org/issueopen.cfm?articleID=1852. Accessed 12 Nov 2015.
19. WHO. Guidance on Prevention of viral hepatitis B and C among people who inject drugs, 2012. http://apps.who.int/iris/bitstream/10665/75357/1/9789241504041_eng.pdf. Accessed 27 Oct 2015.
20. Bristol-Myers Squibb Foundation, USA. http://www.bms.com/foundation/Pages/home.aspx. Accessed 27 Apr 2015.
21. MAMTA Health Institute for Mother and Child, India. www.mamta-himc.org Accessed 27 Apr 2015.
22. United Nations Office on Drugs and Crime, Government of India Ministry of Social Justice and Empowerment. Injecting drug use and HIV in India: an emerging concern. 2004. www.unodc.org/pdf/india/publications/idu_and_HIVAIDS_in_India-Monograph/08_extentofiduhiv-aidsinindia.pdf. Accessed 12 Oct 2015.
23. Government of Punjab. Human Development Report. 2004.
24. Gelberg L, Andersen RM, Leake BD. The Behavioral Model for Vulnerable Populations: application to medical care use and outcomes for homeless people. Health Service Research. 2000;34(6):1273–302.
25. Lewis JH, Andersen RM, Gelberg L. Health care for homeless women: unmet needs and barriers to care. J Gen Intern Med. 2003;18(11):921–8.
26. Stein JA, Andersen RM, Koegel P, Gelberg L. Predicting health services utilization among homeless adults: a prospective analysis. J Health Care Poor Underserved. 2000;11(2):212–30.
27. Stein JA, Andersen RM, Robertson M, Gelberg L. Impact of hepatitis B and C infection on health services utilization in homeless adults: a test of the Gelberg-Andersen Behavioral Model for Vulnerable Populations. Health Psychol. 2012;31(1):20–30.
28. Desai MM, Rosenheck RA. HIV testing and receipt of test results among homeless persons with serious mental illness. Am J Psychiatry. 2004;161(12):2287–94.
29. Government of India, Ministry of Health and Family Welfare. Targeted Intervention of National AIDS Control Program Phase IV (2012-17). http://www.naco.gov.in/upload/NACP%20-%20IV/NACP-IV%20Strategy%20Document%20.pdf. Accessed 22 June 2016.
30. Planning Commission, Government of India. Report of the expert group to review the methodology for measurement of poverty. June 2014. http://planningcommission.nic.in/reports/genrep/pov_rep0707.pdf Accessed 12 Nov 2015.
31. Government of India, Ministry of Health and Family Welfare. Targeted Intervention of National AIDS Control Program Phase IV (2012-17). HRG Registration Form. https://www.google.co.in/url?sa=t&rct=j&q=&esrc=s&source=web&cd=5&cad=rja&uact=8&ved=0ahUKEwjH6P_R_aDKAhULFCwKHc6FCTQQFggsMAQ&url=http%3A%2F%2Fnaco.gov.in%2Fupload%2FNGO%2520%26%2520Targeted%2FMonitoring%2FData%2520Collection%2520Tools%2FTools%2520used%2520by%2520ORW%2FHRG_registration_form.doc&usg=AFQjCNHChoGkkyPeP7A0DGd4SCmnx5bYoQ&sig2=xd56ZMjxfPx9mrhMM3o_5w&bvm=bv.111396085,d.bGg. Accessed 12 Nov 2015.
32. Strathdee SA, Stockman JK. Epidemiology of HIV among injecting and non-injecting drug users: current trends and implications for interventions. Curr HIV/AIDS Rep. 2010;7(2):99–106.
33. Jemima A. Frimpong, Erick G. Guerrero, Yinfei Kong and Gary Tsai. Correlates of HIV testing and receipt of test results in addiction health services in Los Angeles County. Substance Abuse Treatment, Prevention, and Policy 2015; doi:10.1186/s13011-015-0026-1.
34. The UFO Model: An HCV prevention intervention for young adult IDU. http://www.ufomodel.com. Accessed 2 May 2016.

14

A community- based hepatitis B linkage-to-care program: a case study on Asian Americans chronically infected with hepatitis B virus

Chul S. Hyun[1,2*], William R. Ventura[3], Soon S. Kim[4], Soyoung Yoon[4] and Seulgi Lee[2]

Abstract

Background: Hepatitis B is an important disease of ethnic disparity which affects Asian Americans and other minority populations disproportionately. Despite the high prevalence of hepatitis B in Asian Americans, many of them remain unscreened and untreated. A majority of the individuals chronically infected with hepatitis B virus (HBV) are not linked to care, for instance, due to a lack of culturally competent programs. There are many serious barriers preventing linkage to care (LTC), including personal, socio-cultural, and economic issues. The purpose of this study was to evaluate various barriers affecting LTC and to investigate the role and efficacy of a community-based Patient Navigator (PN) program in expediting LTC and in improving health outcomes for hepatitis B patients in a high risk population.

Methods: A total of 45 individuals chronically infected with HBV were identified through community screening events and were subsequently linked to patient navigators (PN), who then arranged for the patients to have a medical evaluation with a provider of their choice in their communities. The navigators kept detailed records of the patients' progress towards goal, and planned follow up visits for each patient. A self-report questionnaire was employed to assess patients' demographics, history of HBV infection, and barriers in accessing health care. Specifically, the levels of importance of the barriers due to language, culture, financial reasons were assessed.

Results: The study revealed that 38 of the 45 HBV infected individuals knew about their infection status from previous screening. Forty two out of 45 HBV infected individuals were linked to care within a 12 month period, demonstrating a high linkage rate. Most significant barriers identified were language and finance, followed by cultural barrier and others.

Conclusion: There are specific barriers to accessing adequate care for the patients affected by chronic hepatitis B (CHB) in Korean American community. The implementation of a PN program in conjunction with the community network of health care providers may help to overcome the barriers and facilitate LTC in hepatitis B.

Keywords: Health disparity, Hepatitis B, Linkage to care, Patient navigator, Community program

* Correspondence: chulhyunmd@gmail.com
[1]Holy Name Medical Center, Teaneck, NJ, USA
[2]Center for Viral Hepatitis, 35 Van Nostrand Avenue, Englewood, NJ 07631, USA
Full list of author information is available at the end of the article

Background

Chronic HBV infection causes the majority of liver related morbidity and mortality throughout the world. Up to 25 % of patients with HBV infection may suffer from liver cirrhosis, liver failure and primary liver cancer [1–3]. There is a marked disparity among racial and ethnic groups in the prevalence of chronic hepatitis B and its complications. For instance, approximately 5–10 % of all Asian Americans have HBV infection compared to 0.2 % of Caucasian Americans [4, 5]. In the United States, an estimated two million Americans are chronically infected with HBV, with a major proportion being Asian Americans. Surprisingly, a majority of these two million chronically infected people are unaware of the fact that they are infected. Furthermore, fewer than 50,000 people are currently receiving antiviral treatment in the United States, demonstrating a large disparity between the number of chronically infected individuals and the number of people receiving treatment [6, 7].

HBV screening and LTC are critical in the Asian American population for a number of reasons. With a recent immigration wave from Asia, this is the fastest growing ethnic group in the United States [8]. Although vaccination can prevent infection, rates of prevention in Asian Americans have been suboptimal [9, 10]. Secondly, not only are Asian Americans disproportionately affected by chronic hepatitis B (CHB), but they are also most likely of any population group in America to develop HBV-related liver cancer [11, 12]. Despite these grim statistics, two thirds of Asian Americans do not know they are infected, exposing a large undiagnosed population to transmission [5, 7, 10].

As hepatitis B remains significantly underdiagnosed, it is also poorly linked to adequate clinical care. The barriers to LTC in Asian Americans are multi-factorial and include personal, socio-cultural, health care system and provider-related issues. Individual obstacles mostly consist of lack of awareness about the disease, linguistic and cultural barriers, and financial issues. Additionally, providers and healthcare systems currently available in the United States lack the understanding of the significance of chronic hepatitis B. As a result, there is a serious lack of adequate health care access available for Asian Americans and other minority populations [7, 10, 13–15].

The challenges met in LTC are most often related to finding community resources, which can provide the affected population with health care services in a culturally and linguistically sensitive manner. Improvements in patient navigation, education, and counseling efforts may also foster empowerment within the community, thereby facilitating LTC from testing sites to HBV-directed medical care [7, 13, 15, 16].

This study focuses on a group of 45 Korean American individuals chronically infected with HBV from New York and New Jersey to examine various barriers in LTC. The results suggest that PN and community-based LTC not only effectively facilitate health care access, but also may address many of the health disparity issues associated with barriers in ethnic minority populations.

Methods

Participants

HBV infected individuals were identified from hepatitis B awareness campaigns held in northern New Jersey and metropolitan New York during the period between January 2014 and December 2014. These campaigns consisted of community-based hepatitis B screening events organized by Center for Viral Hepatitis (CVH) and Korean Community Services (KCS), which are two major non-profit Korean American organizations devoted to promoting hepatitis B screening and linkage to care. A total of 45 HBV infected individuals, who were found to have hepatitis B surface antigen, were identified. Results of the screenings were provided directly to all the individuals. Subsequently, these patients were linked to a patient navigator (PN), who then arranged for the patients to have a medical evaluation with a provider of their choice in their communities. All the HBV infected individuals who were linked to providers had a confirmatory hepatitis B DNA test. Secondly, their attendances at scheduled medical visits were individually confirmed by the PN.

Data collection and measurement

The key variables in this study were measured by a self-report questionnaire, which consisted of three different parts. The first part of the questionnaire included demographic characteristics of gender, age, place of birth, and length of residence in the United States. The second part asked the following five questions: "When were you told you were infected with HBV?", "Were you referred to a physician at the time of diagnosis?", "Did you follow up with a physician after the diagnosis?", "If not, what was the reason?", and "Are you currently seeing a physician for hepatitis B?". The last part of the questionnaire assessed the potential barriers of LTC. Specifically, barriers due to language, culture, and financial reasons were evaluated. In addition, structural barriers due to difficulties in obtaining transport and appointments were evaluated. Thirty six of 45 HBV infected individuals, who understood the nature of the survey, willingly participated. Using 'Levels of Importance' questions with scale of 0 = not at all important to 5 = most important, participants were asked to rate each barrier. The Levels of Importance were assessed for each barrier by obtaining the total number of the respondents selecting each level.

Patient navigation program

The PN program was employed to provide HBV infected individuals with specific information on the management of CHB and to link them to providers who have expertise in hepatitis B care within their community. The PN program offered specific efforts to assist HBV infected individuals to find their way through the health care system by identifying and providing resources for Korean Americans with socioeconomic and communication barriers. There were three PNs employed in the current study. Two had BS degrees in public health, and the other PN had a BS in nursing. The PNs were trained and supervised by a group of GI and primary care physicians within the community. They were employees of community service organizations. They were not affiliated with any hospitals. Periodic quality assessments were made to address issues or problems identified through a comprehensive evaluation and to assess the stability of PN care over time.

Once all the HBV infected individuals were informed of the screening results, the PN met with them to explain the results in greater detail and to recommend a GI physician for their initial consultation. At each initial visit and follow up appointment, the PN met the patients at the providers' office to ensure that they were guided through the process of the entire evaluation. The navigators kept detailed records of the patients' progress towards goal, and planned follow up visits for each patient.

Results

Demographic characteristics of the HBV infected individuals

The sample of 45 HBV infected individuals included 24 men and 21 women whose age range was 26–70, with an average age of 46. There were 30 participants from New York and 15 from New Jersey.

Role of patient navigation in LTC

After being informed of the results, all the HBV infected individuals were linked to PN, who then arranged for the patients to attend their medical evaluation with a provider of their choice within their communities. As a liaison between the physician and the patient, and being the advocate for the patient, the PN helped assess the patients' condition and discuss any issues with the provider and his/her nursing staff. Navigators also played a role in educating and updating the patient and family members, if needed, to implement the care plan. This study showed that 42 out of 45 HBV infected individuals were linked to care within a 12 month period, demonstrating an overall linkage rate of 93 % (Table 1). All these 42 patients had a minimum of two visits to their providers' offices for continuous monitoring and/or treatment. Seventeen of these patients were then started on antiviral medication.

Table 1 Demographic characteristics

	Number of HBV infected	Percentage (%)
Gender		
Male	24	53.3
Female	21	46.7
Total	45	100
Age		
20–29	4	8.9
30–39	8	17.8
40–49	9	20.0
50–59	15	33.3
60–69	6	13.3
70–79	3	6.7
Antiviral medication		
Yes	17	37.8
No	28	62.2
Successful LTC		
Male	22 (out of 24)	91.7
Female	20 (out of 21)	95.2

History of HBV infection in the cohorts

We investigated how many of these HBV infected individuals might have known their infection status prior to the current screening. The survey showed that 38 (84 %) of 45 infected individuals knew about their infection status from previous screening. Only 7 (16 %) discovered that they had chronic hepatitis B from their most recent screening (Table 2).

Of those 38 people who were diagnosed with CHB, 36 have lived in the United States for more than 10 years. Twenty five of them were recommended to see a specialist for further evaluation. Only 4 of these infected individuals went on to see GI specialists, but did not engage in any further work up. Twenty seven (71 %) of them felt they did not seek medical care because they had no symptoms. Twenty four (63 %) said that they were not aware of potential complications of hepatitis B such as cirrhosis and liver cancer.

Barriers in accessing health care

We also evaluated patient-related factors influencing HBV care. The survey revealed that the most significant barriers were language and finance, followed by cultural and other barriers (Table 3). If the levels of importance 3 to 5 (important to most important) are combined, cultural factors (78 %) were as significant as financial factors (72 %) in hindering the HBV infected individuals from seeking medical care. On the other hand, structural

Table 2 Time of diagnosis in HBV Infected Individuals

Year CHB was diagnosed	Number of HBV infected ($n = 45$)	Percentage (%)
Before 1995	13	28.9
1996–2005	14	31.1
2006–2015	18	40.0
At screening events (2014–2015)	7	15.6

barriers due to travel and time factors were not as significant as the other barriers.

Discussion

This study demonstrates a significant lack of CHB LTC in a high prevalence population. The results also suggest that the community-based initiatives, which mobilize local health care providers, and PN program can effectively facilitate HBV infected individuals to access and receive necessary health care services within the community.

Lack of LTC for HBV infected individuals

A majority of Korean American HBV infected individuals identified in community-based screening events may have been previously diagnosed. As shown in Table 2, only 16 % of the HBV infected individuals identified from the current community-based screenings were newly diagnosed. In contrast, a striking 84 % had been previously diagnosed, reflecting a significant failure in LTC in this particular group. These findings are similar to the previous reports which demonstrated that only a minority of the chronically infected patients were successfully linked to care [7, 17–19]. Other investigators have also noted that up to 66 % of the HBV infected individuals screened in hospital settings were referred to care while only 40 % of those screened in community settings were referred to appropriate care [18, 19]. Although the referral percentage was greater in the group screened from the hospital setting as compared to the group screened from the community setting, there was no clear documentation on the sustainability of LTC. This issue of sustainability of LTC is critical in the care of hepatitis B since its management requires a long period of time. Furthermore, it has been frequently noted that many of those referred to the providers in a hospital setting did not continue to follow up with the providers because of various patient-related barriers.

The failure to link the HBV infected individuals to medical care has been attributed to a number of reasons. First, there are language, financial, and cultural barriers. We, therefore, conducted a survey on these HBV infected people to examine the weight of various factors prohibiting health care access in hepatitis B. The results summarized in Table 3 clearly demonstrated that language, finance, and cultural factors were all important in hindering health access in this study population. Second, patients had minimal medical knowledge about hepatitis B and its potential complications. In addition, there may be other barriers due to a lack of knowledge on the providers' part [13].

Community-centered approach for LTC

This study illustrates that LTC can be made successful in a community setting. The Patient Navigator program and mobilization of local health care providers who have expertise in hepatitis B care were instrumental in providing sustainable linkage from the testing site to HBV-directed care. Forty two out of 45 HBV infected individuals were successfully linked to providers within the community, revealing a high LTC rate of 93 %. PNs communicated in Korean and took individual patients through the continuum of care, ensuring that any potential barriers were adequately addressed. They also ensured that HBV infected individuals attended their first and follow up medical evaluations at their provider's office. We learned that these patients looked for the providers, who could speak their languages, within their community. Thus, the challenging tasks in LTC may be most often related to finding qualified providers [7, 16].

There are important limitations to consider in this study. First, the participants, namely Korean American residents in New Jersey and New York, may not be representative of the overall Korean population in the United States. Education level and socioeconomic status are also important factors known to affect patients' behavior towards health access. How these factors might have influenced the results of the current study is

Table 3 Barriers in Accessing Health Care

	Level of importance ($n = 36$)					
Barriers	0*	1*	2*	3*	4*	5*
Language	0 (0 %)	1 (2.8 %)	2 (5.6 %)	5 (13.9 %)	13 (36.1 %)	15 (41.7 %)
Finance	1 (2.8 %)	4 (11.1 %)	5 (13.9 %)	6 (16.7 %)	7 (19.4 %)	13 (36.1 %)
Culture	0 (0 %)	3 (8.3 %)	5 (13.9 %)	16 (44.4 %)	7 (19.4 %)	5 (13.9 %)
Others	17 (47.2 %)	13 (36.1 %)	6 (16.7 %)	0 (0 %)	0 (0 %)	0 (0 %)

*0 = not at all important; 1–5 = increasing degree of importance

unknown. Secondly, the sample size of the HBV infected people is small, and many of our study subjects underwent screening knowing their hepatitis B status. For instance, some of the HBV infected participants could have utilized screening as a way of health access. Whether this would have potentially underestimated the preexisting level of LTC is a possibility. The future studies with a larger number of HBV infected individuals would be necessary to determine a more accurate level of LTC as well as to assess the sustainability of LTC in these patients.

Effective LTC with a successful implementation of PN program in the care of various diseases can enable the community to build up trust among its members, and further empower the community [20, 21]. The health status outcomes can not only help to modify individual's health belief, but they can also influence the community's perception of the need for health services [22]. Successful hepatitis B LTC in the community setting involves full mobilization of resources, including health care professionals who can provide culturally competent health care. Partnering with community organizations and fostering both medical and non-medical personnel are essential to promoting equitable access and improving the community's overall health and wellbeing.

Conclusion

There are important barriers that lead to poor linkage to care in hepatitis B for Asian Americans. The community-based patient navigation program and local health care providers can effectively engage HBV infected patients to access necessary health care services within the community.

Ethics

All procedures performed in studies involving human participants were in accordance with the ethical standards of the institutional and/or national research committee.

Abbreviations

CHB: chronic hepatitis B; HBV: hepatitis B Virus; LTC: linkage to care; PN: patient navigator.

Competing interests

The authors declare that they have no competing interests.

Authors' contributions

CSH conceived of the study, participated in the design of the study, and drafted the manuscript. SSK and SY participated in the design of the study and performed statistical analysis. RWV and SL participated in its coordination and helped with the literature review. All authors read and approved the final manuscript.

Acknowledgements

This study was supported in part by a grant from Gilead Foundation. The authors acknowledge the work by members and volunteers of the Center for Viral Hepatitis and the Korean Community Services.

Author details

[1]Holy Name Medical Center, Teaneck, NJ, USA. [2]Center for Viral Hepatitis, 35 Van Nostrand Avenue, Englewood, NJ 07631, USA. [3]St. Joseph's Regional Medical Center, Patterson, NJ, USA. [4]Korean Community Services, Queens, NY, USA.

References

1. Hollinger FB, Liang TJ. Hepatitis B virus. In: Knipe DM et al., editors. Fields virology. 4th ed. Philadelphia, PA: Lippincott Williams & Wilkins; 2001.
2. Colvin HM, Mitchell AE, editors. Hepatitis and liver cancer: a national strategy for prevention and control of hepatitis b and C. Washington, DC: Institute of Medicine; 2010. Retrieved from http://www.cdc.gov/hepatitis/pdfs/iom-hepatitisandlivercancerreport.pdf. Accessed 2 Oct 2015.
3. McMahon BJ. Natural history of chronic hepatitis B. Clin Liver Dis. 2010;14(3):381–96.
4. Lok AS, McMahon BJ. Chronic hepatitis B: update 2009 AASLD practice guideline. Hepatology. 2009;50(3):661–2.
5. Chang ET, So SK. Ten largest racial and ethnic health disparities in the United States based on healthy people 2010 objectives. Am J Epidemiol. 2007;166:1105–6.
6. Cohen C, Evans AA, London WT, Block J, Conti M, Block T. Underestimation of chronic hepatitis B virus infection in the United States of America. J Viral Hepat. 2008;15(1):12–3.
7. Cohen C, Holmberg S, McMahon BJ, et al. Is chronic hepatitis B being undertreated in the United States? J Viral Hepat. 2011;8(6):377–83.
8. Census Bureau Reports. Asians fastest-growing race or ethnic group in 2012, released June 13, 2013. Retrieved from https://www.census.gov/newsroom/releases/archives/2010_census/cb12-cn22.html. Accessed 2 Oct 2015.
9. Hutton DW, Tan D, So SK, Brandeau ML. Cost-effectiveness of screening and vaccinating Asian and Pacific Islander adults for hepatitis B. Ann Intern Med. 2007;147(7):460–9.
10. Hu KQ, Pan CQ, Goodwin D. Barriers to screening for hepatitis B virus infection in Asian Americans. Dig Dis Sci. 2011;56:3163–71.
11. Wong R, Corley DA. Racial and ethnic variations in hepatocellular carcinoma incidence within the United States. Am J Med. 2008;121:525–31.
12. Miller BA, Chu KC, Hankey BF, Lies LA. Cancer incidence and mortality patterns among specific Asian and Pacific Islander populations in the United States. Cancer Causes Control. 2008;19:227–56.
13. Upadhyaya N, Chang R, Davis C, Conti MC, Salinas Garcia D, Tang H. Chronic hepatitis B: perceptions in Asian American communities and diagnosis and management practices among primary care physicians. Postgrad Med. 2010;122(5):165–75.
14. Philbin MM, Erby LA, Lee S, Juon HS. Hepatitis B and liver cancer among three Asian American sub-groups: a focus group inquiry. J Immigr Minor Health. 2012;14(5):858–68.
15. Chen Jr MS, Fang DM, Stewart SL, et al. Increasing hepatitis B screening for Hmong adults: results from a randomized controlled community-based study. Cancer Epidemiol Biomarkers Prev. 2013;22(5):782–91.
16. Cohen C, Caballero J, Martin M, et al. Eradication of hepatitis B: a nationwide community coalition approach to improving vaccination, screening, and linkage to care. J Community Health. 2013;38(6):1042–9.
17. Cohen C, Chen G, Block J, et al. Chronic hepatitis B in Chinese immigrants: assessing barriers to care [Abstract 199702]. American Public Health Association annual meeting. Philadelphia, PA. November, 2009
18. Nishimura A, Shiono P, Stier, D, et al. Enhanced surveillance for chronic hepatitis B-San Francisco, [abstr OP-57]. Presented at the 13th International Symposium on Viral Hepatitis and Liver Disease, Washington, DC, March 22, 2009.
19. Pollack H, Wan K, Miyoshi T, et al. Management of chronic hepatitis B virus (HBV) infection by primary care physicians in urban hospitals and clinics in New York City [abstract 984]. Hepatology. 2007;46(Suppl):676A.
20. Natale-Pereira A, Enard KR, Nevarez L, Jones LA. The role of patient navigators in eliminating health disparities. Cancer. 2011;117(15 Suppl):3543–52.
21. Farrisi D, Dietz N. Patient navigation is a client-centered approach that helps to engage people in HIV care. HIV Clin. 2013;25(1):1–3.
22. Andersen RM. Revisiting the behavioral model and access to medical care: does it matter? J Health Soc Behav. 1995;36:1–10.

15

Antiretroviral therapy and liver disease progression in HIV and hepatitis C co-infected patients

Alexis Llewellyn[1], Mark Simmonds[1], Will L Irving[3], Ginny Brunton[2] and Amanda J Sowden[1*]

Abstract

Background: HIV co-infection exacerbates hepatitis C disease, increasing the risk of cirrhosis and hepatitis C-related mortality. Combination antiretroviral therapy (cART) is the current standard treatment for co-infected individuals, but the impact of cART and antiretroviral (ARV) monotherapy on liver disease in this population is unclear. We aimed to assess the effect of cART and ARV monotherapy on liver disease progression and liver-related mortality in individuals co-infected with HIV and chronic hepatitis C.

Methods: A systematic review with meta-analyses was conducted. MEDLINE and EMBASE bibliographic databases were searched up to September 2015. Study quality was assessed using a modified Newcastle-Ottawa scale. Results were synthesised narratively and by meta-analysis.

Results: Fourteen observational studies were included. In analyses that adjusted for potential confounders, risk of liver-related mortality was significantly lower in patients receiving cART (hazard ratio/odds ratio 0.31, 95 % CI 0.14 to 0.70). Results were similar in unadjusted analyses (relative risk 0.40, 95 % CI 0.29 to 0.55). For outcomes where meta-analysis could not be performed, results were less consistent. Some studies found cART was associated with lower incidence of, or slower progression of liver disease, fibrosis and cirrhosis, while others showed no evidence of benefit. We found no evidence of liver-related harm from cART or ARV monotherapy compared with no HIV therapy.

Conclusions: cART was associated with significantly lower liver-related mortality in patients co-infected with HIV and HCV. Evidence of a positive association between cART and/or ARV monotherapy and liver-disease progression was less clear, but there was no evidence to suggest that the absence of antiretroviral therapy was preferable.

Keywords: Systematic review, Meta-analysis, Anti-retroviral agents, Hepatitis C, HIV

Abbreviations: ARV, Antiretroviral therapy; cART, Combination antiretroviral therapy; HCV, Hepatitis C virus; HR, Hazard ratio; IDU, Injection drug use; MD, Mean difference; OR, Odds ratio; RR, Relative risk

Background

Hepatitis C is an infectious liver disease caused by the hepatitis C virus (HCV). Hepatitis C infections occur if the virus is able to enter the blood stream and reach the liver. Co-infection with hepatitis C virus (HCV) and human immunodeficiency virus (HIV) is common due to similar modes of transmission. There are an estimated 7 million individuals worldwide co-infected with HCV and HIV [1]. Chronic HCV infection affects approximately 6.2 % of HIV positive individuals, with greater rates in intravenous drug users [2]. HIV co-infection exacerbates HCV disease, increasing the risk of cirrhosis and HCV-related mortality [3].

In high-income countries, the widespread use of monotherapy with an antiretroviral drug (or ARV monotherapy) in the late 80s, followed by combination antiretroviral therapy (cART) since 1996 has resulted in HIV-infected patients living longer, and chronic HCV

* Correspondence: amanda.sowden@york.ac.uk
[1]Centre for Reviews and Dissemination, University of York, York, UK
Full list of author information is available at the end of the article

infection is now the second most common cause of death, after AIDS-related complications, among HIV-infected individuals in areas where cART is available [1]. The effect of cART on the clinical course of HCV infection is not clear. It has been suggested that the HIV viral suppression [4] and immune reconstitution possible with cART are critical factors that slow down the rate of HCV fibrosis progression [5]. However, some studies have reported that cART may adversely affect hepatitis C-related outcomes by increasing HCV viral load, liver toxicity and fibrosis progression [6–8].

Today, most individuals infected with HCV in high-income countries acquire the virus through unsterile drug injecting practices. However, before the introduction of effective blood donor screening, individuals became infected through blood transfusion or therapy with medical products manufactured from donated human blood. It is estimated that blood transfusion resulted in approximately 23,500 HCV transmissions during the 1970s and 1980s in England, [9] and around 28,000 in the UK, [10] before an effective blood donor screening test was introduced in the UK in 1991. More than 4,600 patients with bleeding disorders were also infected via treatment with HCV-contaminated plasma products. Since 2004, those surviving patients who acquired chronic HCV infection through NHS contaminated blood or blood products before donor screening tests or virus inactivation methods were available have received financial help via a UK wide ex-gratia scheme established by the Department of Health [11].

We report the findings from a systematic review that was commissioned by the Department of Health, England [12]. cART is the current standard treatment for this patient group but its impact on liver disease progression and liver related mortality is unclear. Evidence of harm associated with cART and/or ARV monotherapy may have implications for compensation policies for people who acquired HCV through contaminated blood products prior to 1991. The findings from an earlier review examining the association between cART and ARV monotherapy and liver disease outcomes were inconclusive [13]. Since publication of the review in 2007 new primary studies have become available and an up-to-date review of the available evidence is needed.

Methods

We followed the general principles recommended in Centre for Reviews and Dissemination (CRD) Guidance for Undertaking Reviews in Health Care, [14] and the reporting guidance of the PRISMA and MOOSE statements [15, 16].

Search strategy

MEDLINE and EMBASE electronic databases were searched up to September 2015 for studies published in English. We applied no date restrictions or study design filters. Search terms included "hepatitis C", "HIV", "antiretroviral therapy", and "liver disease". The reference lists of relevant published reviews were checked for additional studies [13, 17–19]. A full search strategy is reported in the Additional file 1.

Study selection

Studies evaluating the effect of cART and/or ARV monotherapy in individuals co-infected with HIV and HCV were eligible for inclusion. Studies had to include a comparison group of participants who did not receive the intervention. Studies that measured treatment exposure and outcome at the same point in time were excluded because they were not considered suitable for measuring disease progression.

The two outcomes of interest were liver-related mortality and liver disease progression, and the latter includes progression to/of fibrosis and cirrhosis; decompensated liver disease; end-stage liver disease; and hepatocellular carcinoma. Outcomes had to be measured using liver biopsy or a validated non-invasive method. Studies examining HCV viral load or transaminase/aminotransferase only were excluded. Data had to be presented as, or allow calculation of, relative risks (RR), odds ratios (OR), hazard ratios (HR), or mean differences (MD).

Titles and abstracts were screened by a single reviewer, and full papers were assessed by two reviewers independently, with disagreements resolved through discussion.

Data extraction and risk of bias

Relevant study details and patient characteristics (e.g., age, sex, baseline liver disease severity, mode of HCV/HIV infection; HIV/HCV treatment regimens and history; concomitant treatments) and outcomes were extracted into standardised forms. Where outcomes were reported with different levels of adjustment (e.g., adjusting for age and sex only versus age, sex and time-dependent covariates), data with the greatest number of adjustments were preferred. Risk of bias was evaluated using a modified version of the Newcastle-Ottawa quality assessment tool [20]. Three main domains were considered: participant selection, confounding, and outcome measurement. Further details are reported in the Supporting Information. Data were extracted by a single reviewer and checked by a second, with disagreements resolved through discussion. Where relevant, study authors were contacted for missing data.

Synthesis

Results for liver-related mortality and liver disease progression were pooled in a meta-analysis if at least two studies reported that outcome, and if data were reported consistently enough for analysis to be feasible. Otherwise, results were synthesised narratively. Where meta-analyses were performed, studies were pooled using standard random-effects DerSimonian-Laird meta-analyses [21]. Heterogeneity was assessed through visual inspection of forest plots and using I^2 [22]. When pooling adjusted odds, hazard or risk ratios these were assumed to be equivalent regardless of the specific statistic reported or which covariates were used in adjusted models. Adjusted and unadjusted ratios were pooled using the inverse variance method. Meta-analyses were conducted using R software.

Where participants from several studies were recruited from the same cohorts and significant overlap was suspected, data from only one study with the most reliable reporting were included in the main analyses. The impact of suspected overlap in participants across studies was explored in sensitivity analyses, as was the use of composite outcomes (one study reported end-stage liver disease, hepatocellular carcinoma or death only as a composite outcome [23]).

Where possible, pre-planned subgroup analyses including only studies with a large proportion of patients with haemophilia were conducted. Meta-regression analyses or other subgroup analyses were considered inappropriate due to the small number of studies.

Results

The bibliographic searches yielded a total of 1,943 unique records. From these, 96 studies of potential relevance were identified and 14 studies met our inclusion criteria (see Fig. 1 for further details).

Risk of bias

As would be expected in observational studies, risk of confounding of results due to unmeasured factors was the most frequent quality concern in the included studies, with ten studies classed at moderate or high risk of bias. Risk of bias associated with participant selection was considered unclear due to limited reporting in five studies, and low in nine studies (where the study sample was considered broadly representative of the population of interest, and assessment of HIV/HCV and outcome at baseline were considered appropriate). The risk of bias associated with outcome measurement was considered mostly low, as ten studies measured and reported their outcomes using appropriate methods. Further details about quality criteria and judgments are reported in Table 1 and Additional file 2.

Study characteristics

Most studies were carried out in Europe, with six from Spain, two from Italy and one in each of France, Germany and Austria. Three studies were carried out in the USA. Study dates ranged from 1970 to 2011 and six studies were conducted across the pre-post cART era (before and after 1996) [23–28]. Seven studies followed patients prospectively in time [23, 27, 29–33] and the

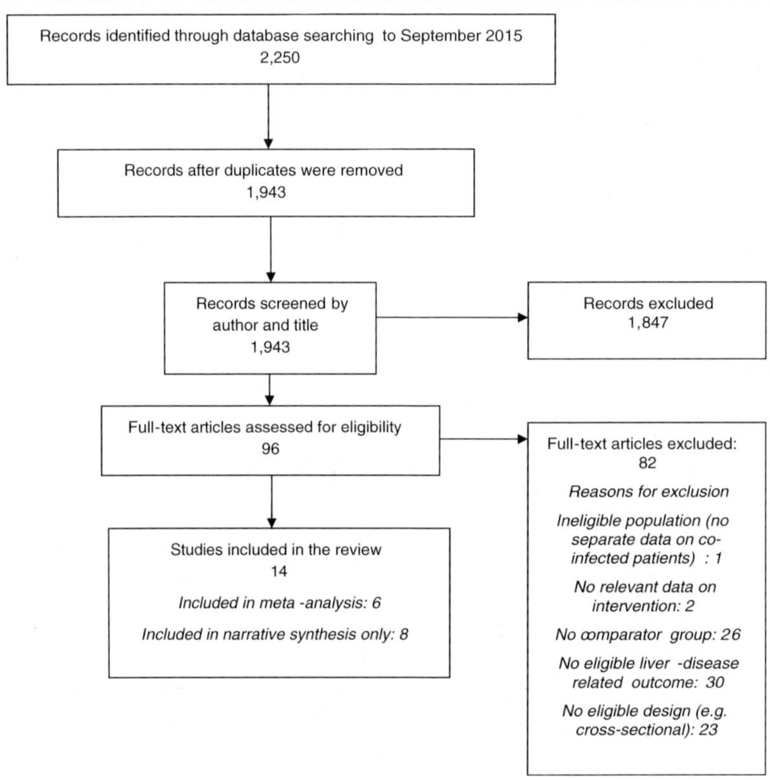

Fig. 1 Flow of studies

Table 1 Risk of bias

	Selection bias	Confounding bias	Outcome measurement bias
Bruno (2007) [34]	Low	Moderate	Low
Giron-Gonzalez (2007) [29]	Unclear	Moderate	Low
Limketkai (2012) [23]	Low	Low	Low
Macias (2006) [25]	Low	Moderate	Low
Macias (2009) [24]	Low	Low	Unclear
Mariné-Barjoan (2004) [35]	Low	High	Low
Mehta (2005) [30]	Unclear	High	High
Merchante (2006) [31]	Unclear	High	Low
Pineda (2009) [32]	Low	Moderate	Low
Qurishi (2003) [26]	Unclear	Low	Low
Ragni (2009) [27]	Low	Low	Unclear
Reiberger (2010) [36]	Low	High	Low
Sanmartin (2014) [33]	Low	High	High
Schiavini (2006) [28]	Unclear	High	Low
Total risk of bias	9 low	4 low	10 low
	0 high	6 high	2 high
	5 unclear	4 moderate	2 unclear

remaining seven studies were classed as retrospective [24–26, 28, 34–36].

Many participants were current or past injection drug users (IDU), with eight studies having IDU rates of 72 % or above. One study focused on patients with haemophilia exclusively [27], and another reported that 81 % of patients had the condition [26]. The other studies failed to report the number of patients with haemophilia. Baseline liver damage severity varied across the studies: ten studies included no or few patients with cirrhosis [23–28, 30, 33, 35, 36]; four studies included only patients with compensated cirrhosis at baseline [29, 31, 32, 34]. Where reported, cART regimens were primarily based on protease inhibitors and non-nucleoside reverse transcriptase inhibitors. Further study characteristics are presented in Table 2.

Seven studies reported data on liver-related mortality, [23, 26, 27, 29, 31, 32, 34] and ten studies reported on liver disease progression [24, 25, 27–30, 32, 33, 35, 36]. Three studies reported separate data on both outcomes [27, 29, 32].

Liver-related mortality

Findings from six of the seven studies on liver-related mortality were combined in meta-analyses [23, 26, 27, 29, 32, 34]. Of those, four studies presented analyses adjusted for potential confounding factors [23, 26, 29, 32]. Figure 2 presents a forest plot of the results from these four studies. cART use was associated with a substantial reduction in liver-related mortality, with a hazard/odds around one-third of that in untreated patients (HR/OR 0.31, 95 % CI 0.14 to 0.70). Heterogeneity was high ($I^2 = 95$ %), likely to be due to the discordant result between two studies [26, 32]. One showed a much larger benefit; most participants in this study had haemophilia, whereas in the other studies a large majority of patients had a history of IDU.

All six studies included in the meta-analysis presented numbers of patients with and without liver-related mortality from which unadjusted relative risks could be calculated. Figure 3 presents a forest plot of the results. cART is associated with a statistically significant lower risk of liver-related mortality (RR 0.40, 95 % CI 0.29 to 0.55). Moderate heterogeneity was found ($I^2 = 24$ %).

Subgroup analysis

Figure 4 presents the forest plot for the two studies which included primarily patients with haemophilia. cART is associated with a reduced risk of liver related mortality (RR 0.28, 95 % CI 0.09 to 0.83), but there is too little data to accurately estimate the effect, or to determine if the effect differs from patients with a history of IDU.

Sensitivity analyses

The number of liver-related deaths per group was not reported in one [23] of the two studies, but it appears that at least 63 % of the events reported across the two study groups were liver-related deaths. Removing this study from the analyses had only a limited effect on the pooled estimates (RR 0.35, 95 % CI 0.21 to 0.57).

Results from one study [31] were not included in the main analyses to avoid the risk of possible double counting with participants from another related study [29]. This study found that the risk of liver-related mortality was significantly lower in cART patients with compensated cirrhosis compared to untreated patients (unadjusted HR 0.5; 95 % CI 0.3 to 0.9). Adding the results of this study to the meta-analysis had a limited effect on the overall findings (RR 0.46, 95 % CI 0.28 to 0.75).

Liver disease outcomes

Liver disease outcomes were reported too diversely, or in too few studies for meta-analysis and we synthesised the findings narratively [24, 25, 27–30, 32, 33, 35, 36]. A summary of the findings from these studies is presented in Table 3.

End-stage liver disease and decompensation events

Three studies reported data on end-stage liver disease or liver decompensation events [27, 29, 32]. Two of these studies found at least one statistically significant effect in favour of cART [27, 29].

Table 2 Intervention and patient characteristics

Study	Country	Start-end date	Total N (I/C)[a]	% with prior HCV therapy	% with concomitant HCV therapy	Age (years)	Male %	Baseline liver damage (%)	Current or past substance abuse (%)
Bruno (2007) [34]	Italy	1999-2004	53 (29/24)	NR	NR	median 37.1	90	100 compensated cirrhosis	NR
Giron-Gonzalez (2007) [29]	Spain	2004-2006	92 (76/22)	19	8	median 40	89	100 compensated cirrhosis	Alcohol: 46 current IDU: 90
Limketkai (2012) [23]	USA	1993-2011	638 (440/198)	NR	NR	median 45.6	66	METAVIR F0-F2: 82 F3: 6 F4: 1	Alcohol: 47 current IDU: 76 past
Macias (2009) [24]	Spain	1986-2008	135 (113/22)	NR	44	mean 37	68	Scheuer F0-F2: 78 F3: 22 F4: 0	Alcohol: 21 current IDU: 90
Macias (2006) [25]	Spain	1991-2005	683 (509/174)	NR	0	median 23[c]	83	Scheuer F0-F2: 68 F3: 18 F4: 14	Alcohol: 23 current IDU: 86 current
Mariné-Barjoan (2004) [35]	France	1997-2000	116 (91/25)	0	0	median 21[c]	67	METAVIR F0-F2: 74 F3-4: 26	Alcohol: 14 current IDU: 72
Mehta (2005) [30]	USA	2001-NR[b]	210 (135/75)	0	NR	median 44.5	67	Ishak F0-F2: 74 ≥F3:26	Alcohol: 39.5 history IDU: 77 current or past
Merchante (2006) [31]	Spain	1997-2004	153 (101/58)	6	NR	median 38	86	100 compensated cirrhosis	Alcohol: 46 current IDU: 88 previous
Pineda (2009) [32]	Spain	1996-2006	154 (145/9)	NR	43	median 39.9	87	100 compensated cirrhosis	Alcohol: 21 IDU: 86 current or previous
Qurishi (2003) [26]	Germany	1990-2002	285 (148/137)	NR	0	median 30	95	No symptomatic liver disease	Alcohol: 12 IDU: 15
Ragni (2009) [27]	USA	1970-2005	85 (60/25)	NR	1	mean 39[d]	100	No cirrhosis	Alcohol: 12 IDU: NR
Reiberger (2010) [36]	Austria	NR-NR	74 (49/25)	0	0	mean 37	77	METAVIR F0-F2: 59 F3-F4: 41	Alcohol: 29 current IDU: NR
Sanmartin (2014) [33]	Spain	1997-2010	162 (149/13)	0	54	mean 37	73	Scheuer F0-F2: 100	Alcohol & IDU: 0 current
Schiavini (2006) [28]	Italy	1985-2002	36 (20/16)	NR	92	median 28	75	Ishak-Knodell F0-2: 75 F3-4: 25	Alcohol: 53 history IDU: NR

ART: 0.279 (0 · 122–0 · 414); untreated: 0.255 (0 · 079–0 · 473); untreated: 145 (SD 43, range 2–610) (time of measurement UC)
[a]I = Intervention, C = Control
[b]Median follow-up 5 years (IQR 2.9-7.5)
[c]At HCV infection
[d]At follow-up

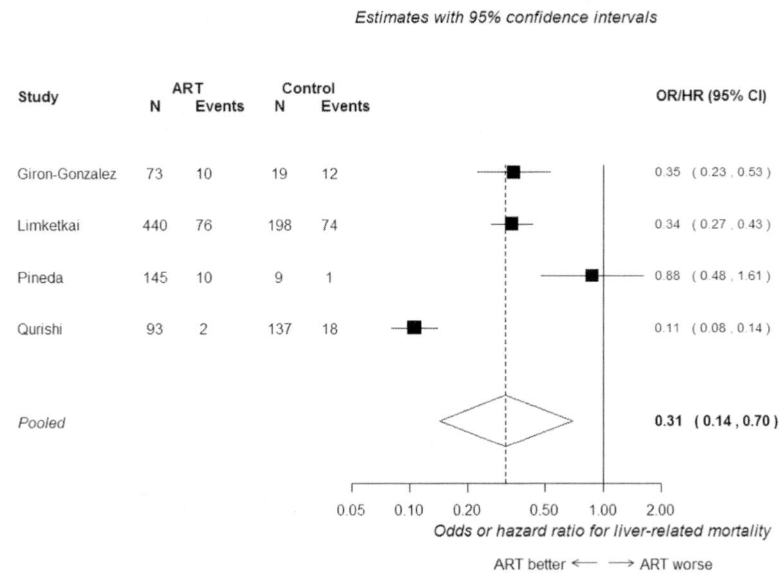

Fig. 2 Adjusted odds or hazard of liver-related mortality in HIV/HCV co-infected patients receiving cART versus no cART. Variables adjusted for: Giron-Gonzalez (2007): HCV viral load, liver disease severity, liver disease progression, decompensation during or before follow-up. Limketkai (2012): Age, sex, race, injection drug use, time-varying CD4 cell count and current cART exposure. Pineda (2009): Not reported. Qurishi (2003): Sex, age, risk category, alcohol misuse, HBV, CD4 count, AAT, AST, cholinesterase bilirubin, platelets count, immunoglobulin concentration

One study [27] found no difference between patients with haemophilia receiving cART and/or ARV monotherapy and untreated patients in the risk of developing end-stage liver disease over 35 years (RR 1.00; 95 % CI 0.37 to 2.71). However, patients receiving cART survived longer before progressing to end-stage liver disease compared with untreated patients (30.3 vs. 20.0 years; HR 3.14; 95 % CI 1.27 to 7.08).

Two studies reported on the risk of liver decompensation in patients with liver cirrhosis [29, 32]. One [29] found a significantly lower risk of a new event of decompensation in cART patients with stable cirrhosis who had experienced decompensation in the past (HR 0.376; 95 % CI 0.161 to 0.883). However, no statistically significant difference was found in the subgroup of patients with no previous decompensation at baseline. Similarly, the other [32] found no significant difference between cART and untreated patients in the risk of decompensation in individuals with cirrhosis.

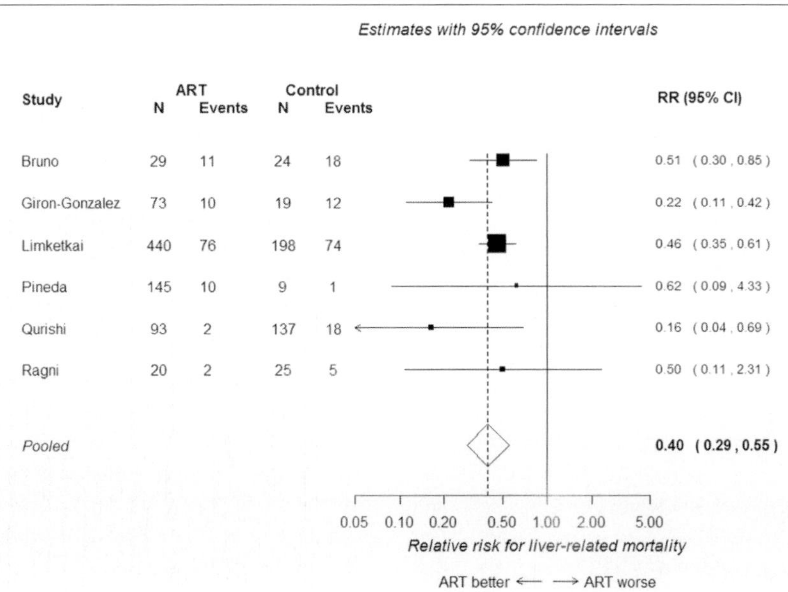

Fig. 3 Unadjusted relative risk of liver-related mortality in HIV/HCV co-infected patients receiving cART versus no cART

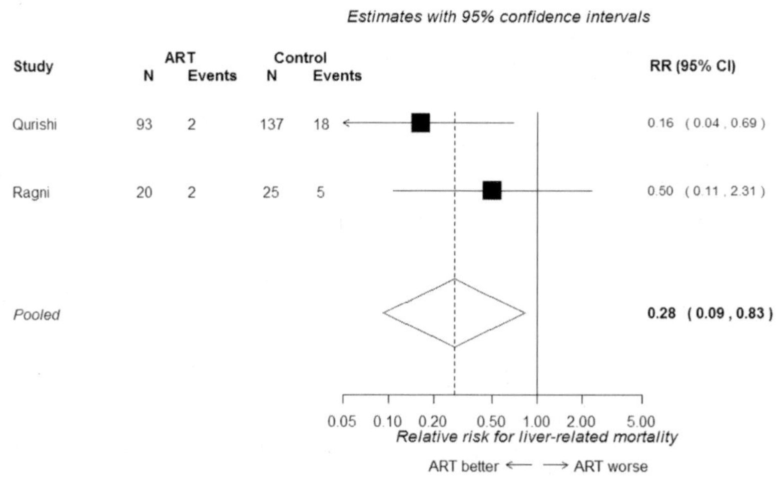

Fig. 4 Unadjusted relative risk for liver-related mortality in HIV/HCV co-infected haemophiliac patients receiving cART versus no cART

Fibrosis progression

Seven studies reported on liver damage in patients with no cirrhosis at baseline, expressed in terms of odds/hazard of fibrosis progression, [24, 25, 28, 30, 33] and/or progression rate [25, 35, 36]. Of the five studies that reported the odds/hazard of fibrosis progression, only one reported a statistically significant difference between intervention and control. This study [25] found significantly lower odds of liver fibrosis progression in patients on cART with protease inhibitors (PI) (OR 0.4; 95 % CI 0.2 to 0.7) and in patients who switched from a PI based regimen to efavirenz during the course of their treatment (OR 0.3; 95 % CI 0.1 to 0.7), but not with other regimens.

Of the three studies that reported fibrosis progression rates, two found a difference in favour of cART [25, 35], and one found no difference between cART and no treatment [36]. One [25] found slower median rates of fibrosis progression in patients treated with cART compared with untreated patients, regardless of regimens used. However, the difference was only statistically significant for some regimens (zidovudine/lamivudine and stavudine/lamivudine). Another [35] found a slower mean rate of fibrosis progression over approximately 15 years in patients undertaking cART at follow-up, although the difference did not reach statistical significance.

Discussion

We included 14 studies evaluating the association between cART and/or ARV monotherapy and liver disease progression and liver-related mortality in patients co-infected with HIV and hepatitis C. In most studies the majority of patients had a history of IDU, except for two studies that included only or mostly participants with haemophilia. cART was found to be associated with a substantial reduction in liver-related mortality, with a chance/hazard around one-third of that in untreated patients. Pooled estimates from unadjusted analyses also showed a clear association in favour of cART for preventing liver-related mortality. A subgroup analysis including nearly all patients with haemophilia also found a reduced incidence of liver related mortality in individuals receiving cART, but there were too little data to provide an accurate estimate or to determine if the effect differed from other populations. Findings for other liver-related outcomes were less consistent, although no studies reported that lack of cART or ARV monotherapy was associated with significantly better liver-disease outcomes.

Strengths and limitations

This systematic review was conducted following the general principles recommended in CRD Guidance for Undertaking Reviews in Health Care, and the reporting guidance of the PRISMA and MOOSE statements [15, 16]. Study quality was assessed systematically and considered when interpreting the findings. Whenever possible, data on treatment effect for individual studies were extracted or calculated, even when quantitative synthesis was not undertaken. The review was completed within a ten-week timeframe to meet the needs of the Department of Health in England and due to time constraints we did not search for conference abstracts, included only English language studies and one reviewer screened titles and abstracts. This means that relevant studies may have been missed, and the risk of publication bias cannot be ruled out. Quantitative assessment of publication bias was considered inappropriate due to the limited number of included studies. Despite the limitations of our searches, we believe it is unlikely that any potential missed studies would

Table 3 Liver fibrosis progression, decompensation and end stage liver disease outcomes

Study	Intervention	Outcome	Follow-up duration	Effect estimate	Statistically significant?[a]	Adjustments
End-stage liver disease (ESLD) and decompensation events						
Giron-Gonzalez (2007) [29]	cART	Decompensation[j]	Median 20 months (IQR 12 to 28)	HR 0.376 (95 % CI 0.161 to 0.883)	Yes. Favours treatment	Liver disease severity
Giron-Gonzalez (2007) [29]	cART	Decompensation[j]	Median 20 months (IQR 12 to 28)	NR	No	None
Pineda (2009) [32]	cART	Decompensation	Mean 36 months (SD 27), range 1 to 131 months	RR 1.06 (95 % CI 0.30 to 3.71)	No	None
Ragni (2009) [27]	cART & ARV monotherapy	ESLD	NR (up to 35 years from HCV infection)	RR 1.00 (95 % CI 0.37 to 2.71)	No	None
Ragni (2009) [27]	cART vs. ARV monotherapy & no ARV[b]	Time to ESLD	NR (up to 35 years from HCV infection)	HR 3.14 (95 % CI 1.27 to 7.08) (30.3 vs. 20.0 Years)	Yes. Favours treatment	Multivariate (covariates NR)
Liver fibrosis progression (dichotomous)						
Macias (2006) [25]	cART with PI	Liver fibrosis progression[d]	Median 1.6 to 7 years	OR 0.4 (95 % CI 0.2 to 0.7)	Yes. Favours treatment	Age at infection, CD4 count
Macias (2006) [25]	cART with PI switched to efavirenz	Liver fibrosis progression[d]	Median 1.6 to 7 years	OR 0.3 (95 % CI 0.1 to 0.7)	Yes. Favours treatment	Age at infection, CD4 count
Schiavini (2006) [28]	cART and ARV monotherapy	Liver fibrosis progression[e]	Median 54 months (IQR 50 to 86)	OR 2.5 (95 % CI 0.64 to 9.65)	No	None
Macias (2009) [24]	cART and ARV monotherapy	Liver fibrosis progression[h]	3 years	OR 0.94 (95 % CI 0.67 to 1.33)	No	Multivariate[k]
Mehta (2005) [30]	ARV monotherapy	Advanced fibrosis or cirrhosis[c]	Median 5 years (IQR 2.9 to 7.5)	OR 0.61 (95 % CI 0.18 to 2)	No	None
Mehta (2005) [30]	cART	Advanced fibrosis or cirrhosis[c]	Median 5 years (IQR 2.9 to 7.5)	OR 0.92 (95 % CI 0.48 to 1.8)	No	None
Sanmartin (2014) [33]	cART	Liver fibrosis progression[i]	Median 7.8 years (IQR 5.5 to 10.0)	HR 1.94 (95 % CI 0.46 to 8.13)	No	None
Liver fibrosis progression (continuous)						
Macias (2006) [25]	cART with: NVP; or efavirenz; or with PI switched to NVP	Fibrosis progression rate[f]	Median 1.6 to 7 years	Median rate 0.087 to 0.115	No	None
Macias (2006) [25]	cART with zidovudine/lamivudine, or with stavudine/lamivudine	Fibrosis progression rate[f]	Median 1.6 to 7 years	Median rate 0.107 and 0.112	Yes. Favours treatment	None
Mariné-Barjoan (2004) [35]	cART	Fibrosis progression rate[f]	Median 19 to 20 years	MD −0.06 (95 % CI −0.14 to 0.01)	No	None
Reiberger (2010) [36]	cART	Fibrosis progression rate[f]	NR	MD 0.01 (95 % CI −0.01 to 0.04)	No	None
Reiberger (2010) [36]	cART	Time to cirrhosis[g] from initial HCV exposure	NR	MD −1.00 (95 % CI −7.26 to 5.26)	No	None

cART combination antiretroviral therapy, *PI* protease inhibitors, *NVP* nevirapine
[a] $p < 0.05$
[b] ARV monotherapy patients formed 62 % of the comparator group in this analysis
[c] Ishak score ≥ F3 measured with liver biopsy
[d] Odds of slower fibrosis proression (fibrosis progression rate ≥0.2 vs <0.2), fibrosis measured with liver biopsy
[e] ≥1 Knodell-Ishak stage increase between two liver biopsies
[f] METAVIR Fibrosis stage (0 to 3) measured by liver biopsy/length of HCV infection
[g] In years, measured with liver biopsy
[h] ≥1 Scheuer stage increase between two liver biopsies spaced by ≥1 year
[i] Liver stiffness value ≥9.5 kPa or died of liver disease
[j] Subgroup without previous decompensation at baseline
[k] Age, undetectable HIV viraemia, genotype 3, ALT and necroinflammatory activity at baseline, time between liver biopsies, HCV treatment response

significantly modify the findings of the main analyses on liver-related mortality and our main conclusions. This is because the observed effect associated with cART is substantial.

Findings from most studies on liver-related mortality were synthesised quantitatively. Adjusted and unadjusted results were pooled separately as an attempt to address potential confounding. Adjusted mortality values could only be combined based on the (inaccurate) assumption that odds and hazard ratios are equivalent, and this approach could create heterogeneity across studies because of different analysis methods used to obtain the adjusted results; therefore these results need to be interpreted with caution. However, the pooled estimates from adjusted and unadjusted values did not differ significantly, and both suggested substantial benefits of cART.

Liver disease outcomes were reported too diversely, or in too few studies for statistical pooling. This limits the strength of the findings on liver disease progression. There were too few studies to conduct meta-regression or further subgroup analyses to explore the moderating effect of several relevant factors, including age, liver disease severity, baseline CD4 count, HBV co-infection, co-intervention with HCV therapy, time since HCV/HIV infection, HIV treatment duration treatment history of HCV infection or alcohol abuse.

Unsurprisingly, no RCTs were identified and all included studies were observational. Given the known overall survival benefits associated with cART, it would be unethical to randomise patients to no cART. Half of the studies adjusted for potential confounders such as age or sex, although the variables accounted for varied across the studies. For instance, only two studies controlled for alcohol misuse in their analyses. Although attempts were made to address the risk of confounding in the analyses, risk of confounding cannot be ruled out. The pooled analyses showed heterogeneity, particularly for the meta-analysis of adjusted results, which limits the strength of the review findings.

Studies might have been affected by a survivorship bias if patients in the intervention group who survived long enough to receive treatment had slower HCV progression, and therefore may have had better HCV-related outcomes [13]. The use of a time-dependent variable or Cox proportional hazards modelling taking HCV duration or progression into account might have remedied this bias. However, no studies reported using this technique. On the other hand, it is possible that comparison groups had levels of immunosuppression that were considered sufficiently high for their treatment to be delayed [37–39]. In this case, patients in the ART group may have had poorer health at treatment initiation, and may therefore have been at higher risk of liver disease progression. Unfortunately, reporting of participant characteristics in the studies was insufficient to support or reject these assumptions.

Reasons for not receiving cART or ARV monotherapy were generally not reported. However, given that cART, and previously ARV monotherapy, would likely be recommended to most HIV/HCV co-infected individuals, particularly those with high HIV viral load, reasons for not receiving treatment were likely influenced by individual patient choice. Those receiving cART may be less likely to be active IDUs (for example, ex-IDUs on methadone programmes) and may have different lifestyles (for example, less alcohol and substance abuse) compared to those who do not receive cART. Reporting of baseline differences between cART/ARV monotherapy and untreated groups was often limited. Although no studies reported significant differences between groups such as current alcohol, IDU or other substance abuse, and although some studies adjusted for these variables in their analyses, it is still possible that those who received treatment for HIV were different to those who did not for reasons that may have influenced liver-related outcomes.

Where reported, most participants had a history of IDU. This should be taken into account when interpreting the results of the review. Most participants included in the studies were under 50 years of age and the burden of other co-morbidities is likely to be higher in older populations. This, in addition to the toxicity of other treatments, may impact differently upon liver disease. This limits the applicability of the findings to older populations, especially given the increasing life expectancy of people with HIV and HCV, and the growing proportion of people with HIV aged 50 years and over.

We identified only studies from high-income countries and note that the applicability of the review findings to low- and middle-income countries is uncertain.

Implications for policy, practice and further research

This systematic review provides an up-to-date synthesis of the available evidence on the effect of cART and ARV monotherapy on liver disease progression and liver-related mortality in individuals co-infected with HIV and hepatitis C. This review, together with another review on quality of life and extrahepatic conditions in individuals with chronic hepatitis C, [40] was commissioned as part of ongoing policy consideration about the shape of support for those affected by hepatitis C or HIV from historic NHS blood treatments before donor screening tests or virus inactivation methods were available in the UK. A public consultation on reform of the existing financial and other support available was announced in January 2016.

The findings of this review support the use of cART in patients co-infected with HIV and HCV as recommended by current guidelines [39, 41]. Given the increased risk of liver-related morbidity and mortality in patients co-infected with HIV and HCV and the limited evidence on the impact of cART on liver disease progression, the need for monitoring liver-disease progression in this population clearly remains. Future management of patients co-infected with HIV and HCV is likely to evolve with the advent of new directly acting antivirals (DAAs) for the treatment of HCV, [42–45] and recent trials have found high sustained virologic response (SVR) rates in non-cirrhotic patients co-infected with HIV and HCV with certain DAA combinations [46, 47].

Few included studies reported data separately for different antiretroviral classes and combinations. Several studies comparing different ARV regimens did not compare cART and/or ARV monotherapy with no HIV treatment and were therefore excluded from our review. Given the ubiquitous use of cART in HIV management, a systematic review on the acute and chronic effect of different cART regimens would be relevant. The mechanisms by which liver disease mortality is reduced with cART are still largely unknown [27]. Further research would clarify whether the effect of cART on liver-disease progression and mortality may occur through immune reconstitution, viral suppression or a combination of both [13].

Conclusions

The use of cART was found to be associated with a significantly reduced risk of liver-related mortality in patients co-infected with HIV and HCV. Evidence of a positive association with liver disease progression is less clear, although there is no evidence to suggest that the absence of cART and/or ARV monotherapy is preferable.

Acknowledgments

We thank members of our advisory group, including Joseph Peaty and Mark Ward from Tainted Blood for providing testimonies on living with HIV, Hepatitis C and haemophilia and undergoing antiretroviral therapy, for suggesting references for inclusion, and for commenting on the draft report. We also thank Professor James Thomas, UCL Institute of Education, University College London, for his advice and support, and Dave Fox, Information Specialist at CRD, University of York, for conducting the bibliographic searches. *Guarantor of the article*: Amanda Sowden

We confirm that the manuscript has not been published previously, in any language, in whole or in part, and is not currently under consideration elsewhere. Please note that a linked report was published on the EPPI Centre website http://eppi.ioe.ac.uk/cms/Default.aspx?tabid=3481.

Funding

This is an independent report commissioned and funded by the Policy Research Programme in the UK Department of Health. The Department of Health approved the design of the study, and played no part in the collection, analysis and interpretation of data, or writing of the manuscript. The views expressed are not necessarily those of the funder.

Authors' contributions

AL, MS, GB and AJS contributed to the protocol development. AL and MS performed the study selection, data extraction, quality assessment, narrative synthesis and contributed to the analyses; MS performed the statistical analyses. WI provided clinical advice throughout the review. AS took overall responsibility for the project and contributed to all aspects. AL wrote the paper, MS, WI, GB and AS revised the manuscript. All authors have contributed to and agreed on the content of the manuscript.

Competing interests

Will Irving has served as a speaker, a consultant and an advisory board member for Janssen Cilag, Bristol-Myers Squibb, and has received research funding from Gilead Sciences, Janssen Cilag and educational grants from Boehringer Ingelheim, Gilead Sciences and MSD. The authors declare they have no other competing interests.

Author details

[1]Centre for Reviews and Dissemination, University of York, York, UK. [2]UCL Institute of Education, University of London, London, UK. [3]Faculty of Medicine & Health Sciences, University of Nottingham, Nottingham, UK.

References

1. Soriano V, Vispo E, Labarga P, Medrano J, Barreiro P. Viral hepatitis and HIV co-infection. Antiviral Res. 2010;85(1):303–15. doi:http://dx.doi.org/10.1016/j.antiviral.2009.10.021.
2. Platt L, Easterbrook P, Gower E, McDonald B, Sabin K, McGowan C et al. Prevalence and burden of HCV co-infection in people living with HIV: a global systematic review and meta-analysis. Lancet Infect Dis. 2016;16(7):797–808
3. de Ledinghen V, Barreiro P, Foucher J, Labarga P, Castera L, Vispo ME, et al. Liver fibrosis on account of chronic hepatitis C is more severe in HIV-positive than HIV-negative patients despite antiretroviral therapy. J Viral Hepat. 2008; 15(6):427–33.
4. Brau N, Salvatore M, Rios-Bedoya CF, Fernandez-Carbia A, Paronetto F, Rodriguez-Orengo JF, et al. Slower fibrosis progression in HIV/HCV-coinfected patients with successful HIV suppression using antiretroviral therapy. J Hepatol. 2006;44(1):47–55.
5. Lange CG, Lederman MM. Immune reconstitution with antiretroviral therapies in chronic HIV-1 infection. J Antimicrob Chemother. 2003;51(1):1–4. doi:10.1093/jac/dkg071.
6. Bonacini M. Liver injury during highly active antiretroviral therapy: the effect of hepatitis C coinfection. Clin Infect Dis. 2004;38 Suppl 2:S104–8.
7. Verma S, Wang CH, Govindarajan S, Kanel G, Squires K, Bonacini M. Do type and duration of antiretroviral therapy attenuate liver fibrosis in HIV-hepatitis C virus-coinfected patients? Clin Infect Dis. 2006;42(2):262–70.
8. Sulkowski MS, Mehta SH, Torbenson M, Afdhal NH, Mirel L, Moore RD, et al. Hepatic steatosis and antiretroviral drug use among adults coinfected with HIV and hepatitis C virus. AIDS. 2005;19(6):585–92.
9. Soldan K, Ramsay M, Robinson A, Harris H, Anderson N, Caffrey E, et al. The contribution of transfusion to HCV infection in England. Epidemiol Infect. 2002;129(3):587–91. doi:10.1017/s0950268802007744.
10. Department of Health, UK. Review of the support available to individuals infected with hepatitis C and/or HIV by NHS supplied blood transfusions or blood products and their dependants. London: Department of Health; 2011. https://www.gov.uk/government/uploads/system/uploads/attachment_data/file/215828/dh_125977.pdf
11. The Skipton Fund website. http://www.skiptonfund.org. Accessed 6 Aug 2013.
12. Llewellyn A, Simmonds M, Brunton G, Sowden A. Impact of antiretroviral therapy on liver disease progression and mortality in patients co-infected with HIV and hepatitis C. Systematic review and meta-analysis. London: EPPI-Centre, Social Science Research Unit, UCL Institute of Education, University College London; 2015.
13. Kramer JR, Giordano TP, El-Serag HB. Effect of human immunodeficiency virus and antiretrovirals on outcomes of hepatitis C: a systematic review

from an epidemiologic perspective. Clin Gastroenterol Hepatol. 2007;5(11):1321–8.e7.
14. Centre for Reviews and Dissemination. Systematic reviews: CRD's guidance for undertaking reviews in health care. York: Centre for Reviews and Dissemination, University of York; 2009.
15. Moher D, Liberati A, Tetzlaff J, Altman DG, Grp P. Preferred reporting items for systematic reviews and meta-analyses: the PRISMA statement. BMJ. 2009;339:b2535. doi:10.1136/bmj.b2535.
16. Stroup DF, Berlin JA, Morton SC, et al. Meta-analysis of observational studies in epidemiology: A proposal for reporting. JAMA. 2000;283(15):2008–12. doi:10.1001/jama.283.15.2008.
17. Thein HH, Yi Q, Dore GJ, Krahn MD. Natural history of hepatitis C virus infection in HIV-infected individuals and the impact of HIV in the era of highly active antiretroviral therapy: a meta-analysis. AIDS. 2008;22(15):1979–91.
18. Chen T, Ding E, Seage Iii G, Kim A. Meta-analysis: increased mortality associated with hepatitis C in HIV-infected persons is unrelated to HIV disease progression. Clin Infect Dis. 2009;49(10):1605–15.
19. Hua L, Andersen J, Daar E, Glesby M, Hollabaugh K, Tierney C. Hepatitis C virus/HIV coinfection and responses to initial antiretroviral treatment. AIDS. 2013;27(17):2725–34.
20. Wells G, Shea B, O'Connell D, Peterson J, Welch J, Losos M, et al. The Newcastle-Ottawa Scale (NOS) for assessing the quality of nonrandomised studies in meta-analyses. Ottawa: Ottawa Hospital Research Institute; 2014. http://www.ohri.ca/programs/clinical_epidemiology/oxford.asp. Accessed 6 Aug 2014.
21. DerSimonian R, Laird N. Meta-analysis in clinical trials. Control Clin Trials. 1986;7(3):177–88.
22. Higgins JPT, Green S (editors). Cochrane Handbook for Systematic Reviews of Interventions Version 5.1.0 [updated March 2011]. The Cochrane Collaboration, 2011. Available from www.handbook.cochrane.org.
23. Limketkai BN, Mehta SH, Sutcliffe CG, Higgins YM, Torbenson MS, Brinkley SC, et al. Relationship of liver disease stage and antiviral therapy with liver-related events and death in adults coinfected with HIV/HCV. JAMA. 2012;308(4):370–8. doi:http://dx.doi.org/10.1001/jama.2012.7844.
24. Macias J, Berenguer J, Japon MA, Giron JA, Rivero A, Lopez-Cortes LF, et al. Fast fibrosis progression between repeated liver biopsies in patients coinfected with human immunodeficiency virus/hepatitis C virus. Hepatology. 2009;50(4):1056–63. doi:http://dx.doi.org/10.1002/hep.23136.
25. Macias J, Mira JA, Lopez-Cortes LF, Santos I, Giron-Gonzalez JA, Gonzalez-Serrano M, et al. Antiretroviral therapy based on protease inhibitors as a protective factor against liver fibrosis progression in patients with chronic hepatitis C. Antivir Ther. 2006;11(7):839–46.
26. Qurishi N, Kreuzberg C, Luchters G, Effenberger W, Kupfer B, Sauerbruch T, et al. Effect of antiretroviral therapy on liver-related mortality in patients with HIV and hepatitis C virus coinfection. Lancet. 2003;362(9397):1708–13.
27. Ragni MV, Nalesnik MA, Schillo R, Dang Q. Highly active antiretroviral therapy improves ESLD-free survival in HIV-HCV co-infection. Haemophilia. 2009;15(2):552–8. doi:http://dx.doi.org/10.1111/j.1365-2516.2008.01935.x.
28. Schiavini M, Angeli E, Mainini A, Zerbi P, Duca PG, Gubertini G, et al. Risk factors for fibrosis progression in HIV/HCV coinfected patients from a retrospective analysis of liver biopsies in 1985–2002. HIV Med. 2006;7(5):331–7.
29. Giron-Gonzalez JA, Brun F, Terron A, Vergara A, Arizcorreta A. Natural history of compensated and decompensated HCV-related cirrhosis in HIV-infected patients: a prospective multicentre study. Antivir Ther. 2007;12(6):899–907.
30. Mehta SH, Thomas DL, Torbenson M, Brinkley S, Mirel L, Chaisson RE, et al. The effect of antiretroviral therapy on liver disease among adults with HIV and hepatitis C coinfection. Hepatology. 2005;41(1):123–31.
31. Merchante N, Giron-Gonzalez JA, Gonzalez-Serrano M, Torre-Cisneros J, Garcia-Garcia JA, Arizcorreta A, et al. Survival and prognostic factors of HIV-infected patients with HCV-related end-stage liver disease. AIDS. 2006;20(1):49–57.
32. Pineda JA, Aguilar-Guisado M, Rivero A, Giron-Gonzalez JA, Ruiz-Morales J, Merino D, et al. Natural history of compensated hepatitis c virusrelated cirrhosis in HIV-infected patients. Clin Infect Dis. 2009;49(8):1274–82. doi:http://dx.doi.org/10.1086/605676.
33. Sanmartin R, Tor J, Sanvisens A, Lopez J, Jou A, Muga R, et al. Progression of liver fibrosis in HIV/hepatitis C virus-coinfected individuals on antiretroviral therapy with early stages of liver fibrosis at baseline. HIV Med. 2014;15(4):203–12. doi:http://dx.doi.org/10.1111/hiv.12105.
34. Bruno R, Sacchi P, Puoti M, Maiocchi L, Patruno S, Carosi G, et al. Natural history of compensated viral cirrhosis in a cohort of patients with HIV infection. J Acquir Immune Defic Syndr. 2007;46(3):297–303.
35. Marine-Barjoan E, Saint-Paul MC, Pradier C, Chaillou S, Anty R, Michiels JF, et al. Impact of antiretroviral treatment on progression of hepatic fibrosis in HIV/hepatitis C virus co-infected patients. AIDS. 2004;18(16):2163–70.
36. Reiberger T, Ferlitsch A, Sieghart W, Kreil A, Breitenecker F, Rieger A, et al. HIV-HCV co-infected patients with low CD4+ cell nadirs are at risk for faster fibrosis progression and portal hypertension. J Viral Hepat. 2010;17(6):400–9. doi:http://dx.doi.org/10.1111/j.1365-2893.2009.01197.x.
37. Williams I, Churchill D, Anderson J, Boffito M, Bower M, Cairns G, et al. British HIV Association guidelines for the treatment of HIV-1-positive adults with antiretroviral therapy 2012 (Updated November 2013. All changed text is cast in yellow highlight.). HIV Med. 2014;15 Suppl 1:1–85. doi:10.1111/hiv.12119.
38. Nunez M. British HIV, guidelines for the management of hepatitis B and C in HIV-coinfected patients. AIDS Rev. 2005;7(3):181.
39. Brook G, Main J, Nelson M, Bhagani S, Wilkins E, Leen C, et al. British HIV Association guidelines for the management of coinfection with HIV-1 and hepatitis B or C virus 2010. HIV Med. 2010;11(1):1–30. doi:http://dx.doi.org/10.1111/j.1468-1293.2009.00781.x.
40. Brunton G, Caird J, Sutcliffe K, Rees R, Stokes G, Oliver S, et al. Depression, anxiety, pain and quality of life in people living with chronic hepatitis C: a systematic review and meta-analysis. London: EPPI-Centre, Social Science Research Unit, UCL Institute of Education, University College London; 2015.
41. Rockstroh JK, Bhagani S, Benhamou Y, Bruno R, Mauss S, Peters L, et al. European AIDS Clinical Society (EACS) guidelines for the clinical management and treatment of chronic hepatitis B and C coinfection in HIV-infected adults. HIV Med. 2008;9(2):82–8. doi:http://dx.doi.org/10.1111/j.1468-1293.2007.00535.x.
42. European Medicines Agency (EMA). Sovaldi 400 mg film-coated tablets. Annex I summary of product characteristics. [s.l.]: EMA[s.a.]. https://www.medicines.org.uk/emc/medicine/28539.
43. European Medicines Agency (EMA). OLYSIO 150 mg hard capsules. Annex I summary of product characteristics. [s.l.]: EMA[s.a.]. https://www.medicines.org.uk/emc/medicine/28888.
44. Gilead Sciences Ltd. Summary of Product Characteristics: Harvoni 90 mg/400 mg film-coated tablets. electronic Medicines Compendium (eMC), Leatherhead, Surrey. 2015. http://www.medicines.org.uk/emc/medicine/29471. Accessed 27 Aug 2015.
45. AbbVie Limited. Summary of Product Characteristics: Viekirax 12.5 mg/75 mg/50 mg film-coated tablets. electronic Medicines Compendium (eMC), Leatherhead, Surrey. 2015. https://www.medicines.org.uk/emc/medicine/29784. Accessed 27 Aug 2015.
46. Osinusi A, Townsend K, Kohli A, Nelson A, Seamon C, Meissner EG, et al. Virologic response following combined ledipasvir and sofosbuvir administration in patients with HCV genotype 1 and HIV co-infection. JAMA. 2015;313(12):1232–9.
47. Sulkowski M, Hezode C, Gerstoft J, Vierling JM, Mallolas J, Pol S, et al. Efficacy and safety of 8 weeks versus 12 weeks of treatment with grazoprevir (MK-5172) and elbasvir (MK-8742) with or without ribavirin in patients with hepatitis C virus genotype 1 mono-infection and HIV/hepatitis C virus co-infection (C-WORTHY): a randomised, open-label phase 2 trial. Lancet. 2015;385(9973):1087–97. doi:10.1016/s0140-6736(14)61793-1.

16

Hepatitis B knowledge among women of childbearing age

Swati Jha[1*], Divyesh Devaliya[1], Susan Bergson[2] and Shripad Desai[1]

Abstract

Background: More than 17 million people in India are chronically infected with the hepatitis B virus (HBV). Approximately one million of the 26 million children born in India annually will develop chronic HBV infection in the course of their lives. Studies have put the HBsAg prevalence rate among pregnant women in India between 0.9 % and 3.1, indicating a considerable need for public health interventions aimed at protecting their offspring from infection. The PAHAL project in Mumbai, India, conducted an HBV knowledge survey among women of childbearing age in three local slum communities preparatory to planning a comprehensive HBV education intervention targeting this population.

Methods: Female health workers approached all households in three designated slum neighborhoods: one each in the eastern suburbs (ES), western suburbs (WS) and Island City (IC). Female residents aged 18–45 were invited to participate in the study, and those who agreed to participate responded to a questionnaire that was administered in the form of an oral interview. The five sections of the questionnaire addressed demography, hepatitis B knowledge, personal risk related to hepatitis B, pregnancy and childbearing history, and the participant's most recent pregnancy. A descriptive statistical analysis was performed.

Results: Health workers submitted 6571 interview forms that were suitable for analysis (ES, 28 %; WS, 34 %; IC, 38 %). Large proportions of study participants were married (89 %), were not employed (94 %) and had completed less than 12 years of school (87 %). Only 240 (3.6 %) women answered yes when asked if they knew about hepatitis B. Among those women, there were high levels of accurate knowledge regarding some modes of hepatitis B transmission but low levels of accurate knowledge regarding other modes. Twenty-two percent of 739 women who had given birth within the previous 36 months reported that they had been tested for HBV during pregnancy. While 70 % of these women reported that their children had received three doses of hepatitis B vaccine, reported vaccination levels varied greatly across the three study areas.

Conclusions: Despite the availability of a safe HBV vaccine, which is free for newborns and infants in many parts of India, preventing mother-to-child transmission of HBV remains a major challenge. Low awareness of HBV among women of childbearing age in Mumbai-area slums indicates a need for educational interventions targeting this population.

Keywords: Hepatitis B, Pregnant women, Women of child bearing age, Hepatitis B testing, Hepatitis B transmission

* Correspondence: sjha@americares.org
[1]AmeriCares india Foundation, Mumbai, India
Full list of author information is available at the end of the article

Background

An estimated 240 million people globally are chronically infected with the hepatitis B virus (HBV), with a great deal of geographical variation in disease prevalence [1]. The World Health Organization (WHO) has reported that India's chronic HBV prevalence level is between 3 % and 4.2 % [2], while a recent systematic review found a lower prevalence level of approximately 1.5 % [3]. India appears to have lower chronic HBV prevalence than many countries in Asia and the Pacific, but the sheer size of the population translates into a large disease burden. To put the numbers in perspective, the 1.5 % prevalence estimate noted in the systematic review represents an infected population of more than 17 million [3].

It is estimated that approximately one million of the 26 million children born in India annually will develop chronic HBV infection in the course of their lives [4]. The natural history of the disease is such that acquiring HBV at birth or in childhood results in a higher chance of developing chronic infection compared to acquiring it in adulthood [1]. Based on the similar prevalence of infection in different age groups in the under-age-five population, a study in the outpatient department of a large hospital in India concluded that most of the hepatitis B cases encountered in the subjects were the result of vertical transmission [5]. Studies from different parts of India have put the HBsAg prevalence rate among pregnant women between 0.9 % and 3.1 % [6–8], suggesting that there is a considerable need for public health interventions aimed at protecting their offspring from infection.

Universal vaccination with screening of pregnant women plus the administration of hepatitis B immunoglobulin to the children of HBV-infected women at birth is the most effective strategy for reducing, and ultimately, eradicating hepatitis B, but insufficient financial resources and health system constraints prevent some countries from fully implementing this strategy. India introduced universal immunization against hepatitis B in 10 states in the year 2002, and in 2011, scaled up this intervention to target the entire country. WHO and UNICEF estimate that India had 8 % national coverage of hepatitis B birth-dose immunization in 2011, and that national coverage of the three-dose vaccine was 44 % in the same year [9]. Although pregnant women in India can undergo free HBV testing at government testing sites in major cities, those who learn that they have HBV may be unable to take measures to protect their newborns from infection as a result of financial barriers or other reasons.

In this context, AmeriCares India and United Way India collaborated to establish the PAHAL project to provide HBV prevention education in three slum communities in the Mumbai metropolitan area. The word *pahal,* which means "new beginning" in Hindi, was chosen because the project sought to promote community awareness of a disease that has received little attention from the Indian government and Indian medical community despite its heavy impact.

Slums in Mumbai are typically built illegally on government land, and sometimes on private land, and are characterized by a shortage of living space and inadequate water and sanitation facilities. PAHAL was planned as a comprehensive educational intervention to promote targeted hepatitis B screening, hepatitis B immunization, medical care and related interventions among women of childbearing age in slum communities, particularly pregnant women. Before the intervention, a survey was undertaken to determine what these populations already knew about hepatitis B. PAHAL planners also sought to establish whether women of childbearing age in the three targeted communities had similar or different needs in relation to HBV prevention education. This paper reports on the baseline survey that was conducted to inform decision-making about the PAHAL intervention.

Methods

Study setting and study population

The city of Mumbai is divided into three large informal geographical regions: the Island City (IS), the eastern suburbs (ES) and the western suburbs (WS). Since PAHAL was to be implemented in all three regions, one slum neighborhood from each region was chosen to serve as a study site. A female health worker was assigned to each slum. This person visited all lanes in the slum during the 1-year data collection period (April 2013 to April 2014). She approached every household in every lane to invite female residents of childbearing age to participate in the study. Women were eligible to participate if they were between the ages of 18 and 45 and were willing to provide oral consent. In households with more than one woman who met this requirement, only one woman was asked to participate. Usually the first woman who met the eligibility criteria was the one selected.

Data collection

The health workers collected data from study participants using a questionnaire that they administered as an interview in the local language, which is Hindi. The questionnaire was prepared in English and translated into Hindi, then checked using English back-translation. The study was piloted in a community similar to the study communities. Based on the pilot experience, researchers simplified the questionnaire. Several questions were deleted, most relating to risk factors, and other questions were modified. Researchers also made the decision to limit study participation to only one eligible woman from households with more than one member who met study inclusion criteria.

The questionnaire was made up of five sections. Section A was on demography (13 questions); section B, hepatitis B knowledge (4 questions); section C, personal risk related to hepatitis B (7 questions); section D, pregnancy and childbearing history (10 questions); and section E, details of most recent pregnancy (7 questions). With respect to hepatitis B knowledge, a screening question was first asked regarding whether the person had heard about hepatitis B. If the reply was yes, then the hepatitis B knowledge-related questions were asked. If the reply was no, the interviewer proceeded to the next section of the questionnaire. Information about the most recent pregnancy was collected only from women who had given birth within the previous 36 months. If a woman's youngest child was older than 36 months, the woman was not asked to respond to this section of the questionnaire.

At the time of the interview, study participants' names and addresses were entered in a register so that implementers of the planned hepatitis B prevention education program would be able to follow up with them at a later date. For data management purposes, each study participant was assigned an area code number and a unique identifying code, both of which were recorded on the paper study interview forms used by the health workers. No personal identifying information was recorded on the interview forms.

Data analysis

The same data entry operator entered all data from the interview forms into Microsoft Excel. A descriptive data analysis was performed using Microsoft Excel 2007 (Redmond, WA). Simple two-by-two tables were created and respondents' answers to survey questions were summed and expressed as percentages. For all but one section of the survey, disaggregated findings for the eastern suburbs, western suburbs and Island City were also reported. Responses to questions about hepatitis B knowledge were not disaggregated by geographical area because of the relatively small number of women who reported knowing about hepatitis B.

Research ethics

The health workers provided all prospective study participants with information about the study and about the hepatitis B prevention education program that was to be carried out in the community following the study. Before administering the questionnaire, the health workers obtained oral consent from women who agreed to be in the study. No identifying information was collected on the interview form. Following the interview, each study participant was given a leaflet in Hindi about hepatitis B and was invited to participate in the hepatitis B prevention education program that followed. Eligible women who did not want to be in the study were still given leaflets and invited to participate in the program. Since the study posed minimal risk to participants, no ethics committee was asked for formal approval.

Results

The health workers visited 11,527 households and conducted interviews with 6794 women. Among the completed interview forms submitted by the health workers, 6571 forms were found to be suitable for analysis.

Demographics of study participants

The participation of women in absolute numbers was lowest from eastern suburbs, followed by the western and then the Island city (ES = 28 %, WS = 34 %, IC = 38 %) (Table 1). Of all the women interviewed, more than 64 % were below the age of 30 years, the percentages being similar across all three areas (ES = 64 %, WS = 65 %, IC = 66 %). The vast majority (89 %) of the women were married (ES = 91 %, WS = 89 %, IC = 87 %); the lowest percentage of married women was from the Island City. A larger proportion (94 %) of women were not employed anywhere (ES = 89 %, WS = 94 %, IC = 96 %); the Island City had the largest percentage of women with no employment. Most women (87 %) reported that their highest level of schooling was below grade 12, with considerable variation between the eastern suburbs cohort and the other two cohorts (ES = 78 %, WS = 92 %, IC = 90 %). More than 20 % of women in the eastern suburbs reported that they had studied in college. A household size of three to five people was the most common; most households (83 %) had five or fewer members. More than a quarter of women from the eastern suburbs reported a household size larger than five, whereas a much smaller percentage reported this household size from the other regions (ES = 28.5 %, WS = 11.7 %, IC = 9.6 %). More than 84 % of households included only one woman aged 18–45. More than one-fifth of women in the eastern suburbs reported having more women of childbearing age in their households, while the other areas had fewer families with more than one woman of childbearing age (ES = 21.4 %, WS = 13.1 %, IC = 11.7 %).

Hepatitis B knowledge

Of all respondents who were asked whether they knew about hepatitis B, only 240 (4 %) replied in the affirmative (ES = 4 %, WS = 8 %, IC = 0.1 %). These 240 women were then asked further about modes of disease transmission, symptoms of acute HBV and conditions caused by chronic HBV (Table 2).

Table 1 Study participant demographics *(N:6571)*

	Total *N = 6571* *n*	Percentage	Eastern suburbs *N = 2238* *n (%)*	Western suburbs *N = 1808 n(%)*	Island City *N = 2525* *n (%)*
Age group					
≤20	728	11.1	257 (11.5)	154 (8.5)	317 (12.6)
21–25	1713	26.1	605 (27.0)	436 (24.1)	672 (26.6)
26–30	1807	27.5	616 (27.5)	506 (28.0)	685 (27.1)
31–35	1009	15.4	349 (15.6)	279 (15.4)	381 (15.1)
≥36	1314	20.0	411 (18.4)	433 (23.9)	470 (18.6)
Marital status					
Single	716	10.9	236 (10.6)	153 (8.5)	327 (13.0)
Married	5847	89.0	1999 (89.4)	1652 (91.4)	2196 (87.0)
Divorced	4	0.1	1 (0.0)	1 (0.1)	2 (0.1)
No response	4	0	2 (0.0)	2 (0.1)	0 (0.0)
Employment status					
Employed	417	6.3	232 (10.4)	99 (5.5)	85 (3.4)
Unemployed	6150	93.6	2003 (89.6)	1707 (94.5)	2438 (96.6)
No response	7	0.1	3 (0)	2 (0)	2 (0.1)
Highest level of education					
Did not attend school	576	8.8	254 (11.4)	89 (4.9)	233 (9.2)
Highest level of schooling was below grade 10	2603	39.6	461 (20.6)	1125 (62.3)	1015 (40.2)
Highest level of schooling was below grade 12	2551	38.8	1066 (47.7)	456 (25.2)	1028 (40.7)
Highest level of education was simple graduation or less (equivalent to three years in college)	838	12.8	453 (20.3)	136 (7.5)	249 (9.9)
No response	6	0	4 (0.1)	2 (0.1)	0 (0.0)
Household Size					
≤2	1019	15.5	155 (6.9)	352 (19.5)	511 (20.2)
3–5	4461	67.9	1444 (64.6)	1244 (68.8)	1771 (70.1)
6–8	908	13.8	523 (23.4)	173 (9.6)	212 (8.4)
≥9	183	2.8	114 (5.1)	38 (2.1)	31 (1.2)
No response	3	0	3 (0)	1 (0)	0 (0)
Number of women aged 18–45 in the household					
1	5555	84.6	1756 (78.5)	1571 (86.9)	2228 (88.2)
2	687	10.5	294 (13.1)	170 (9.4)	223 (8.8)
3	257	3.9	148 (6.6)	52 (2.9)	57 (2.3)
4	50	0.8	34 (1.5)	10 (0.6)	6 (0.2)
>4	19	0.3	4 (0.2)	4 (0.2)	11 (0.4)
No response	3	0	2 (0)	1 (0)	0 (0)

Hepatitis B transmission

Eighty-four percent of respondents knew that eating contaminated food does not cause hepatitis B. Transfusion of blood was identified correctly as a method of acquiring hepatitis B by 55 %. A smaller proportion (22 %) knew that hepatitis B can be transmitted through sexual contact and the same percentage was aware of its spread from a mother to her baby. Only 6 % of respondents knew that hepatitis B can be spread through tattooing or body piercing. The same small proportion of respondents was aware of the potential for hepatitis B to be transmitted by sharing needles or other injection equipment. No respondent correctly answered all six of the questions, and only four respondents correctly answered five of them.

Table 2 Hepatitis B knowledge ($N = 240$)

Do you know how hepatitis B spreads?	Yes	No	Do not know
Eating contaminated food*	10 %	84 %	6 %
Tattoo or body piercing	6 %	87 %	7 %
Sharing needles or other injection equipment	6 %	86 %	8 %
Transfusion of infected blood	55 %	40 %	4 %
Sexual contact	20 %	73 %	7 %
Mother-to-infant transmission during childbirth	20 %	73 %	6 %
** All "yes" answers in this section are correct with the exception of this one, for which "no" is the correct answer.*			
Do you know the symptoms of acute hepatitis B?†	Yes	No	Do not know
Weakness and fatigue	43 %	53 %	4 %
Loss of appetite	65 %	32 %	3 %
Nausea and vomiting	39 %	55 %	6 %
Upper abdominal discomfort	53 %	42 %	5 %.
Tea-coloured urine	46 %	50 %	5 %
Yellowing of skin	43 %	52 %	5 %
† All "yes" answers in this section are correct.			
Which of the following conditions may arise from chronic hepatitis B infection?‡	Yes	No	Do not know
Liver cirrhosis	14 %	78 %	8 %
Liver cancer	30 %	63 %	7 %
Liver failure	8 %	83 %	10 %
‡ All "yes" answers in this section are correct.			
Should a mother with hepatitis B breastfeed her baby?§	Yes	No	Do not know
	35 %	60 %	5 %
§ The correct answer is "yes."			

* All "yes" answers in this section are correct with the exception of this one, for which "no" is the correct answer
† All "yes" answers in this section are correct
‡ All "yes" answers in this section are correct
§ The correct answer is "yes"

Symptoms of hepatitis B

Sixty-five percent of respondents could identify the symptom of loss of appetite correctly, 53 % identified abdominal discomfort correctly, and 46 % knew about tea-colored urine. Less than half (43 %) were aware of the symptoms of weakness and fatigue, and the same percentage knew about yellowing of skin being a symptom in acute cases. Similarly, nausea/vomiting was identified as a symptom by only 39 % of the respondents. Twenty-one respondents (9 %) correctly identified all symptoms.

Complications of chronic hepatitis B infection

Thirty percent of respondents were aware that hepatitis B in its chronic phase can cause liver cancer, 14 % knew about liver cirrhosis and 8 % identified liver failure as a complication of the disease. Six respondents (3 %) gave correct answers regarding all three complications.

On being asked if they knew whether a hepatitis B-positive mother should breastfeed her baby, only 35 % of respondents correctly answered in the affirmative, whereas 60 % replied in the negative and 5 % did not know the answer.

Hepatitis B and most recent pregnancy

Only women whose youngest child was no older than 36 months were asked questions about their most recent pregnancy. A total of 739 (11.2 %) women met this condition (Table 3).

More than half of the 739 women had given birth to their last child in the previous year, while mothers of children older than age two formed a very small percentage of the cohort (2 %). Twenty-two percent of women reported that they had taken a hepatitis B test during pregnancy, with responses varying considerably across the three study areas (ES = 18 %, WS = 37 %, IC = 7 %). Among women who reported being tested for hepatitis B, two indicated that they were hepatitis B-positive.

A large majority of children (81 %) had been delivered in the city of Mumbai, with the highest percentage from

Table 3 Pregnancy behavior among women[a] ($N = 739$)

	Total number n (%)	Eastern suburbs n (%)	Western suburbs n (%)	Island City n (%)
Age of most recent child				
12 months or less	440 (60)	144 (62)	168 (60)	128 (56)
13–24 months	281 (38)	87 (37)	110 (40)	84 (37)
25–36 months	18 (2)	3 (1)	0 (0)	15 (7)
Tested for hepatitis B during pregnancy?				
Yes	162 (22)	43 (18)	103 (37)	16 (7)
No	267 (36)	165 (71)	73 (26)	29 (13)
No reply	310 (42)	26 (11)	102 (37)	182 (80)
Hepatitis B status of those tested ($N = 162$)				
Positive	2 (1)	2 (5)	0	0
Negative	158 (98)	41 (95)	103 (100)	14 (88)
Not known	2 (1)	0	0	2 (12)

[a]Women who reported giving birth within the previous 36 months

Island City (ES = 71 %, WS = 84 %, IC = 89 %) (Table 4). Eighty-one percent of women reported that their children had received the first dose of the hepatitis B vaccine before leaving the hospital as newborns. Island City stood apart from the other two study sites in regard to this question, with only 56 % of Island City women reporting administration of the first dose, while 44 % did not know what their child's vaccination status had been upon leaving the hospital. Seventy percent of children went on to receive three complete doses of the vaccine, according to their mothers' reports. The eastern suburbs had the highest level of vaccination, and Island City, the lowest (ES = 84 %, WS = 74 %, IC = 52 %). A large proportion (43 %) of Island City mothers were unaware of the current vaccination state of their children.

Discussion

The present study was conducted to assess HBV knowledge levels among women of childbearing age in three Mumbai slums in order to help determine how their HBV-related needs should be addressed through a prevention education program. Among 6571 study participants who were asked if they knew about this disease, less than five percent answered yes. The 240 women in this subset demonstrated high levels of correct knowledge about some modes of transmission and disease

Table 4 Hepatitis B vaccination status of children[a] as reported by their mothers ($N = 739$)

	Total number n (%)	Eastern suburbs n (%)	Western suburbs n (%)	Island City n (%)
Place of delivery				
Mumbai	602 (81)	165 (71)	234 (84)	203 (89)
Outside	103 (14)	61 (26)	22 (8)	20 (9)
No answer	34 (5)	8 (3)	22 (8)	4 (2)
Newborn hepatitis B vaccination status upon leaving hospital				
Vaccinated before leaving hospital	599 (81)	216 (92)	257 (92)	126 (56)
Not vaccinated before leaving hospital	4 (1)	4 (2)	0 (0)	0 (0)
Do not know	119 (16)	9 (4)	10 (4)	100 (44)
No reply	17 (2)	5 (2)	11 (4)	1 (0)
Child's current hepatitis B vaccination status				
Three complete doses	520 (70)	197 (84)	206 (74)	117 (52)
Partially vaccinated	80 (11)	18 (8)	51 (18)	11 (5)
Do not know	122 (17)	14 (6)	10 (4)	98 (43)
No reply	17 (2)	5 (2)	11 (4)	1 (0)

[a]Children born within the previous 36 months

symptoms, but low levels of correct knowledge about other modes of transmission and disease symptoms. Small proportions of this subset knew that chronic hepatitis B may cause liver cancer, liver cirrhosis and liver failure. Less than one-quarter of 739 study participants with children aged 36 months or younger reported undergoing a hepatitis B test during pregnancy. On the other hand, more than two-thirds of women indicated that their children had received the recommended three doses of HBV vaccine.

Other studies conducted in various populations elsewhere in India and around the world have revealed less than optimal awareness of hepatitis B and the presence of misconceptions about the disease [10–14]. For example, a study conducted among 430 women of childbearing age in rural Pakistan reported that less than half of women had correct knowledge about HBV vaccination, with especially poor knowledge among women of lower socioeconomic status [14]. Our study results further substantiate concerns about a lack of public awareness and knowledge being a major driver of ongoing mother-to-child transmission of HBV globally, while at the same time indicating a need for setting-specific interventions in Mumbai. Consideration should be given to investigating reasons for the lack of knowledge about HBV within our study communities, including whether different health care providers might have different approaches to communicating with women about how to protect themselves and their children from HBV.

There was more correct knowledge about some modes of HBV transmission than others in our study population. Only one-fifth of women knew about sexual contact as a mode of transmission, and the same proportion knew that infants could acquire HBV from infected mothers during childbirth. Also important from a program planning perspective was the finding that more than half of women wrongly thought that a mother with hepatitis B should not breastfeed her baby. Given the poor breastfeeding numbers prevalent in urban areas, especially Mumbai [15], inaccurate beliefs of this nature are potentially harmful to an already at-risk newborn's health. HBV prevention education thus also serves as an opportunity to contribute to the broader child health agenda.

Our study findings raised additional concerns about the nature of the HBV prevention efforts in India. Only 22 % of study participants with children aged 36 months or younger indicated that they had been tested for hepatitis B during pregnancy. Seventy percent of the same subset of women indicated that their children had received three doses of hepatitis B vaccine, but reported vaccination levels varied greatly across the three study areas. The World Health Organization recommends administering the first dose of HBV vaccine to all newborns within 24 h of birth regardless of their mothers' HBV status [16]. Furthermore, the likelihood of the hepatitis B vaccine schedule being completed—along with other immunizations—is found to improve when vaccination is initiated at birth [17]. Study results thus suggest that there is considerable work to be done in terms of making women more aware of testing procedures and the implications of the results, along with accepted recommendations for vaccination. This is particularly true in Island City, where the largest proportion (56 %) of mothers with children under 12 months reside. At the same time, other types of research are needed to acquire insight into the roles of health service providers in facilitating or hindering the uptake of HBV screening and prevention recommendations by women during pregnancy and delivery and afterwards.

Study limitations

The survey was conducted for the express purpose of determining community needs in relation to a planned HBV education intervention and also to gauge the size of the potential target audience for the intervention. It was not designed with scientific publishing in mind. No systematic sampling was carried out, as the mandate was to include all willing subjects in the target group. Although care was taken to train the health workers in administering the survey questions, there may have been some observer bias. Additionally, since the survey was administered over a year-long period, there may have been some information transfer from the women surveyed earlier to those surveyed later. The study was a simple survey to assess knowledge levels. It did not include a data analysis plan to test for statistical significance; the absolute information obtained was used to inform the activities of the project. Although sociodemographic information was collected, survey findings were not analyzed on the basis of age or education levels. Further research may be able to throw light on the relevance of these variables in designing HBV education interventions.

The information obtained regarding whether study participants were tested for hepatitis B during pregnancy was not, in most cases, supported by actual evidence in the form of the test reports. Similarly, in the absence of vaccination cards for verification, information on the percentage of childhood vaccinations administered was also as per the mother's memory and comprehension. The likelihood of misreporting may have been reduced because interviewers sought to help study respondents avoid confusing the hepatitis B vaccine and the bacille Calmette-Guerin vaccine by describing the injection site (the left lateral thigh, for the former, or the left deltoid, for the latter).

Conclusion

Despite the availability of a safe HBV vaccine that is free for newborns and infants in many parts of India, preventing mother-to-child transmission of HBV remains a major challenge. Low awareness of HBV among women of childbearing age in Mumbai-area slums indicates a need for educational interventions targeting this population. Additional research is needed to further elucidate the barriers to implementing key HBV control measures, such as screening pregnant women and achieving universal HBV vaccination coverage, including administration of the first dose of vaccine within 24 h of birth.

Abbreviations

ES: eastern suburbs; IC: Island City; HBsAg: hepatitis B surface antigen; HBV: hepatitis B virus; UNICEF: The United Nations Children's Fund; WHO: World Health Organization; WS: western suburbs.

Competing interests

The authors declare that they have no competing interets.

Authors' contributions

SJ took part in the conception, design, acquisition of data, data analysis, and was the primary person in drafting the manuscript. DD took part in the conception, design and analysis of the data. SB took part in the analysis of data. All authors read and approved the final manuscript. SD was involved in the conception and design of the program.

Acknowledgements

We thank the HMAP journal and the BMSF for bringing out the supplement featuring work of BMSF grantees.We especially thank Prof. Jeffrey Lazarus of the HMAP for his team's invaluable help with the editing of the manuscript. We gratefully acknowledge the support of Bristol-Myers Squibb Foundation for its support through the entire program. Last but not the least, we want to thank all the field workers and staff related to the PAHAL project for tirelessly working to make this study and the resultant work possible.

Financial support

This work was a part of the project supported by the Bristol-Myers Squibb Foundation (grant #1204).

Author details

[1]AmeriCares india Foundation, Mumbai, India. [2]AmeriCares, Stamford, CT, USA.

References

1. World Health Organization. Guidelines for the prevention, care and treatment of persons with chronic hepatitis B infection. 2015. http://apps.who.int/iris/bitstream/10665/154590/1/9789241549059_eng.pdf?ua=1&ua=1. Accessed 28 Dec 2015.
2. World Health Organization Regional Office for South-East Asia. Regional strategy for the prevention and control of viral hepatitis. 2013. http://www.searo.who.int/entity/emerging_diseases/topics/CD_282.pdf. Accessed 28 Dec 2015.
3. Schweitzer A, Horn J, Mikolajczyk RT, Krause G, Ott JJ. Estimations of worldwide prevalence of chronic hepatitis B virus infection: a systematic review of data published between 1965 and 2013. Lancet. 2015;386(10003):1546–55. doi:10.1016/S0140-6736(15)61412-X. Epub 2015 Jul 28.
4. Ministry of Health and Family Welfare, Government of India. Operational guidelines for Hepatitis B vaccine introduction in UIP. 2011. http://www.searo.who.int/india/topics/routine_immunization/Operational_Guidelines_for_HepatitisB_vaccine_introduction_in_UIP_2011.pdf?ua=1. Accessed 28 Dec 2015.
5. Chakravarti A, Rawat D, Jain M. A study on the perinatal transmission of the hepatitis B virus. Indian J Med Microbiol. 2005;23(2):128 30.
6. Pande C, Sarin SK, Patra S. Prevalence, risk factors and virological profile of chronic hepatitis B virus infection in pregnant women in India. J Med Virol. 2011;83:962–7. http://www.ncbi.nlm.nih.gov/pubmed/21503907. Accessed 28 Dec 2015.
7. Dwivedi M, Misra SP, Misra V, Pandey A, Pant S, Singh R, et al. Seroprevalence of hepatitis B infection during pregnancy and risk of perinatal transmission. Indian J Gastroenterol. 2011;30:66–71.
8. Khakhkhar VM, Bhuva PJ, Bhuva SP, Patel CP, Cholera MS. Sero- prevalence of hepatitis B amongst pregnant women attending the antenatal clinic of a tertiary care hospital, Jamnagar (Gujrat). Natl J Med Res. 2012;2(3):362–5.
9. World Health Organization. India: WHO and UNICEF estimates of immunization coverage: 2014 revision. http://www.who.int/immunization/monitoring_surveillance/data/ind.pdf. Accessed 28 Dec 2015.
10. Taylor VM, Jackson JC, Chan N, Kuniyuki A, Yasui Y. Hepatitis B knowledge and practices among Cambodian American women in Seattle, Washington. J Community Health. 2002;27(3):151–63.
11. Gulfareen H, Ambreen H. Awareness of women regarding hepatitis B. J Ayub Med Coll Abbottabad. 2008;20(4):141–4.
12. Misra B, Panda C, Das HS, Nayak KC, Singh SP. Study on awareness about Hepatitis B viral infection in coastal Eastern India. Hep B Annual. 2009;6:19–28.
13. Pathoumthong K, Khampanisong P, Quet F, Latthaphasavang V, Souvong V, Buisson Y. Vaccination status, knowledge and awareness towards hepatitis B among students of health professions in Vientiane, Lao PDR. Vaccine. 2014; 32:4993–9.
14. Noreen N, Kumar R, Shaikh BT. Knowledge about hepatitis B vaccination among women of childbearing age: a cross-sectional study from a rural district of Punjab, Pakistan. East Mediterr Health J. 2015;21(2):22. -26,129–33.
15. District level household and facility survey IV: Mumbai Suburban. https://nrhm-mis.nic.in/DLHS4/State%20and%20District%20Factsheets/Maharasthra/District%20Factsheets/Mumbai%20Suburban.pdf. Accessed 28 Dec 2015.
16. World Health Organization. Hepatitis B vaccines. Wkly Epidemiol Rec. 2009; 84(40):405–20.
17. Yusuf HR, Daniels D, Smith P, Coronado V, Rodewald L. Association between administration of hepatitis B vaccine at birth and completion of the hepatitis B and 4:3:1:3 vaccine series. JAMA. 2000;284:978–83.

17

Hepatitis C in Eastern Europe and Central Asia: a survey of epidemiology, treatment access and civil society activity in eleven countries

Ludmila Maistat[1*], Natalija Kravchenko[1] and Amulya Reddy[2]

Abstract

Introduction: The 16 countries of the Eastern Europe and Central Asia (EECA) region are home to 6.6 million people in need of treatment for chronic hepatitis C virus (HCV) infection. Because of transformational change in HCV treatment, global efforts to address HCV are accelerating. Given its large regional burden, the EECA needs to ensure its inclusion in and benefit from any new developments.

Methods: Our 2015–16 survey aimed to collect and report on epidemiology, treatment access (including drug registration and prices, national HCV guidelines and treatment program coverage) and pertinent civil society organization (CSO) activities in 11 countries in the EECA.

Results: Major gaps in epidemiological data exist; reported anti-HCV prevalence ranged from 1.5 to 7.5% for the general population, 22.7 to 70–95% for people who inject drugs (PWID) and 18 to 80% for people living with HIV (PLHIV). Ten countries (91% of the sample) have registered one or more of the second-generation, direct-acting antiviral medications (DAA) for potential interferon-free treatment. However, intellectual property issues and prices limit access to these drugs. In 2014, HCV programs in the surveyed countries covered only 0.15% of the total number of people in need of treatment. CSO-driven, international donor-funded programs are starting to fulfill needs of PWID and PLHIV.

Conclusions: As feasible curative HCV treatment is now available, and given the significant regional disease burden, EECA countries need to ensure HCV surveillance and DAA availability at affordable prices in order to expand treatment and prevent the onward transmission of the infection. EECA CSOs have demonstrated their capacity to play a crucial role in advancing HCV issues, and they should continue leveraging these issues for the benefit of individual patients and public health in general.

Keywords: Hepatitis C, Civil society, Access to treatment, Direct-acting antivirals, Treatment, Vulnerable groups, Eastern Europe and Central Asia

* Correspondence: maistat@aph.org.ua
[1]Alliance for Public Health, Kiev, Ukraine
Full list of author information is available at the end of the article

Background

According to a 2014 (updated in 2015, 2016 and 2017) systematic review, the 16 countries of Eastern Europe and Central Asia (EECA) are home to approximately 11.3 million people who are antibody-positive for the hepatitis C virus (HCV). HCV antibody positive (anti-HCV) prevalence estimates are 3.3% for Eastern Europe and 5.4% for Central Asia, respectively [1]. The EECA region represents almost 10% of the total global anti-HCV positive population of approximately 115 million people. Based on the estimated regional viremia prevalence of 2.5%, 6.6 million people are in need of treatment for chronic HCV. Because HCV is a blood-borne pathogen, people who inject drugs (PWID) are disproportionately affected globally. In the EECA, prevalence estimates among PWID are as high as 90% in some regional cohorts [2, 3]. HCV is known to have mutually detrimental effects with the human immunodeficiency virus (HIV) in co-infected individuals, including increased risk of death from acquired immunodeficiency syndrome and early-onset advanced liver disease. The EECA has low antiretroviral therapy (ART) coverage, estimated at 21%. This makes people living with HIV (PLHIV) in this region particularly vulnerable [4–8].

In recent years, several important developments have increased attention to viral hepatitis in general and to HCV in particular. In May 2014, the World Health Assembly, the decision-making body of the World Health Organization (WHO), passed a resolution committing WHO and its Member States to urgent action on the prevention, diagnosis and treatment of viral hepatitis. This followed the April 2014 publication of the first *WHO Guidelines for the Screening, Care and Treatment of Persons with Hepatitis C Infection*, a multi-organizational collaboration with a focus on low- and middle-income countries (LMICs) [9, 10]. Major international donors (e.g. the Global Fund, Open Society Foundations and Unitaid) are now supporting HCV programs on a much larger scale, including in EECA countries [11–13]..

Transformational change in HCV treatment is an impetus to action: new direct-acting antivirals (DAAs) allow all-oral curative protocols of significantly shorter duration. DAAs obviate the need for lengthy parenteral interferon (IFN) schedules and the extensive auxiliary resources they entail. The rapidly moving pipeline has already introduced second generation DAAs and has withdrawn first generation products. Nonetheless, DAA accessibility and costs remain major issues [14, 15]. Prices, which have been as high as 84,000 USD for a 12-week sofosbuvir course, have headlined extensive media coverage and stakeholder discussions, including United States Senate hearings [16–19].

Global efforts to address HCV diagnosis and treatment are accelerating and, given the large regional disease burden, the EECA needs to ensure its inclusion in and benefit from any new developments. EECA civil society organizations (CSOs) have already demonstrated notable achievement in the HCV arena. Greater involvement of CSOs will be a powerful force for reaching more people in need of services.

In our survey, we queried 17 CSOs in 11 EECA countries: Armenia, Azerbaijan, Belarus, Georgia, Kazakhstan, Kyrgyzstan, Moldova, Russia, Tajikistan, Ukraine and Uzbekistan. Our objective was to elucidate and report on HCV epidemiology, treatment access (including drug registration and prices, national HCV guidelines and treatment program coverage) and pertinent CSO activities. In this summary article, we report and discuss key results of this survey and propose recommendations for further action.

Methods

Between March and April 2015, the Alliance for Public Health (Alliance, Ukraine) in collaboration with the Saint Petersburg-based ITPCru (International Treatment Preparedness Coalition) surveyed 17 CSOs in the 11 aforementioned EECA countries [20, 21]. Given the fast-changing HCV arena, the survey was repeated between March and September 2016 to update information.

Participant countries were selected between November and December 2014 on the basis of their membership on the EECA Community Advisory Board, which engages in viral hepatitis treatment access activism [22]. CSOs were chosen based on their experience in hepatitis and HIV advocacy in their respective countries. The survey instrument contained nine open-ended questions with sub-questions covering country-level HCV epidemiology among the general population, PWID and PLHIV, availability and content of HCV treatment guidelines, government and donor-funded HCV program coverage, and CSO activities. Blank tables were included for listing of HCV epidemiology data, testing, care and prevention strategies, drug registration and prices. We conducted Skype or telephone interviews with all participants to follow up on written responses, particularly regarding CSO activities.

We cross-referenced data obtained from CSOs with open-source information wherever available. We used national-source 2016 total population numbers, European Association for the Study of the Liver (EASL) and WHO HCV treatment protocols and calculated prices using June 2016 USD-local currency exchange rates listed on the www.cal-c.ru website unless respondents provided USD amounts. Additional patent information was obtained from WHO and the Initiative for Medicine, Access and Knowledge analyses and from CSOs involved in activities such as patent opposition (e.g. in Russia, Ukraine) [23–25]..

Results

Between one and three CSOs in each EECA country received the questionnaire on epidemiology, treatment access (drug registration and prices, national HCV guidelines and

Table 1 HCV prevalence data by country

Country (2016 total population)	National anti-HCV prevalence estimate (%)	Adult anti-HCV prevalence Gower, et al. (%)	Estimated number of anti-HCV+ people	Estimated anti-HCV prevalence among PWID (%)	Estimated anti-HCV prevalence among PLHIV (%)	Key populations specified
Armenia (2994400)	4		120,000	52.1	17.9	Migrants, PWID
Azerbaijan (9705600)	3.2	3.1	300,800	62.8	5.9	PWID
Belarus (9498700)	2–3	1.3	250,000	70–95		PWID
Georgia (3720400)	7.5		208,800	57–74	4.8	PWID, MSM, healthcare workers
Kazakhstan (17753200)	1.5–3	3.3	255,000–510,000	% not available (estimated 6049 people)	4.5	
Kyrgyzstan (6019500)	4	2.5	220,000	45.2	80	
Moldova (3553100)	1.7–4	4.5	60,000–142,000	35.3–65.4	4.6	PWID
Russia (146544710)	4	4.1	5,900,000	69	27	PWID
Tajikistan (8547000)	2.3	3.1	200,000	22.7–49.3	25.6% among HIV+ PWID	PWID
Ukraine (42708647)	5		2,135,000	55		PWID; hemophiliacs, hemodialysis patients; MSM; PMTCT clients
Uzbekistan (31575300)	6.5		1,800,000	36		Healthcare workers, PWID, patients receiving invasive treatment

Table 2 Direct-acting antiviral drug registration in surveyed countries (September 2016)

Country	sofosbuvir	sofosbuvir generic	sofosbuvir/ ledipasvir	sofosbuvir/ ledipasvir generic	daclatasvir	daclatasvir generic	ombitasvir/ paritaprevir/ ritonavir/ dasabuvir (Viekira Pak)	ombitasvir/ paritaprevir/ ritonavir	dasabuvir	simeprevir	asunaprevir	narlaprevir	boceprivir	telaprevir
Armenia													Yes	Yes
Azerbaijan		Yes				pending	Yes						Yes	Yes
Belarus							Yes						Yes	Yes
Georgia	Yes		Yes			pending							Yes	Yes
Kazakhstan			pending				Yes			Yes			Yes	Yes
Kyrgyzstan		Yes	Yes	Yes		pending								
Moldova		Yes						Yes	Yes	Yes			Yes	Yes
Russia	Yes				Yes		Yes			Yes	Yes	Yes	Yes	Yes
Tajikistan		Yes												
Ukraine	Yes	Yes	Yes			pending	Yes	Yes	Yes	Yes			Yes	Yes
Uzbekistan		Yes								humanitarian			Yes	

treatment program coverage) and pertinent activities; the response rate was 17/17 (100%).

The submitted HCV prevalence data (Table 1) show a general national population anti-HCV prevalence range of 1.5 to 7.5%, with Kazakhstan and Georgia having the lowest and highest rates, respectively. Using 2016 population figures from national sources, total numbers of HCV-positive people are highest in Russia (5.9 million), Uzbekistan (1.8 million) and Ukraine (2.1 million). Prevalence among PWID ranges from 22.7% (Tajikistan) to 70–95% (Belarus). Since only small studies were available, ranges are shown for Belarus, Georgia, Moldova and Tajikistan. For PLHIV, prevalence ranges from 17.9% (Armenia) to 80% (Kyrgyzstan). PWID are specified as a key population in nine countries (82%); healthcare workers and patients undergoing invasive/hospital-level procedures are specified in three (27%).

With respect to treatment access, one or more second generation DAAs are registered in 10 (91%) of 11 countries (Table 2). This includes generic sofosbuvir in six countries, combination sofosbuvir/ledipasvir in three countries and combination ombitasvir/paritaprevir/ritonavir/dasabuvir in six. For daclatasvir, the original product is registered in Russia; generic registration is pending in Kyrgyzstan; and generic manufacture and sale without royalty payments will occur in Azerbaijan, Georgia and Ukraine under an agreement between Bristol-Myers Squibb and the Medicines Patent Pool. Simeprevir is registered in five countries and available through a humanitarian aid program in Uzbekistan.

The first generation DAAs boceprivir and telaprivir, which are no longer recommended, are registered in nine (82%) and eight (73%) countries, respectively. Additionally, older pegylated interferon (PEG-IFN) original and/or biosimilar products are available in all countries.

Reported DAA prices vary among countries and procurement sources (public and private). Twelve-week generic sofosbuvir treatment price ranges in cost from USD 780 in Kyrgyzstan to USD 2805 in Ukraine; donor-supported supported programs lead by the Government in Georgia and run by ICF "Alliance for Public Health" in Ukraine are simultaneously providing it free of charge. Combination ombitasvir/paritaprevir/ritonavir/dasabuvir costs USD 16,749 per 12-week course in Belarus. A 12-week course of originator simeprevir ranges from USD 9840 (Russia) to USD 25,407 (Moldova). Armenia, Belarus, Kazakhstan, Kyrgyzstan, Russia, Ukraine and Uzbekistan reported "buyers' clubs" that arrange "personal-use" importation of primarily Indian and Egyptian generic sofosbuvir, sofosbuvir/ledipasvir and daclatasvir for their members. Prices for sofosbuvir obtained through the "buyers' club" range from 465 USD per 12-week course in Belarus and Ukraine (versus USD 2805 for registered generic in the latter) and USD 390/12-week course in Uzbekistan (versus USD 825 for registered generic). Table 3 shows lowest available September 2016 prices by country.

PEG-IFN is still used for treatment of HCV in some countries, prices range from USD 3038 to USD 13,300 for a 48-week course, with ribavirin ranging from USD 250 to 3500.

Additional activities to improve treatment access were reported: Sofosbuvir patent opposition is in progress in Russia and Ukraine. Kyrgyzstan has amended its laws on intellectual property to better accommodate trade-related aspects of intellectual property rights (TRIPS). DAA patents have been issued for daclatasvir and simprevir by the Eurasian Patent Organization (EAPO), which includes Armenia, Azerbaijan, Belarus, Kazakhstan, Kyrgyzstan, Russia, Tajikistan and Turkmenistan; for ABT-450, daclatasvir, simeprevir and sofosbuvir by Russia; and for ombitasvir by Ukraine.

HCV treatment guidelines are available in nine countries (82%). Armenia has an adapted WHO version of guidelines for only HCV-HIV co-infection, and Tajikistan reported using the Russian guidelines. PEG-IFN is listed as a first-line medication in all existing EECA guidelines. Kazakhstan, Moldova, Russia and Ukraine also include first-generation DAAs that are no longer recommended. Georgia added sofosbuvir with the launch of its donor-funded program in 2015 and is in the process of updating its national guidelines, as are Azerbaijan and Belarus.

Regarding access to HCV treatment services, in 2014, programs covered a regional total of 10,000 people (0.15% of the total 6.6 million estimated in need of treatment), mainly in Kazakhstan and Russia, using IFN-based regimens. In 2015, donor-funded programs using combination DAA-IFN protocols were

Table 3 Lowest direct-acting antiviral drug prices in surveyed countries - USD per 12-week course (September 2016)

Country	sofosbuvir generic	sofosbuvir generic 'buyers' club'	ombitasvir/ paritaprevir/ dasabuvir/ ritonavir	simeprevir	daclatasvir	asunaprevir
Azerbaijan	1011		15,000	7200		
Belarus		465	16,749			
Kyrgyzstan	780					
Russia		360	13,770	9840	5556	558
Ukraine	2805	465				
Uzbekistan	825	390				

Table 4 Civil society organization HCV activity summary

Category	Activities			
Awareness raising	National campaigns to inform decision makers and the general public	Patient 'schools' on access to treatment and other HCV issues	Media notices on HCV	Educational videos
Mobilization	Establishing networks of individuals and organizations to advocate HCV issues	Implementing letter writing/petition signing campaigns, e.g. a 'Treatment Waiting List' and lower price requests to pharmaceutical companies	Organizing research and reporting on HCV needs	Organizing CSOs to meet with pharmaceutical companies
Advocacy	Encouraging national treatment programs and guideline development	Organizing campaigns aiming to bring about favorable policy and response from governments, industry and donors	Negotiating lower prices with pharmaceutical companies	Specific opposition to pharmaceutical patent applications and support for alternate licensing
Testing and treatment	Conducting screening test campaigns to identify HCV- antibody positive people (that also raise awareness and provide evidence for advocacy)	Implementing treatment programs integrated into existing services, particularly for the disproportionately affected/marginalized, e.g. PWID	Seeking donor funding for expanded treatment programs using updated protocols	Providing community-level and technical input on national program planning and guideline committees

EECA Civil Society Involvement in HCV Work

expected to cover 5000 people in Georgia and 1500 in Ukraine. Gilead Sciences, Inc. (developer of sofosbuvir) reportedly plans future expansion to provide 20,000 treatment courses per year in Georgia [26].

CSO activities included HCV awareness raising, mobilization, advocacy, testing and treatment to promote patient rights and appropriate policy and service provision. Formal evaluation/quantitative results were generally not available. Activities are categorized and highlighted in Tables 4 and 5.

Discussion

Chronic untreated HCV infection progresses to conditions such as cirrhosis and hepatocellular carcinoma, which eventually lead to death. Despite an overall decline in new infection incidence globally, mortality due to chronic HCV is still high and may increase in coming years due to existing high infection rates and lack of connection to diagnosis and treatment [27, 28]. However, with treatment, chronic HCV infection is curable [29, 30]. Different combinations of available DAAs allow oral, IFN-free treatment for different HCV genotypes, while the new sofosbuvir/velpatasvir is pan-genotype [31, 32]. DAAs, especially broad coverage/pan-genotype combinations, simplify chronic HCV infection diagnosis and treatment such that it can be delivered through a range of service platforms to increase accessibility for PWID, PLHIV and the general population in comparison to complicated IFN-based protocols. DAA treatment has also been shown to have a reduced cost when compared to long-term treatment of chronic HCV infection complications [33, 34]. Thus, access to DAAs is particularly important for EECA countries with high HCV burdens. Our survey has identified specific information gaps as well as valuable knowledge, which can be utilized in EECA countries to advance DAA-based HCV treatment towards national and global hepatitis control objectives.

In the 11 countries we surveyed, HCV epidemiological data that is required to define response and plan services, including commodities procurement, are lacking. Anti-HCV prevalence data are more often available while HCV viremia confirmation data, as well as details on genotyping and staging, are less forthcoming. Georgia is an exception with its comprehensive prevalence surveys and viremia confirmation testing protocols. Overall, the data submitted by CSOs in this survey are consistent with cited regional estimates, i.e. anti-HCV prevalence in Eastern Europe is 3.3% (range 1.6–4.5%) and is 5.4 (range 3.5–6.8%) in Central Asia. The infection prevalence rates among PWID and PLHIV are, as expected, consistently higher than general population rates [1]. Survey data support the hypothesis that initial decision-making based on published estimates is a reasonable starting point to fill epidemiological information gaps.

Table 5 Selected civil society organization HCV activity examples

Category	Activity	Organization(s) involved	Results and/or comments
Awareness raising	National campaign using mass media and celebrities in Georgia	Concerted effort by Georgian Harm Reduction Network, OSF Georgia, Georgia CAB, Medecins du Monde, Hepa+, New Vector and others	Large-scale treatment program implemented
	"Demand treatment!" campaign in Ukraine	Concerted effort of 90 CSOs led by Alliance for Public Health	Community-level HCV screening to document prevalence; subsequent national and regionally/locally-funded HCV treatment programs
Mobilization	HCV advocacy and policy brief research and dissemination in 11 countries	Eurasian Harm Reduction Network; Kyrgyz Harm Reduction Network; Andrey Rylkov Foundation (Russia; Treatment Preparedness Coalition (Russia); Alliance for Public Health	Evidence compiled for awareness-raising and advocacy activities
	Drug registration, pricing, clinical trial and early access issue negotiation at EECA level	EECACommunity Adivsory Board meetings addressing AbbVie, BMS, Gilead, Janssen and Merck Sharp & Dohme	Inclusion of simeprevir on the Russian "List of Vital and Essential Medicines" and removal of telapravir, which was included due to industry price reduction (market segmentation) despite being obsolete
Advocacy	DAA price reduction negotiation in Ukraine	Alliance for Public Health	USD 750 for a 12-week sofosbuvir course; USD 900 for a 12-week sofosbuvir/ledipasvir course
	National treatment guideline modification and program endorsement advocacy neogtiations		Inclusion of DAAs in national treatment guidelines and establishment of a national and over 15 regional treatment programs; government procurement of sofosbuvir
Testing and treatment	HCV treatment for HIV-HCV coinfected PWID implementation in harm reduction programs in Ukraine	Alliance for Public Health	Global Fund support and DAAprice reduction (above) obtained
	Contribution to national HCV guideline development/revision and strategic planning	Multiple CSOs inAzerbaijan, Georgia, Kazakhstan, Kyrgyzstan, Moldova and Ukraine	Supports appropriate policy and program implementation

All surveyed countries need to address DAA registration and pricing promptly in order to implement HCV treatment per current international guidelines. The rapid pace at which products are introduced leaves registration lagging. At the same time, pharmaceutical company maneuvers, such as market segmentation with telaprevir and simprevir in Russia (Table 5), have caused further delay in the establishment of affordable optimal treatment protocols. Patented products and their associated high prices also act as barriers to access as exemplified in Russia, where sofosbuvir patent opposition is in progress and only buyers' club supplies are available at this time. Countries must negotiate with manufacturers for voluntary licensing agreements (which the Medicines Patent Pool can facilitate) and the key TRIPS flexibility of compulsory licensing as needed to facilitate generic production, which has been projected to cost as little as USD 100–250 per 12-week DAA treatment course with two or three drug combinations [35–37].

There has been progress in the past year based on the first and second rounds of our survey, with more countries registering second generation DAAs. Notably, the majority now have an IFN-free DAA regimen option for most HCV genotypes. Several surveyed countries also achieved increased availability of generic DAAs and lower prices, albeit some through personal use imports via buyers' clubs. Generic daclatasvir manufacture in several EECA countries has been agreed upon with Medicines Patent Pool involvement. In Ukraine, successful negotiations with manufacturers yielded prices much closer to projected targets – sofosbuvir is USD 750 and sofosbuvir/ledipasvir is USD 900 per 12-week course (Table 5).

A survey of HCV guidelines in the participating countries indicated that there are generally guidelines for first-line treatment with IFN- and/or first generation DAA-based protocols. WHO, EASL and the American Association for the Study of Liver Diseases all recommend second-generation oral DAA-based regimens [10, 23, 38]. Up-to-date national guidelines will underpin policy and program development and anticipate appropriate drug registration and supply. Countries should seek technical support as needed to stay up-to-date with current knowledge; for example, CSOs have recently been an important source of expertise in Azerbaijan, Georgia, Kazakhstan, Kyrgyzstan, Moldova and Ukraine.

Treatment programs in the surveyed countries have had minimal coverage rates, i.e. a total of 0.15% of the population in need in 2014. Donor-supported programs in Georgia and Ukraine are introducing second-generation DAAs. While these services currently target the disproportionately affected, they can also serve as examples for healthcare workers, hospital-treated patients and other groups who are at risk for iatrogenic HCV transmission in settings of suboptimal infection control such as those of the EECA and other LMIC healthcare systems. Substantial treatment program scale-up through domestic and international collaboration is needed. Implementation partners who can expand their services by integration of HCV care into existing platforms can fulfill priority needs with the added advantage of established knowledge of and acceptance from "hard-to-reach" and high-risk people, as seen in Ukrainian harm reduction programs.

CSOs in the surveyed countries have executed awareness raising and advocacy campaigns that have gathered HCV data and improved treatment access in terms of increased DAA availability, reduced medication prices, updated guidelines and expanded services. EECA CSOs should also capitalize on global experience with HIV ART patent opposition and price reduction that has informed HCV activities in Brazil, Egypt, the European Union and India, where as a result, one DAA patent has been revoked. Based on survey information, recommendations for further CSO action are listed in Table 6.

Conclusions

Highly effective curative HCV treatment is now available, and given the significant regional burden, EECA

Table 6 Recommendations for stakeholders

Based on this survey, we recommend that CSOs:

- conduct HCV epidemiology studies in key populations;
- integrate HCV services in PWID and PLHIV programs;
- monitor PWID access to HCV treatment; document, disseminate and, if appropriate, pursue legal and media options for any cases of service denial;
- advocate for inclusion of PWID in national HCV guidelines and programs;
- advocate for HCV medication price reductions through stakeholders and the media;
- monitor the drug registration landscape and maintain pressure on pharmaceutical companies and governments for prompt registration of new drugs;
- partner with international organizations to oppose barriers and leverage TRIPS flexibilities;
- work with governments on regulatory measures to ensure lower prices for generics;
- advocate for government disclosure of prices, purchase volumes and relevant treatment program details to allow independent expert evaluation;
- participate on national HCV program advisory committees;
- participate in advocacy related to keeping WHO guidelines updated;
- include HCV testing and treatment in project proposals, with focus on key populations but also considering the general population;
- document and disseminate CSO-led HCV program best practices.

countries need to establish epidemiologic surveillance and initiate appropriate response, including ensuring DAA availability at affordable prices in order to implement programs with updated treatment guidelines and expanded coverage, particularly for PWID and PLHIV.

Eastern European and Central Asian Civil Society Organizations have demonstrated capacity to play a crucial role in advancing HCV issues, which they should continue leveraging for individual patient and global health benefit.

Abbreviations
ABT-450: Paritaprevir; anti-HCV: HCV antibody positive; ART: Antiretroviral therapy; CSO: Civil society organization; DAA(s): Direct-acting antiviral medication(s); EAPO: Eurasian patent organization; EASL: European Association for the Study of the Liver; EECA: Eastern Europe and Central Asia; HCV: Hepatitis C virus; HIV: Human immunodeficiency virus; IFN-free: Treatment regimen without interferon; LMIC: Low- and middle-income countries; PEG-IFN: Pegylated interferon; PLHIV: People living with HIV; PWID: People who inject drugs; TRIPS: Agreement on trade-related aspects of intellectual property rights; WHO: World Health Organization

Acknowledgements
Sergey Golovin and Tatyana Khan (ITPCru), Maka Gogia (GHRN), Akmal Aliyev (Community of People Living with HIV, Uzbekistan), Anahit Harutyunyan (NGO Armenian Network of Positive People), Tatyana Barnard (ICF Alliance for Public Health), Stela Bivol (PAS Center, Moldova), Sergey Biryukov (NGO AGEP'C, Kazakhstan), Pascal Boulet (Medicines Patent Pool), Kiromiddin Gulov (Equal Opportunities CSO, Tajikistan), Pulod Jamolov (NGO SPIN plus, Tajikistan), Yuliya Dragunova (Treatment Preparedness Coalition, Russia), Ihor Kilchevskyi (League of People Living with HIV, Moldova), Aleksandr Kurashov (Positive Initiative, Moldova), Saida Mamedli (Research Institute of Obstetrics and Gynecology, Baku, Azerbaijan), Zulfia Mustafaeva (NGO Legal Development and Democracy, Azerbaijan), Ehtiram Pashaev (NGO To Fight AIDS Azerbaijan), Dmitry Proskurnin (Together Against Hepatitis, Belarus), Paata Sabelashvili (independent consultant, Georgia), Rita Seicas (PAS Center, Moldova), Aibar Sultangaziev (Partner Network, Kyrgyzstan), Sergey Tolstolychenko (Youth for the Right to Life, Moldova), Ludmila Trukhan (Belarus NGO Positive Movement), Liudmyla Untura (league of People Living with HIV, Moldova), Kamila Fatyhova (Uzbekistan), Mari Chokheli (Open Society Foundation, Georgia), Olga Holubovska (Ministry of Health of Ukraine).

Funding
Funding for collection, analysis, interpretation of data and in writing the manuscript was received from Levi Strauss Foundation.

Authors' contributions
All authors were involved in teamwork during analysis, interpretation of the data. All authors read and approved the final manuscript.

Competing interests
The authors declare that they have no competing interests.

Author details
[1]Alliance for Public Health, Kiev, Ukraine. [2]London, UK.

References

1. Gower E, Estes C, Blach S, Razavi-Shearer K, Razavi H. Global epidemiology and genotype distribution of the hepatitis C virus infection. J Hepatol. 2014; 61:S45–57.
2. Paintsil E, Vervochkin SV, Dukhovlinova E, et al. Hepatitis C virus infection among drug injectors in St Petersburg, Russia: social and molecular epidemiology of an endemic infection. Addiction. 2009;104(11):1881–90.
3. Nelson P, Mathers B, Cowie B, Hagan H, Des Jarlais D, Horyniak D, et al. The epidemiology of viral hepatitis among people who inject drugs: results of global systematic reviews. Lancet. 2011;378(9791):571–83.
4. Koziel MJ, Peters MG. Viral hepatitis in HIV infection. NEJM. 2007;356(14):1444–54.
5. Chen T-YY, Ding EL, Seage Iii GR, Kim AY. Meta-analysis: increased mortality associated with hepatitis C in HIV-infected persons is unrelated to HIV disease progression. Clin Infect Dis. 2009;49(10):1605–15.
6. Deng L-P. Impact of human immunodeficiency virus infection on the course of hepatitis C virus infection: a meta-analysis. World J Gastroenterol. 2009;15(8):996–1003.
7. Van der Helm J, Geskus R, Sabin C, Meyer L, et al. Effect of HCV infection on cause-specific mortality after HIV seroconversion, before and after 1997. Gastroenterology. 2013;144:751–60.
8. UNAIDS Fact sheet global and regional statistics. http://www.unaids.org/en/resources/campaigns/2014/2014gapreport/factsheet. Accessed 1 Aug 2016.
9. WHO Media centre "World Health Assembly approves resolution on hepatitis and mechanism to coordinate noncommunicable disease response". http://www.who.int/mediacentre/news/releases/2014/WHA-20140522/en/. Accessed 1 Aug 2016.
10. Guidelines for the screening, care and treatment of persons with hepatitis C infection. WHO; 2014. Available at: http://www.who.int/hiv/pub/hepatitis/hepatitis-c-guidelines/en/. Accessed 1 Aug 2016.
11. Global Fund Board Decisions GF/B32/DP07. https://www.theglobalfund.org/media/4141/bm32_22-hepc_report_en.pdf. Accessed 1 Aug 2016.
12. Open Society Foundations Hepatitis C Treatment. https://www.opensocietyfoundations.org/publications/hepatitis-c-treatment-price-profits-and-barriers-access. Accessed 1 Aug 2016.
13. UNITAID World Hepatitis Day: Why UNITAID is investing in hepatitis C. https://www.unitaid.eu/news-blog/unitaid-sees-access-hepatitis-c-treatments-diagnostics-top-priorities/. Accessed 1 Aug 2016.
14. Hepatitis C Medicines Technology and Market Landscape. UNITAID. 2015. Available at: http://www.unitaid.org/assets/Hepatitis_C_Medicines_Technology_and_Market_Landscape__Update.pdf. Accessed 1 Aug 2016.
15. Andrieux-Meyer I, Cohn J, Affonso de Araujo ES, Hamid SS. Disparity in market prices for hepatitis C virus direct-acting drugs. Lancet Glob Health 2015;3(11):e676-e677.
16. United States Senate Committee on Finance "Wyden-Grassley Sovaldi investigation finds revenue-driven pricing strategy behind $84,000 hepatitis drug". http://www.finance.senate.gov/ranking-members-news/wyden-grassley-sovaldi-investigation-finds-revenue-driven-pricing-strategy-behind-84-000-hepatitis-drug. Accessed 1 Aug 2016.
17. Scientific American "We now have the cure for hepatitis C, but can we afford it?". http://www.scientificamerican.com/article/we-now-have-the-cure-for-hepatitis-c-but-can-we-afford-it/. Accessed 1 Aug 2016.
18. Forbes "Sovaldi and the cost-innovation paradox". http://www.forbes.com/sites/natesadeghi/2014/03/27/breaking-the-bank-the-innovation-cost-paradox-of-us-healthcare/#ae5f93993dab. Accessed 1 Aug 2016.
19. HEP "U.S. Senate opens investigation on price of Hep C drug Sovaldi". https://www.hepmag.com/article/senate-investigates-sovaldi-price-25943-716124207. Accessed 15 Aug 2016.
20. ITPCru website. http://itpcru.org/. Accessed 15 Aug 2016.
21. Alliance for Public Health "eastern europe and central asia – response to hepatitis C epidemic. http://aph.org.ua/en/news/good-news-hcv-treatment-is-becoming-more-accessible/. Accessed 15 Aug 2016.
22. EECA Community advisory board website. http://eeca.cab/en/. Accessed 1 Aug 2016.

23. EASL "Management of hepatitis C virus infection – revised version". http://www.easl.eu/research/our-contributions/clinical-practice-guidelines/detail/management-of-hepatitis-c-virus-infection-revised-version. Accessed 15 Aug 2016.
24. WHO patent update reports. http://www.who.int/phi/implementation/ip_trade/ip_patent_landscapes/en/. Accessed 15 Apr 2015.
25. Initiative for Medicines, Access & Knowledge. I-MAK Hepatitis C Patent Landscape. 2013. Available at: http://essentialdrugpatents.com/hepcdatabase.php. Accessed 15 Apr 2015.
26. WHO Regional Office for Europe "Georgia sets sights on eliminating hepatitis C". http://www.euro.who.int/en/health-topics/communicable-diseases/hepatitis/news/news/2015/07/georgia-sets-sights-on-eliminating-hepatitis-c. Accessed 1 Aug 2016.
27. Lozano R, Naghavi M, Foreman K, Lim S, Shibuya K, Aboyans V, et al. Global and regional mortality from 235 causes of death for 20 age groups in 1990 and 2010: a systematic analysis for the Global Burden of Disease Study 2010. Lancet. 2012;380(9859):2095–128.
28. GBD 2013 Mortality and Causes of Death Collaborators. Global, regional, and national age–sex specific all-cause and cause-specific mortality for 240 causes of death, 1990–2013: a systematic analysis for the global burden of disease study 2013. Lancet. 2015;385:117–71.
29. Strader DB, Seef LB. A brief history of the treatment of viral hepatitis C. Clin Liver Dis. 2012;1(1):6–11.
30. Perlman BL, Traub N. Sustained virologic response to antiviral therapy for chronic hepatitis C virus infection: a cure and so much more. Clin Infect Dis. 2011;52(7):889–900.
31. Feld JJ, Jacobson IM, Hezode C, et al. Sofosbuvir and Velpatasvir for HCV genotype 1, 2, 4, 5, and 6 infection. NEJM. 2015;373:2599–607.
32. Pol S, Corouge M, Vallet-Pichard A. Daclatasvir-sofosbuvir combination therapy with or without ribavirin for hepatitis virus infection: from the clinical trials to real life. Hepat Med. 2016;8:21–6.
33. Kim DD, Hutton DW, Raouf AA, Salama M, Hablas A, Seifeldin IA, et al. Cost-effectiveness model for hepatitis C screening and treatment: implications for Egypt and other countries with high prevalence. Glob Public Health. 2015;10(3):296–317.
34. Razavi H, ElKhoury AC, Elbasha E, Estes C, Pasini K, Poynard T, et al. Chronic Hepatitis C Virus (HCV) disease burden and cost in the United States. Hepatology. 2013;57(6):2164–70.
35. I-MAK paper entitled "Voluntary licensing: optimizing global efforts and measuring impact." 2012. Avaiable at: http://apps.who.int/medicinedocs/en/d/Js19791en/. Accessed 19 Sept 2016.
36. Nicol D, Owoeye O. Using TRIPS flexibilities to facilitate access to medicines. Bull World Health Organ. 2013;91:533–9.
37. Hill A, Khoo S, Fortunak J, Simmons B, Ford N. Minimum costs for producing Hepatitis C Direct Acting Antivirals, for use in large-scale treatment access programs in developing countries. Clin Infect Dis. 2014;58(7):926–36.
38. AASLD Practice Guidelines. http://www.aasld.org/publications/practice-guidelines-0. Accessed 15 Aug 2016.

18

Achieving a hepatitis C cure: a qualitative exploration of the experiences and meanings of achieving a hepatitis C cure using the direct acting antivirals

Jacqueline A. Richmond[1,2,3*], Jeanne Ellard[4], Jack Wallace[1,2], Rachel Thorpe[1], Peter Higgs[2,5], Margaret Hellard[2,6,7] and Alexander Thompson[8,9]

Abstract

Background: Universal access to the hepatitis C direct acting antiviral (DAAs) regimens presents a unique opportunity to eliminate hepatitis C in Australia. Large numbers of Australians have already been cured using these treatments, however, the numbers presenting for treatment have begun to plateau. This study explored how people experienced and understood being cured of hepatitis C, with the aim of informing interventions to increase uptake of DAA treatment among people with hepatitis C.

Methods: This qualitative study used semi-structured interviews to explore the experiences of people with hepatitis C taking DAAs accessing both hospital and community clinics. Interviews were conducted 12 weeks after treatment completion. Participants were asked to reflect on their experience of living with hepatitis C, their reasons for seeking treatment, and their experience of, DAA treatments. Participants were also asked to reflect on the meaning of being cured, and how they shared this experience with their peers. Interviews were transcribed verbatim and key themes were identified using inductive thematic analysis.

Results: Twenty participants were interviewed. While participants described a range of physical health benefits of achieving a hepatitis C cure it was an improved sense of psychological wellbeing that had the most significant impact on participants' lives. The majority described their relief about no longer living with the burden of an uncertain future due to anxiety about developing liver disease or cancer, as well as fear of infecting others. Participants who had a past history of injecting drug use, described being cured as a way to break the connection with their past. Participants who were current injectors raised concerns about re-infection.

Conclusion: Feeling "normal" and not infectious allows people to live with reduced psychological distress, in addition to the physical benefits of no longer being at risk of developing serious liver disease. Future engagement strategies targeting people who are not accessing hepatitis health care need to promote the lived experience of being cured and the substantial psychological, and physical health benefits, offered by achieving a cure. Interventions aimed at people who are currently injecting also need to highlight the availability of re-treatment in conjunction with primary prevention strategies.

Keywords: Hepatitis C, Cure, Qualitative, Lived experience

* Correspondence: J.Richmond@latrobe.edu.au
[1]Australian Research Centre in Sex, Health and Society, La Trobe University, Bundoora, Victoria, Australia
[2]Disease Elimination, The Burnet Institute, Prahran, Victoria, Australia
Full list of author information is available at the end of the article

Background

The universal, government funded access to direct acting antiviral (DAA) treatments for hepatitis C in Australia presents a unique opportunity to eliminate hepatitis C. The Australian Government [1], in line with the World Health Organization (WHO) [2], has set the ambitious target of eliminating hepatitis C as a public health threat by 2030. During the first 15 months of access, an estimated 43,360 people initiated DAA treatment in Australia [3]. However, an estimated 200,000 Australians remain infected with hepatitis C and data suggests the number of people presenting for treatment in Australia plateaued in 2017 [3]. The decline in number of people accessing DAA treatment compared to 2016 reflects the clearing the of the so called "treatment warehouse" where patients were regularly engaging with clinical services while waiting for the DAAs, and highlights the importance of ongoing vigilance regarding testing and linkage to care. The reason for the plateau in number of people presenting for treatment is thought to be multifactorial: lack of knowledge about hepatitis C, [4, 5] the asymptomatic nature of the disease and the negative perceptions of previous interferon-based treatment mean that many people with hepatitis C do not prioritise the treatment [6]. Additionally, the social marginalisation related to current or past injecting drug use and the stigma and discrimination associated with injecting drug use, have been shown to act as significant barriers to accessing hepatitis C testing and treatment [7, 8].

Hepatitis C infection has been associated with multiple extrahepatic manifestations such as depression and diabetes [9], which can have a profound impact on quality of life [10, 11]. The clinical impact of achieving a sustained virological response (SVR) measured at 12 weeks after treatment completion, and now referred to as hepatitis C cure, [12] has been widely reported to reduce the risk of liver-related morbidity and mortality, [13, 14] and the risk of developing extrahepatic manifestations, [15–17] and is associated with improved quality of life [18]. From the patients' perspective cure of hepatitis C is associated with improved energy levels, reduced uncertainty about the future, a more positive outlook on life, and improved personal relationships [19, 20].

While the public health approach to hepatitis C treatment focuses on population level elimination, [12] understanding the impact of cure for individuals and affected communities and communicating these experiences to people with hepatitis C and service providers is central in persuading others to access treatment services. This qualitative study explores experiences of being cured of hepatitis C; the findings contribute new knowledge to inform interventions to promote access to hepatitis C treatment.

Methods

Recruitment

Ethics approval for this study was granted by the St Vincent's Hospital Melbourne, Low and Negligible Risk Human Research and Ethics Committee (LRR-209/15). Participants were recruited through one Melbourne metropolitan tertiary hospital-based liver clinic and three affiliated community-based clinics between October 2016 and April 2017. The three community-based clinics were located in inner and northern metropolitan Melbourne and staffed by medical specialists and nurses employed by the tertiary hospital to offer an outreach specialist service including access to hepatitis C testing, liver diseases assessment and DAA treatment. Nursing staff from each clinic invited consecutive patients who had achieved an SVR, 12 weeks after treatment completion to contact the researcher (JR), who provided a participant information statement and consent form. If the individual decided to proceed, written informed consent was obtained prior to the interview. Interviews were conducted by author JE and were conducted either face to face at the hospital liver clinic or on the phone. Interviews lasted between 20 and 45 min. Participants were offered a $AUD30 gift voucher after the interview.

Data collection

Semi-structured interviews were conducted to explore the experiences of people who achieved an SVR after taking DAA treatment. Participants were asked to:

- Identify the barriers and enablers to treatment success from their perspective
- Explore the meaning of 'cure'
- Describe the ways they shared knowledge and experiences of treatment within their peer networks
- Describe adherence strategies they used while taking the DAAs.

Analysis

Interviews were transcribed verbatim and imported and coded in NVivo Pro, a qualitative data analysis computer software package. A thematic analysis was undertaken by authors JR and RT to identify text relating to the key themes associated with the research questions and informed the development of a coding framework. New themes identified after repeated close reading of the transcripts were added to the coding framework. Memos were used to record ideas about connections between the themes and to the overarching concept of cure.

Results

Participants

Twenty participants were interviewed during the study, with their characteristics presented in Table 1. Equal

Table 1 Characteristics of participants interviewed for the study

Transcript	Gender	Year of diagnosis	Previous Interferon-based treatment	DAA Treatment location
1	Female	2005	No	Hospital
2	Female	2001	No	Community
3	Female	2007	No	Community
4	Male	2007	No	Community
5	Female	1997	No	Hospital
6	Male	2003	No	Community
7	Male	1997	Yes	Hospital
8	Male	2002	Yes	Hospital
9	Female	2015	No	Hospital
10	Male	2002	No	Hospital
11	Female	2010	Yes	Hospital
12	Male	1997	No	Hospital
13	Male	2013	No	Hospital
14	Female	2001	Yes	Community
15	Female	2005	No	Hospital
16	Male	2010	No	Community
17	Female	2000	Yes	Hospital
18	Female	1990	Yes	Hospital
19	Female	2012	No	Community
20	Male	1990	Yes	Community

numbers of men ($n = 10$) and women ($n = 10$) were interviewed. Twelve participants attended the tertiary hospital liver clinic, with the remaining eight participants attending one of three community-based clinics. Participants reported being diagnosed with hepatitis C between two to twenty-seven years ago. Two participants reported being diagnosed with cirrhosis and a further two participants reported they had test results that indicated severe liver disease. Seven participants had completed interferon-based therapy prior to this course of the DAAs. For the remaining 13 participants, this course of the DAAs was their first hepatitis C treatment experience.

The meaning of achieving a 'hepatitis C cure'

Psychological impact

Participants discussed their understanding of being cured in several ways. The most frequently identified outcome of achieving a 'cure' was being relieved of the psychological burden of living with hepatitis C, and this outcome was often prioritised over that of physical symptoms. Most participants reported experiencing few symptoms prior to commencing treatment, and as such, were often unaware of any physical burden of living with hepatitis C:

> *It hasn't changed my life that much because I never really had any symptoms... The biggest change is just...emotionally...you go from being someone with a chronic disease that has the potential to cut your life short to being free* (Participant 18, female).

Three participants were excited about not having to worry about their health and instead being able to plan for their future and old age, with a more positive outlook:

> *It's like a real weight has just been lifted from you. I probably believed that one day it would get me because you just think oh, liver cancer, it's such an insidious nasty thing. If you get that, you're buggered* (Participant 5, female).

Reduced uncertainty and fear

While some participants associated being cured with less uncertainty and fear about the future, others highlighted that being cured allowed them to clarify the physical effects of hepatitis C infection, which reduced their uncertainty related to their general health. Four participants noted that while they lived with hepatitis C, they were never sure whether to attribute illness or fatigue to their hepatitis C infection or another illness, or ageing. Since being cured, participants reported being more certain about the cause of other physical conditions or illnesses:

> *It's hard to tell what it's actually doing to you and whether the fatigue or ill health is related to it because it was never very clear what* [hepatitis C] *did to you* (Participant 7, male).

Another participant described no longer worrying about whether symptoms were underlying signs of a more serious health condition:

> *The fact that that's not there anymore, like if I get sick or I'm ill means all I've got is that. I've just got the 'flu ... It's not that it's my liver's fricking packing up on me or something* (Participant 5, female).

"Feeling normal"

The experience of the cure also related to participants reporting they no longer felt infectious, particularly in the context of their family or people they lived with. This was often expressed in a marked shift in how they thought about themselves. For many the implied meaning of feeling "normal" was not being "dirty" or "infectious":

*I feel normal again ... I don't feel different to everyone else (*Participant 6, male).

For some, no longer being infectious meant they could change their behaviour and personal interactions because they did not have to worry about transmission:

At my house, with toothbrushes and razors and stuff, it's been something that I've had to be really, really vigilant with, with children in the house and with my partner ... it's really nice to know that I don't have that in me anymore, and there aren't those risks there of passing it on to anyone else (Participant 6, male).

However, one participant continued long term habits in avoiding physical contact to prevent possible transmission:

I've got issues where I can't kiss anyone or I won't let anyone take a drag of my cigarette...I still can't, because it's been years like I've been doing that, so I still can't stop doing that (Participant 2, female).

One participant discussed the impact of cure on their interactions with health providers such as dentists and pathology collectors:

I love not being infectious...That for me has probably been the biggest thing – not having to feel guilty every time I had a blood test done that I might infect somebody, going to the dentist is nowhere near as stressful (Participant 17, female).

Breaking a connection to the past

Several participants who contracted hepatitis C through sharing injecting equipment, and who no longer injected, described a sense of guilt and shame about their past injecting; feelings which persisted years after they had stopped injecting. These participants explained that hepatitis C was an ongoing marker of their injecting history and that being cured broke that connection:

It's like the last mark ... is now gone. All the rest is just memories that I don't have to think about (Participant 6, male).

Participants reflected on the ways being cured shifted their sense of self self-perception, and some felt that no longer having the disease would enable a break with the past:

It does make me feel more normal in a community sense ... that I don't have appointments or doctors are going to find out or my daughter's friends are going to find out. That's very liberating (Participant 2, female).

Others expected they would continue to experience guilt in relation to their past drug use:

I still feel guilty about it...about having used drugs when I was younger, about having contracted the hepatitis C... It's just a bit of a mental scar that I suppose I'm going to carry for a long time (Participant 16, male).

Physical impact

While many participants had not felt they had physical symptoms before commencing treatment, some described experiencing improved physical health as a result of being cured. Three participants explicitly attributed their improved physical health to being cured of hepatitis C, while others were uncertain whether their perception that their health had improved was directly related to hepatitis C or a result of the psychological benefits that flowed from no longer living with the virus:

I don't know how much of that is psychological. I don't think it's all psychological. I'm sure there is a physical element ... I have more energy, I am sleeping better, just a whole range of things (Participant 16, male).

One participant with hepatitis C-related liver damage noted that even after being cured, she needed to undergo regular monitoring for liver disease. However, her concern about one day dying of liver disease was reduced:

Because I am cirrhotic I still have to have regular FibroScans and liver function tests. In some ways those things haven't changed. I think it is just more that my outlook has changed (Participant 17, female).

For many participants the physical effects of living with hepatitis C only became apparent post cure. For those participants with significant liver damage, the ongoing need to monitor the liver for complications was a reminder of the physical damage inflicted by living with the virus for a long time.

Adherence strategies

In addition to exploring the impact and meaning ascribed by participants to achieving a cure, the interviews explored the experiences of taking the DAAs. Overall, participants reported that adherence to the DAAs was easy and unproblematic. One reason cited for the ease of adherence was a strong desire to be hepatitis C free and a belief that inconsistent adherence to the treatment would affect their chance of being cured.

I just made sure I did what the doctors recommended to beat this bloody thing (Participant 3, female).

The most common adherence strategy described by participants was taking the tablet(s) at the same time every day, and either by establishing a new routine or fitting the DAAs into an established routine. Participants who were already taking daily medication commonly discussed incorporating the DAAs into this routine and taking the DAAs at the same time as the other medication, most often in the morning:

In the morning with my contraceptive pill. As soon as I wake up ... that's usually what I do, the pill, brush my teeth, shower (Participant 15, female).

Those who were not already taking medication discussed incorporating the DAAs into other daily routines:

It was straightforward for me and I think that's why it was good to do them at night. I had them by the bed and I'd have a drink of water and I'd plug my phone in ... I built it into that kind of a routine (Participant 5, female).

One participant, taking up to five DAA tablets a day, used a dosette box to support adherence while another used a calendar, and others mentioned checking each dose off on a chart that had come with the DAA packaging. Another who was not accustomed to taking daily medication recalled finding it difficult to remember to take the DAAs, and set a daily mobile phone alarm as a reminder.

Fourteen participants reported forgetting to take one or two doses, which in some cases made them feel extremely anxious as they were concerned it would influence the efficacy of the treatment. This episode motivated those participants to take the tablets as soon as they remembered:

A couple of days I thought, you know, at lunchtime, oh, strewth, I haven't taken my pills. (Laughs)... no, no, no, no. And I mean, it was so important. I mean, my future sort of rode on it (Participant 18, female).

Other participants checked with their doctors regarding the recommended strategy for missed doses:

I told the doctor and he said that'd be fine as long as I made sure that I kept everything, you know, spot on from then on, and I did (Participant 6, male).

Overall, participants reported ease with adhering to the DAA regimen and developed individual strategies to support their daily administration.

Barriers and enablers to taking DAA treatment

The challenges associated with using DAA regimens related to individual circumstances, such as pharmaceutical management of existing medical conditions and lack of awareness among health professionals of the DAAs. One participant discussed the need to cease taking existing medication to manage a mental health condition and this required closer monitoring while she was on the course of DAAs. Another participant replaced one medication with another as her liver enzymes had risen.

In terms of side effects, one participant reported experiencing high blood pressure from taking the DAAs, which caused side effects throughout the duration of the treatment:

I still didn't have an easy time because my specialist told me it would lower my blood pressure and it didn't. It made my blood pressure go higher ... it wasn't fun for me at all (Participant 14, female).

Inexperience and lack of confidence amongst health professionals regarding DAAs and potential drug interactions was highlighted by several participants as a potential barrier to access. One participant identified that their doctor was unwilling to prescribe the DAAs given their lack of knowledge:

When I'd decided and rocked up to my appointment to ask her about it and she told me that she wasn't prepared to prescribe because she hadn't got her head around it, that was just a huge blow...if people aren't even prepared to prescribe it, well, why are we doing this? (Participant 19, female).

Another participant was disappointed about their doctor's lack of understanding about potential drug interactions:

[A Nurse] *...told me about this website from ... a hospital that listed all the interactions of the hepatitis C drugs with existing drugs. I'd gone right through that and checked what I was taking against all that and that was how I realised that I shouldn't actually be taking* [the medication]. *So I spoke to my GP about it and we sorted that out ... It was really only the fact* *that* [the nurse] *was so on the ball that we ended up getting it sorted out* (Participant 16, male).

However, most participants reported being supported by health professionals during treatment. One participant, who was currently injecting drugs discussed difficulties in treatment adherence as their life was "a bit chaotic", and described how the health professionals in a community-based service supported adherence.

Another participant discussed that the anticipation of side effects was a barrier to their commencing treatment; the fear of potential side effects was worse than the experience.

I approached it with a degree of trepidation but as it turned out I just simply got stuck into it and had very minimal side-effects (Participant 5, female).

Most participants were treated through specialist services either in a tertiary hospital or in an outreach clinic in the community; only three participants were prescribed their DAA course by a General Practitioner (GP). As interviews were conducted at the beginning of the implementation phase of the DAAs in Australia when few GPs were involved in prescribing DAAs and awareness raising activities had not officially commenced, the experiences of participants with GPs may have been be less than ideal.

Sharing knowledge with peers

All participants reflected on their positive experiences of the treatment and being cured by recommending that people with hepatitis C seek advice from their doctor about taking DAAs:

I have told a few people and other people have asked me ... I recommend it (Participant 1, female).

I'm reasonably medically aware I suppose and cautious, but with that background I would urge anybody with hep C to very much be confident about getting onto this drug to cure themselves (Participant 12, male).

While all participants emphasised the positive aspects of being cured, some also thought that it was important to inform prospective patients of the potential side effects:

The only thing was that I really would be reluctant to tell people that these medications are side-effect free ... there's a 2% chance that anyone would have the reaction I did (Participant 17, female).

One participant said that although they would like to share their experiences of being cured with peers and the broader community, they remained cautious about telling people about their experience of living with hepatitis C given the stigma associated with contracting the virus through injecting drugs:

One part of me wants to sort of yell it at the top of my voice and say, look, this is an amazing, miraculous cure out there. Please, anyone that's got hep C, go and get involved with it. But then the other part of me, sort of I suppose the conservative – but ... I still feel guilty about it (Participant 16, male).

There was a strong sense that the DAAs needed to be distinguished from interferon-based treatments with participants emphasising the need to advertise that DAAs were more effective and had fewer side effects than interferon-based treatment, and were simple to take:

I'd tell them, no matter what your experience with past drugs ... this is totally different (Participant 18, female).

The two participants who identified as current injecting drug users were positive about their treatment experience and said they would encourage peers to seek treatment. One participant shared her experiences formally as a peer educator:

I'd already started working as a peer educator, so part of that was an obligation to other users and needing to know what I was trying to tell people and encourage people to do... if I'm going to tell another user to do something I want to at least have experienced it, so I know what the hell I'm telling them (Participant 19, female).

While the current injectors were positive about taking the DAAs, they identified potential barriers facing other people who inject, including the potential for re-infection. One participant was concerned that re-infection would become a new source of stigma:

I think that there's also something to be said about the stigma and the guilt that goes along with re-infection. That's a whole new monster that we're going to have to deal with soon (Participant 19, female).

This same participant also proposed that some current injectors would continue to hold off on treatment because they conceptualised treatment as something to embark upon after they finished injecting drugs:

Author details
[1]Australian Research Centre in Sex, Health and Society, La Trobe University, Bundoora, Victoria, Australia. [2]Disease Elimination, The Burnet Institute, Prahran, Victoria, Australia. [3]Department of General Practice, The University of Melbourne, Parkville, Victoria, Australia. [4]Kirby Institute, University of New South Wales, Kensington, New South Wales, Australia. [5]Department of Public Health, La Trobe University, Bundoora, Victoria, Australia. [6]Department of Epidemiology and Preventive Medicine, Monash University, Melbourne, Australia. [7]Department of Infectious Diseases, Alfred Health, Melbourne, Australia. [8]Department of Medicine, University of Melbourne, Melbourne, Australia. [9]Department of Gastroenterology, St Vincent's Hospital, Melbourne, VIC, Australia.

References

1. The Hon Sussan Ley MP. Minister for Health. In: Press release: Turnbull Govt invests over $1 billion to cure hep C. Canberra: ACT; 2015
2. World Health Organization. Combating hepatitis B and C to reach elimination by 2030. Geneva, Switzerland. 2016
3. The Kirby Institute. Monitoring hepatitis C treatment uptake in Australia (Issue 8). The Kirby Institute, UNSW Sydney, Sydney, NSW, Australia; 2017. Available at: https://kirby.unsw.edu.au/report/monitoring-hepatitis-c-treatment-uptake-australia-issue-8-december-2017
4. Whiteley D, Whittaker A, Elliott L, Cunningham-Burley S. Hepatitis C in a new therapeutic era: Recontextualising the lived experience. J Clin Nurs. 2017
5. Mah A, Hull MW, DeBeck K, et al. Knowledge of hepatitis C and treatment willingness amongst people who inject drugs in an era of direct acting antivirals. Int J Drug Policy. 2017;47:137–43.
6. Whiteley D, Whittaker A, Elliott L, Cunningham-Burley S. The lived experience of interferon-free treatments for hepatitis C: a thematic analysis. Int J Drug Policy. 2016;38:21–8.
7. Anti-Discrimination Board of New South Wales. C change. In: Report of the enquiry into hepatitis C related discrimination. Sydney, Anti-Discrimination Board of New South Wales; 2001. Retrieved from http://www.antidiscrimination.justice.nsw.gov.au/Documents/hepc_report.pdf.
8. Dowsett LE, Coward S, Lorenzetti DL, MacKean G, Clement F. Living with hepatitis C virus: a systematic review and narrative synthesis of qualitative literature. Can J Gastroenterol Hepatol. 2017;2017:3268650.
9. Younossi Z, Park H, Henry L, Adeyemi A, Stepanova M. Extrahepatic manifestations of hepatitis C: a meta-analysis of prevalence, quality of life, and economic burden. Gastroenterology. 2016;150(7):1599–608.
10. Lee MH, Yang HI, Lu SN, R.E.V.E.A.L.-HCV study group, et al. Chronic hepatitis C virus infection increases mortality from hepatic and extrahepatic diseases: a community-based long-term prospective study. J Infect Dis. 2012;206(4): 469–77.
11. Negro F, Forton D, Craxì A, Sulkowski MS, Feld JJ, Manns MP. Extrahepatic morbidity and mortality of chronic hepatitis C. Gastroenterology. 2015;149(6):1345–60.
12. Wallace J, Richmond JA, Ellard J, Power J, Lucke J. Eradicating hepatitis C: the need for a public health response. Global Public Health. 2017:1–11.
13. Bonkovsky HL, Woolley JM. Reduction of health-related quality of life in chronic hepatitis C and improvement with interferon therapy. The Consensus Interferon Study Group Hepatology. 1999;29:264–70.
14. Gonzalez HC, Duarte-Rojo A. Virologic cure of hepatitis C: impact on hepatic fibrosis and patient outcomes. Curr Gastroenterol Rep. 2016;18(7):32.
15. Arase Y, Suzuki F, Suzuki Y, et al. Sustained virological response reduces incidence of onset of type 2 diabetes in chronic hepatitis C. Hepatology. 2009;49:739–44.
16. Byrnes V, Miller A, Lowry D, et al. Effects of anti-viral therapy and HCV clearance on cerebral metabolism and cognition. J Hepatol. 2012;56:549–56.
17. Hsu YC, Ho HJ, Huang YT, et al. Association between antiviral treatment and extrahepatic outcomes in patients with hepatitis C virus infection. Gut. 2015;64:495–503.
18. Younossi ZM, Stepanova M, Esteban R, et al. Superiority of Interferon-Free Regimens for Chronic Hepatitis C: The Effect on Health-Related Quality of Life and Work Productivity. Medicine (Baltimore). 2017;96(7):e5914.
19. Lane S, Cline S, Szabo S, Beusterien K, Hautamaki E, Bernstein D, Liu Y et al. P20: Understanding the impact of a cure for hepatitis C from the patient perspective. Journal of Viral Hepatitis - Special Issue: Abstracts for the Viral Hepatitis Congress 2013, 26–28 September 2013, Frankfurt, Germany; 20(Suppl s3):27–28.
20. Goutzamanis S, Doyle JS, Thompson A, Dietze P, Hellard M, Higgs P. The impact of hepatitis C-related uncertainty on self-reported stress in people who inject drugs living with hepatitis C. J Virus Eradication. 2017;3(S2):17.
21. Harris M. Managing expense and expectation in a treatment revolution: problematizing prioritisation through an exploration of hepatitis C treatment 'benefit'. Int J Drug Policy. 2017;47:161–8.
22. Treloar C, Rance J, Backmund M. Understanding barriers to hepatitis C virus care and stigmatization from a social perspective. Clin Infect Dis. 2013;57(Suppl 2):S51–5.
23. Australian Injecting and Illicit Drug Users League (AIVL). We live with it almost every day of our lives – an AIVL report into experiences of Stigma & Discrimination. Canberra: AIVL; 2015.
24. Hajarizadeh B, Grebely J, McManus H, et al. Chronic hepatitis C burden and care cascade in Australia in the era of interferon-based treatment. J Gastroenterol Hepatol. 2017;32(1):229–36.
25. Konerman MA, Thomson M, Gray K, et al. Impact of an electronic health record alert in primary care on increasing hepatitis c screening and curative treatment for baby boomers. Hepatology. 2017;66(6):1805–13.
26. Rogers, E. Diffusion of Innovations. 2003, 5th edition. Simon and Schuster, New York.
27. Grebely J, Knight E, Genoway KA, et al. Optimizing assessment and treatment for hepatitis C virus infection in illicit drug users: a novel model incorporating multidisciplinary care and peer support. Eur J Gastroenterol Hepatol. 2010;22(3):270–7.
28. Bonnington O, Harris M. Tensions in relation: how peer support is experienced and received in a hepatitis C treatment intervention. Int J Drug Policy. 2017;47:221–9.
29. Crawford S, Bath N. Peer support models for people with a history of injecting drug use undertaking assessment and treatment for hepatitis C virus infection. Clin Infect Dis. 2013;57(suppl 2):S75–9.
30. Norman J, Walsh NM, Mugavin J, et al. The acceptability and feasibility of peer worker support role in community based HCV treatment for injecting drug. Harm Reduct J. 2008;5:8.
31. Richmond JA, Sheppard-Law S, Mason S, Warner SW. The Australasian Hepatology association consensus guidelines for the provision of adherence support to patients with hepatitis C on direct acting antivirals. Patient Preference and Adherence. 2016;10:2479–89.
32. Goutzamanis S, Doyle J, Thompson A, Hellard M, Higgs P. Direct-acting antiviral treatment for HCV. The Lancet – Infectious Diseases. 2016;16(12):1325–6.

Uptake of hepatitis B-HIV co-infection screening and management in a resource limited setting

Musomba Rachel[1*], Castelnuovo Barbara[1], Claire Murphy[2], Charlene Komujuni[1], Patience Nyakato[1], Ponsiano Ocama[1], Mohammed Lamorde[1], Philippa Easterbrook[3] and Rosalind Parkes Ratanshi[4]

Abstract

Background: WHO hepatitis B guidelines recommend testing all new HIV patients, treating them accordingly or providing immunization. At the Infectious Diseases Institute (IDI) following an audit done in 2012, only 46% patients had been screened for hepatitis B with variable management plans therefore new internal guidelines were implemented. This study describes the uptake of hepatitis B screening and management of patients with hepatitis B and HIV con-infection after the implementation.

Methods: Data included for all HIV positive patients in care at IDI by October 2015. Data are expressed as median with interquartile range (IQR) and percentages were compared using the chi square test. Statistical analysis was performed using STATA version 13. The IDI laboratory upper limit of normal for alanine aminotransferase (ALT) and aspartate aminotransferase (ASTs) was 40 IU/ml.

Results: Number of hepatitis B screening tests increased from 800 by 2012 to 1400 in 2015. By 2015 8042/8604(93.5%) patients had been screened for hepatitis B. Overall hepatitis B positive were 359 (4.6%). 166 (81.4%) hepatitis B positives were switched to a tenofovir (TDF) containing regimen.

Conclusion: Our study confirms the importance of screening for hepatitis B and of using ART regimens containing tenofovir in hepatitis B co-infected patients. Whilst our program has made improvements in care still 18.6% of patients with hepatitis B were not on tenofovir regimens, 98.1% had no hepatitis B viral loads done. Clinicians should recognize the potential for hepatitis B in HIV positive patients and the importance of early diagnosis and treatment to ensure optimal management of cases and follow up.

Keywords: Hepatitis B, HIV/AIDs, Resource limited setting

Background

Chronic viral hepatitis is an increasing cause of morbidity and mortality among HIV confected persons, including those on ART, as persons with HIV continue to live longer [1–3]. The consequences of coinfection include higher rates of chronicity, less spontaneous clearance, accelerated fibrosis progression with increased risk of cirrhosis and hepatocellular carcinoma, higher liver-related mortality, and decreased treatment response [4–6]. Other challenges with coinfection include cross-resistance between HIV and hepatitis B drugs, [7–9] and increased rates of hepatoxicity [10, 11].

Chronic hepatitis B virus infection affects 5–20% of the 36 million people living with HIV worldwide, and the burden of HIV- hepatitis B co-infection is greatest in low and middle income countries, particularly in sub-Saharan Africa. Globally it is estimated that 2.6 million are HIV- hepatitis B co-infected [12]. The World Health Organization (WHO) in an effort to prevent and control hepatitis B Infection has developed a global action framework with four strategic axes: 1) raising awareness, promoting partnerships, and mobilizing resources 2) evidence-based policy and data for action 3) prevention of transmission 4) screening, care and treatment. These

* Correspondence: rmusomba@idi.co.ug
[1]Infectious Diseases Institute, Makerere University, Mulago Hospital, P.O. Box 22418, Kampala, Uganda
Full list of author information is available at the end of the article

strategies offer a global vision for the prevention and control of viral hepatitis [13, 14].

Uganda is highly endemic for hepatitis B infection, with a seroprevalence for hepatitis B positivity of around 10%, based on a national hepatitis serosurvey in 2005 [15, 16]. As with most of Sub-Saharan Africa, the majority of infection is acquired at birth or during early childhood (Franco E, 2012). In 2002, Uganda adopted a policy of providing hepatitis B vaccination to all infants [17] . Uganda has also adopted the 2013 WHO guidelines [18] that recommend hepatitis B testing in all HIV infected patients,and particularly those with elevated alanine aminotransferase (ALT), with linkage to care and treatment, and vaccination if Hepatitis B negative. Additionally knowledge of Hepatitis B serostatus allows optimal selection of antiretroviral drug (ARV) regimen to one that includes tenofovir plus lamivudine or emtricitabine (TDF/3TC or FTC) to ensure additional activity against hepatitis B [18, 19]. During the study period, the Ugandan Ministry of Health recommendations were for immediate initiation of ART for all patients with a CD4 count less than 350 cells, and less than 500 for those with hepatitis B HIV co-infection [20].

Whilst access to HIV care is becoming widely available in Sub-Saharan Africa, in diagnosis and treatment of viral hepatitis co-infection there remains a big disparity between resource rich and poor settings. Limitations such as the availability of further investigations and medication can be challenging in these settings to provide individualized care for more complex patients, such as those with co-infection [21–24].

An audit conducted in September 2012 among newly registered patients at the Infectious Diseases Institute – a large urban HIV clinic in Kampala, Uganda showed a low uptake of hepatitis B screening and variable management of those diagnosed Hepatitis B positive [25]. In response; a new specialty clinic was set up with the aim of identifying and appropriately care for patients co-infected with HIV and hepatitis B.

This study describes the impact on uptake of hepatitis B testing, assesses whether new guidelines and the introduction of the hepatitis B specialty clinic increased hepatitis B screening uptake and improved clinical management.

Methods

Study site and development of hepatitis B clinic services and policies

The Infectious Diseases Institute (IDI) is an HIV center of excellence [26] located in Mulago National referral hospital in Kampala, Uganda. IDI was one of the first HIV care and treatment organizations in Uganda; the IDI clinic began providing HIV care in 2002, while free antiretroviral treatment has been provided since April 2004. In 2015 there were more than 8000 HIV infected patients in active care.

Timescale of key activities relating to delivery of hepatitis B testing and treatment at IDI

1. In 2010, routine hepatitis B testing was first introduced, followed in 2012 by establishment of a dedicated hepatitis B clinic and clinic guidelines. The new guidelines were written by a team of three doctors, the quality manager and approved by the senior Physician who is also the head of the Prevention, Care and Treatment (PCT) department. One staff training session was conducted and the guidelines were implemented starting 1st September 2012. The hepatitis B clinic is held every Friday, staffed by doctors, nurses, counselors, laboratory technician, and pharmacist.
2. IDI has an electronic patient management system (ICEA) [27] and since the new guidelines were introduced in 2012, an electronic alert on the system that reminds clinicians to request hepatitis B tests for patients who have not been screened were further developed, the reminder prompted clinicians to request for the test. Samples were tested for hepatitis B using the hepatitis B surface antigen. Those with a positive test were termed hepatitis B positive. Routine hepatitis core antigen testing was not available.
3. Since September 2012, in accordance with the new IDI clinic guidelines, all newly registered HIV patients are tested for hepatitis B surface antigen, while those already registered in care are tested during their routine clinic appointments. ART naive hepatitis B positive patients are prepared to start ART with two pre-ART counselling sessions. In hepatitis B positive patients already on a zidovudine (AZT) based ART regimens, zidovudine (AZT) is substituted for tenofovir (TDF) if the viral load is undetectable, or switched to a second line regimen containing tenofovir (TDF), if viral failure is confirmed. Free hepatitis B testing and treatment is provided, but additional investigations including hepatitis B DNA viral load and fibro scan to help stage liver disease and monitor response to treatment; ultrasonography and alpha-fetoprotein measurement to screen for hepatocellular carcinoma; and endoscopy to screen and manage varices due to hepatitis B infection related complications need to be paid for by the patient. However, these are expensive and beyond the financial means of many of our patients.

Study population and data collection

This analysis includes all adult (≥18 years) HIV patients in current care at IDI from January 2002 to October 2015, with censorship at lost to follow up (LFU), transfer, or death. For each patient we recorded demographic, clinical, ART status, hepatitis B status, liver function test results, clinical management decisions regarding use of tenofovir containing ART regimen, and clinical outcomes (death, LFU, transfer etc). We also describe the number of patients tested each year, and compared the clinical characteristics and outcomes between those who tested hepatitis B positive and negative.

Two audits were undertaken for this study; the first was done in September 2012 and looked at newly enrolled patients, the second was undertaken in October 2015 following the establishment of the hepatitis B-HIV clinic.

Statistical analysis

We describe the number of patients tested each year and compared baseline characteristics (age, gender, WHO stage) in hepatitis B positive and negative patients and described the clinical outcomes in hepatitis B positive patients. Data are expressed as median with interquartile range (IQR) or number and percentages as appropriate for (CD4 count at hepatitis B test, ART status, current ART regimen, time in days from ART start to hepatitis B test). Proportion of hepatitis B co-infected patients already on a TDF containing ART regimen at the time of test are described. To show trends of for patients tested before and after guideline implementation, we used proportion of patients tested for hepatitis B compared to the number of patients who registered in the period. *P* values were found using Cochran-Armitage test for trend. We used an IDI laboratory upper limit of normal for alanine aminotransferase (ALT) and aspartate aminotransferase (ASTs) of 40 IU/ml. We used the t test for comparison of parametric continuous variables, Wilkinson rank sum test for non-parametric variables and chi square and fisher's exact tests for categorical variables. Statistical analysis was performed using STATA version 13.

Results

In the first audit, 1753 patients were reviewed. Of these only eight hundred seven patients (46%) received hepatitis B testing. Twenty-nine (3.6%) of those tested were hepatitis B positive, of which 8/29 (27.6%) were not started on ART; of note five of those had CD4 count < 500 cells/μL. Of 21 who started ART, eighteen (62.1%) were prescribed TDF-3TC containing regimens, three (10.3%) on ART regimens not known to have activity against hepatitis B. 19/29 (65.5%) patients had baseline liver function tests (LFTs) checked. No patients had follow up LFTs.

During the repeat audit in October 2015, there were 8042 (93.5%) active HIV infected patients screened for hepatitis B at IDI. Of these,2984(37.1%) were male, with median age 31 years (IQR: 26–35), majority in WHO stage 3 and 4; 4608(57.3%). 7416(92.2%) were initiated on ART and were on first line ART regimen 6930 (86.2%). There has been a marked increase in the uptake of testing per year from 611 tests in 2010, to 909 in 2012 and now 1500 in 2015. Overall, 8042 (93.5%) of 8604 current HIV infected patients have been screened for hepatitis B with the largest number of patients being screened between 2014 and 2015. Figure 1 shows the number of hepatitis B tests done each year over the last twelve years.

The proportion of patients screened for hepatitis B compared to the number of patients newly registered in the clinic was higher after the implementation of the new guidelines (2141(79.3%) of 2700 versus 5901 (28.4%) of 20,774 before the guidelines $p < 0.001$).

Characteristics of HIV-infected persons with and without hepatitis B infection as of October 2015

Table 1 shows the descriptive characteristics of 359 (4.6%) hepatitis B positive patients compared to the 7083 hepatitis B negative.

Those who were hepatitis B positive, were more likely to be male (52.6%) versus (36.4%) ($P < 0.0001$) and to have a lower median CD4 count at hepatitis B test (423 cells/μL) (IQR 269–600) versus 483 cells/μL (IQR 325–657). In addition, hepatitis B positive had been on ART for shorter period (days 74 (IQR 27, 399) vs (105 (IQR 28, 596) days) at the time of the hepatitis B test.

There was no difference in median age at 38 (IQR) or in WHO stage 3 and 4 (61.3%). Three hundred thirty-seven (93.9%) of the hepatitis B positives ever used ART with a median time on ART seventy-four days from hepatitis B test (IQR 27–399). Two hundred fifty-four (75.4%) patients started ART before the hepatitis B test date, eighty-one (24.1%) after the test and two (0.5%) on the day of the test. The proportion of deaths (6.5%) was higher among the hepatitis B positives as compared to the hepatitis B negative population (2.3%) (p value < 0.0001).

The median time from testing positive for hepatitis B test to death was 143 days (IQR 15–242). Hepatitis B positive patients were on ART for shorter period prior to testing (days 74 (IQR 27, 399) as compared to the hepatitis B negative patients (105 (IQR 28, 596) days) at the time of the hepatitis B test. Hepatitis B positive had lower CD4 count: 423 cells/μL, (IQR: 269–600) compared to hepatitis B negative patients 483 cells/μL (IQR:325, 657), p value < 0.0001).

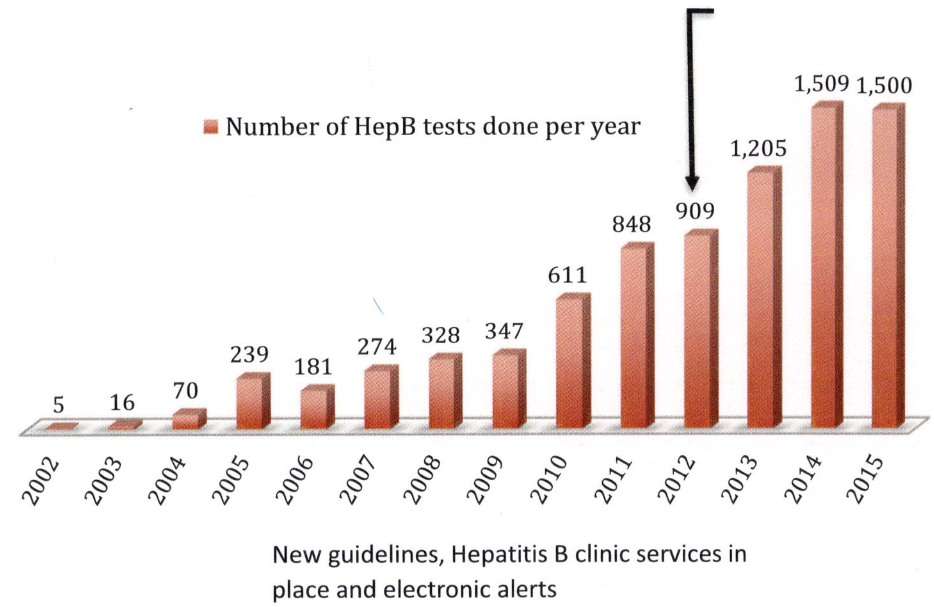

Fig. 1 Number of hepatitis B tests done performed per each year in IDI from January 2002 to October 2015

Clinical management

Figure 2. Management sequence for the 359 HIV-hepatitis B positive persons, as of October 2015

ART management

337 (93.9%) had been started on ART, while 22 (6.1%) had not been started not on ART at the time of the analysis. Of the 22 not on ART - most died (8, 36.4%), four (18.2%) were lost to follow up, seven (31.8%) had been transferred out while three (13.6%) were active in care. One patient of those active in care had documented evidence that they refused to initiate ART while two had results returned before their scheduled return clinic appointments date. Overall 259(76.9%) had been initiated on ART prior to their hepatitis B test, and 78 (23.105%) after.

One hundred thirty-three of 337 (39.4%) patients were already on a TDF containing ART regimen at the time of test, 166 of 337 (49.3%) were subsequently switched to TDF within median of 3.7 months (IQR 1.8–6.3) from hepatitis B test, and 38 (11.2%) were never switched. The most commonly documented reason for not switching was that the viral load was 1000 copies/ml for 24 (92.3%) hepatitis B patients.

Table 1 Demographic and clinical characteristics among hepatitis B positive and negative patients

Characteristics	Hepatitis B positive $N = 359$	Hepatitis B negative $N = 7683$	P value
Male gender N (%)	189 (52.6%)	2795 (36.4%)	<0.0001
Median Age (IQR) in years	38 (32, 45)	39 (32, 46)	0.119
WHO stage N (%) 3&4	220 (61.3%)	4388 (57.1%)	0.156
Median CD4 count at hepatitis B test (IQR) cells/μL	423 (269, 600)	483 (325, 657)	<0.0001
Ever used ART	337 (93.9%)	7079(92.1%)	0.231
Current ART regimen N (%)			
First line	316 (88.0%)	6569 (85.5%)	0.101
Second line ART	20 (5.6%)	507 (6.6%)	
Third line ART	1 (0.3%)	1 (0.01%)	
Median time (days, IQR) from ART start to hepatitis B test	74 (27, 399)	105 (28, 596)	< 0.0001
Active	289 (83.2%)	6801 (88.5%)	<0.0001
Dead	23 (6.5%)	179 (2.3%)	
Lost	5 (1.4%)	118 (1.5%)	
Transferred out	33 (9.6%)	585 (7.7%)	

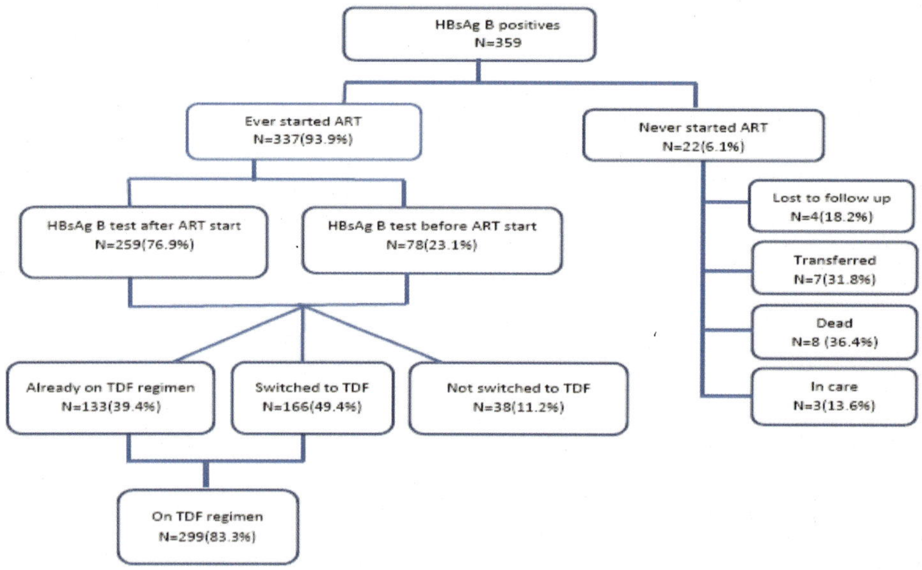

Fig. 2 Summarizes the management sequence for the 359 HIV infected persons identified as hepatitis B positive, as of October 2015

By October 2015, two hundred ninety nine (83.3%) of 359 patients were on a TDF based regimen.

Investigations and status of liver disease

Overall 285 (79.6%) hepatitis B positives had an HIV viral load done with 253 (70.7%) of patients with viral load VL 1000 copies/ml. Patients who never had an HIV viral load done 74(20.4%), 24 (32.9%) patients were active in care, 17 (23.4%) were dead, 4 (5.5%) were lost from care while twenty eight (38.4%) had been transferred out to other health care providers.

Liver enzymes tests (ALTs) were done for 249 (69.4%) patients with 205 (82.3%) of patients having normal alanine aminotransferase levels. Patients with Aspartate transaminase (ASTs) test done were 86 (24%) most of which (61.6%) had results in normal ranges.

Patients with hepatitis B DNA viral loads done were 7(1.9%) while 250 (69.6%) patients had an ultra sound scan done.

Clinical outcomes

Overall twenty three (6.5%) of the hepatitis B positives died, of these 9(39%) were those who had never been initiated on ART.

Discussion

Our findings show the striking impact of the introduction and implementation of a series of clinic activities to support the provision of effective hepatitis B care in an HIV clinic. There was a progressive increase in the uptake of hepatitis B testing particularly over the preceding four years 79.3%, with now almost universal testing of all HIV infected patients at IDI. It also shows the direct impact of knowledge of hepatitis B status on ART regimen choice with 299(83.3%) of 359 patients who were identified as positive on a TDF regimen as recommended in WHO guidelines [15] and consistent with other studies in the region [28].

This scale up and response was largely achieved as a result of results through actions taken in response to the findings of the first audit in 2012 showing a low uptake of testing [25]. These actions were the creation of a hepatitis B dedicated clinic at the facility; the development of specific guidelines; provision of, intensive training of health care worker staff on the current guidelines; and creation of a hepatitis B dedicated clinic at the facility. Further systems like the development of electronic alerts on the patient management systems (ICEA) [27] to remind clinicians to request for testing on all patients not yet tested.

Our study showed that hepatitis B occurred in 359(4.6%) patients; slightly lower than the general hepatitis B seroprevalence for Kampala regions (5.3%) reported in the 2005 national serosurvey [16, 29, 30]. Additional reasons for the lower prevalence maybe the impact of effective ART with TDF and 3TC/FTC containing regimens which may have resulted in hepatitis B clearance. This concurs with other data from the multicenter AIDS cohort study showing that hepatitis B was significantly lower in the ART era than in the pre-ART (IRR, 0.2 [CI, 0.1 to 0.4]), and that effective ART is associated with lower incidence of hepatitis B infection [31, 32].

Analysis of our study population showed that there were more deaths 23 (6.5%) among the hepatitis B positives compared to the negatives patients 179 (2.3%, *p* value <0.0001). (Table 1) These results are similar to findings from other studies. [2, 3, 33–36].

Further investigations and management of hepatitis B patients is still a challenge. IDI has access to hepatitis B, hepatitis C and E testing only. Further investigations that would be standard in resource rich settings are not available. Additional tests including liver function tests and ultra sound scans for hepatitis B patients were not done for all the patients. Only 1.9% of patients were able to have a hepatitis B DNA viral load. In Uganda generally extensive medical investigations are expensive and beyond the financial means of IDI and many of the patients. In our settings, diagnosing chronic liver disease and hepatitis infection is currently a challenge without external funding and availability of appropriate diagnostic investigations. There are also limited drug combinations for those with drug resistance and for more complex patients, such as those with co-infection.

Conclusion

Clinicians should recognize the potential for hepatitis B in HIV positive patients and the importance of early diagnosis and treatment to ensure optimal management of cases and follow up. Effective prevention and treatment of hepatitis B virus infection is an important public health priority with effective ART being associated with lower incidence of hepatitis B infection.

The Ugandan government is making progress in prioritizing hepatitis B screening. We advocate for further budgetary allocation for the implementation of hepatitis B treatment, management and long term screening for liver cancer. In the future additional funding is still required to increase management for complex patients with HIV-hepatitis B co-infection and its complications.

Abbreviations

ART: Antiretroviral therapy; ASTs: Aspartate aminotransferase; DNA: Deoxyribonucleic acid; IDI: Infectious Diseases Institute; LFTs: Liver function tests

Acknowledgements

An abstract to this paper has been presented as a poster at ISPOR 2016 program. Poster number PHS2.

Funding

This study was self-funded.

Authors' contributions

RM wrote the first draft of the manuscript. CM and CK conducted the first audit and were involved in the implementation of the hepatitis B clinic. PN extracted and analyzed the data. BC, PE, ML and PO reviewed the manuscript. RP overall conceived and supervised the study. All authors have reviewed and approved the manuscript.

Competing interests

All authors declare that they have no competing interests.

Author details

[1]Infectious Diseases Institute, Makerere University, Mulago Hospital, P.O. Box 22418, Kampala, Uganda. [2]Centre for Communicable Diseases, Queen Elizabeth University Hospital, Glasgow, Scotland. [3]World Health Organizations, Geneva, Switzerland. [4]Cambridge Institute of Public Health, Cambridge, UK.

References

1. Motamedifar MP, et al. The prevalence and risk factors of Hepatitis Delta virus in HIV/HBV co-infected patients in shiraz, Iran, 2012. Iran J Med Sci. 2015;40(5):448–53.
2. Soriano V, et al. Emerging challenges in managing hepatitis B in HIV patients. Curr HIV/AIDS Rep. 2015;12(3):344–52.
3. Chen G, et al. Chronic hepatitis B virus infection and mortality from non-liver causes: results from the Haimen City cohort study. Int J Epidemiol. 2005;34(1):132–7.
4. El-Serag HB. Epidemiology of viral hepatitis and hepatocellular carcinoma. Gastroenterology. 2012;142(6):1264–73.
5. Baran B, et al. Treatment failure may lead to accelerated fibrosis progression in patients with chronic hepatitis C. J Viral Hepat. 2014;21(2):111–20.
6. Uto H, et al. Increased rate of death related to presence of viremia among hepatitis C virus antibody–positive subjects in a community-based cohort study. Hepatology. 2009;50(2):393–9.
7. Kumar R, Singla V, Kacharya S. Impact and management of hepatitis B and hepatitis C virus co-infection in HIV patients. Trop Gastroenterol. 2008;29(3): 136–47.
8. Puoti M, et al. Hepatitis B virus co-infection in human immunodeficiency virus-infected subjects. AIDS Rev. 2002;4(1):27–35.
9. Matthews GV, et al. Characteristics of drug resistant HBV in an international collaborative study of HIV-HBV-infected individuals on extended lamivudine therapy. AIDS. 2006;20(6):863–70.
10. Sulkowski MS, et al. Hepatotoxicity associated with antiretroviral therapy in adults infected with human immunodeficiency virus and the role of hepatitis C or B virus infection. JAMA. 2000;283(1):74–80.
11. den Brinker M, et al. Hepatitis B and C virus co-infection and the risk for hepatotoxicity of highly active antiretroviral therapy in HIV-1 infection. AIDS. 2000;14(18):2895–902.
12. Prevalence and burden of HCV co-infection in people living with HIV: a global systematic review and meta-analysis. Platt L, Easterbrook P, Gower E, McDonald B, Sabin K, McGowan C, Yanny I, Razavi H, Vickerman P. Lancet Infect Dis. 2016 Jul;16(7):797–808. doi: https://doi.org/10.1016/S1473-3099(15)00485-5. Epub 2016 Feb 25. Review.PMID: 26922272.
13. Chen, D.S., et al., Report from a viral hepatitis policy forum on implementing the WHO framework for global action on viral hepatitis in North Asia: J Hepatol 2013 Nov;59(5):1073–1080. doi: https://doi.org/10.1016/j.jhep.2013.06.029. Epub 2013 Jul 12.
14. WHO, Prevention and Control of Viral Hepatitis Infection: Framework for Global Action. 2012: p. 28.
15. Ocama P, et al. Hepatitis B and HIV co-infection is still treated using lamivudine-only antiretroviral therapy combination in Uganda. Afr Health Sci. 2015;15(2):328–33.
16. Bwogi J, et al. Hepatitis B infection is highly endemic in Uganda: findings from a national serosurvey. Afr Health Sci. 2009;9(2):98–108.
17. UNEPI, Uganda National Expanded Program on immunisation. 2002. http://www.nationalplanningcycles.org/sites/default/files/country_docs/Uganda/uganda_epi_cmyp_2012-2016_update_2013.pdf
18. WHO, Consolidated Guidelines on the Use of Antiretroviral Drugs for Treating and Preventing HIV Infection: Recommendations for a Public Health Approach. Vol.. 2013: PMID: http://www.who.int/hiv/pub/guidelines/arv2013/en/
19. WHO, World Health Organization (WHO) guidelines for the prevention, care and treatment of persons living with chronic hepatitis B (CHB) infection 2015.
20. MOH guidelines, The 2013 Uganda Ministry of ART Health guidelines 2013 (http://www.who.int/hiv/amds/uganda_moh_treatment_guidelines.pdf).
21. Stockdale AJ, Geretti AM, Chronic h B. Infection in sub-Saharan Africa: a

grave challenge and a great hope. Trans R Soc Trop Med Hyg. 2015 Jul; 109(7):421–2. https://doi.org/10.1093/trstmh/trv044.

22. Lemoine M, Eholie S, Lacombe K. Reducing the neglected burden of viral hepatitis in Africa: strategies for a global approach. J Hepatol. 2015;62(2): 469–76.
23. Nwokediuko SC. Chronic hepatitis B: management challenges in resource-poor countries. Hepat Mon. 2011;11(10):786–93.
24. Lacombe K, et al. HIV/hepatitis B virus co-infection: current challenges and new strategies. J Antimicrob Chemother. 2010;65(1):10–7.
25. Claire Murphy, E., Challenges of hepatitis B-HIV co-infection screening and management in resource limited settings. BHIVA, Abstract 2012(www.bhiva.org/documents/Conferences/.../HIVMedicine12.pdf).
26. Nwaka S, et al. Analysis of pan-African Centres of excellence in health innovation highlights opportunities and challenges for local innovation and financing in the continent. BMC Int Health Hum Rights. 2012;12(11):12–1.
27. Castelnuovo B, et al. Implementation of provider-based electronic medical records and improvement of the quality of data in a large HIV program in sub-Saharan Africa. PLoS One. 2012;7(12):17.
28. Wandeler G, et al. Hepatitis B infection, viral load and resistance in HIV-infected patients in Mozambique and Zambia. PLoS One. 2016;11(3)
29. Teshale EH, et al. Hepatitis B virus infection in northern Uganda: impact of pentavalent hepatitis B vaccination. Vaccine. 2015;29(15):01334–1.
30. Macro, M.o.H.U.a.O., Uganda HIV/AIDS Sero-behavioural Survey 2004–2005. Calverton, Maryland, USA, 2006: p. 114–116.
31. Falade-Nwulia O, et al. Incident hepatitis B virus infection in HIV-infected and HIV-uninfected men who have sex with men from pre-HAART to HAART periods: a cohort study. Ann Intern Med. 2015;163(9):673–80.
32. Marcellin P, et al. Effectiveness and safety of Tenofovir Disoproxil fumarate in chronic hepatitis B: a 3-year, prospective, real-world study in France. Dig Dis Sci. 2016;28:28.
33. Nikolopoulos GK, et al. HBV-DNA levels predict overall mortality in HIV/HBV coinfected individuals. J Med Virol. 2015;19(10):24357.
34. Kim JH, Psevdos G Jr, Sharp V. Five-year review of HIV-hepatitis B virus (HBV) co-infected patients in a new York City AIDS center. J Korean Med Sci. 2012; 27(7):830–3.
35. van Meer S, et al. Hepatocellular carcinoma in cirrhotic versus noncirrhotic livers: results from a large cohort in the Netherlands. Eur J Gastroenterol Hepatol. 2015;1:1.
36. Kubo S, et al. Management of hepatitis B virus infection during treatment for hepatitis B virus-related hepatocellular carcinoma. World J Gastroenterol. 2015;21(27):8249–55.

20

Re-evaluation of chronic hepatitis B and hepatitis C patients lost to follow-up

N. Beekmans* and M. Klemt-Kropp

Abstract

Background: Many persons infected with Hepatitis B virus (HBV) and Hepatitis C virus (HCV) in the past are now lost to follow-up. The aim of the Northern Holland Hepatitis Retrieval Project (NHHRP) is to retrieve and re-evaluate persons previously diagnosed with HBV or HCV and bring them back into care. Chronic HBV infection was defined as two positive Hepatitis B surface antigen (HBsAg) tests within 6 months and chronic HCV infection with 2 positive HCV RNA tests by polymerase chain reaction (PCR).

Methods: Data files of the local public health services and microbiology laboratory were explored to identify all registered HBV and HCV cases in the Alkmaar region, the Netherlands, for the past 15 years. Identified cases were compared with patients currently known in our hospital. Patients without follow-up in primary or hospital care were approached via their primary health care physician and invited for evaluation at our hospital

Results: In total, 552 cases of HBV were identified. 356 (64.5%) had no follow-up. Only 113/356 (31.7%) were eligible for retrieval and 44.2% were evaluated in our hospital resulting in a change of management in 22/50 (44%) of patients. Four hundred ninety nine cases of HCV were identified, 150/499 (30.1%) were lost to follow-up. Only 20/150 (13.3%) were eligible for retrieval and 4/20 (20%) were evaluated at our clinic. Resulting in a change of management in 3/4 (75%).

Conclusion: Only a limited part of HBV and HCV persons lost to follow-up is eligible for retrieval, nonetheless re-evaluation of these persons will lead to a change of management in the majority of persons.

Keywords: Hepatitis B, Hepatitis C, Viral hepatitis elimination, Public health

Background

Infection with hepatitis B virus (HBV) and hepatitis C virus (HCV) is present worldwide and a leading cause of liver-related morbidity and mortality. It is estimated that 257 million persons worldwide are living with chronic HBV infection and 71 million persons with chronic HCV infection [1]. The World Health Organization (WHO) estimates that viral hepatitis was responsible for 1.34 million deaths in 2015, 96% of these deaths were due to long-term complications of untreated HBV and HCV infection [1].

In high-endemic HBV areas, such as sub-Saharan Africa and East-Asia, perinatal transmission is the most common mode of infection resulting in chronic HBV in more than 90% of infected neonates. In low-endemic countries such as Western Europe and North-America the majority of acute HBV infections occur during adolescence or adulthood and predominantly via sexual activity or intravenous drug use. In immunocompetent adults, less than 1% of acute HBV infections will progress to chronic HBV infection [2]. Acute HCV infection however, will lead to chronic infection in 55-80% of patients [3]. The predominant forms of transmission of HCV are unsafe therapeutic injections and blood transfusion in developing countries. In developed countries, injection drug use and unsafe

* Correspondence: n.beekmans@nwz.nl
Department of Gastroenterology and Hepatology, Northwest Clinics, Alkmaar, The Netherlands

sexual activities of HIV positive are the main forms of transmission [4].

In order to prevent long-term complications, it is important to achieve an adequate viral suppression or even elimination. Successful antiviral therapy can delay progression to cirrhosis and hepatocellular carcinoma and improve survival [2, 5, 6]. In chronic HBV infection, antiviral therapy is indicated if levels of HBV DNA are elevated, elevated alanine aminotransferase (ALT) values and/or at least moderate liver necroinflammation or fibrosis [7]. .The main goals of antiviral treatment are long-term suppression of HBV replication and hepatic inflammation and thereby preventing progression to cirrhosis and hepatocellular carcinoma. Treatment with antiviral therapy in HBV is often lifelong. In patients without an direct indication for treatment it is required to check ALT levels and viral load every 6-12 months in order to monitor and prevent progression to cirrhosis and hepatocellular carcinoma [7].

The primary goal of treatment in HCV infection is to cure HCV infection. The endpoint of therapy is a sustained viral response defined as undetectable HCV RNA 12 weeks after treatment completion [8]. Every patient with HCV infection has an indication for antiviral therapy according to the Dutch Hepatitis C guideline [9]. If cirrhosis already is present, even after curation, regular follow-up is necessary to screen for hepatocellular carcinoma.

The WHO set the ambitious goal to eliminate HBV and HCV as public health threat by 2030.

To accomplish this goal it is important to detect all persons infected with HBV or HCV. Several screening strategies are deployed in high-risk and low-risk population to detect infected persons. However, many persons previously diagnosed with HBV or HCV are lost to follow-up in primary and/or hospital care. This is an important target group. After all, the chance of spontaneous clearance is low and therefore an indication for antiviral treatment or strict follow-up might exist.

The goal of the Northern Holland Hepatitis Retrieval Project (NHHRP) is to focus on persons previously diagnosed with chronic HBV or HCV who are now lost to follow-up. We aimed to retrieve these persons and bring them back into care. To the best of our knowledge this is the first structured retrieval project within a geographic region. Furthermore, we aim to create a frame-work for other local or even nationwide retrieval programmes.

Methods

Data files of the local public health services and the local microbiology laboratory were explored to identify all registered cases of chronic HBV and HCV in our region for the past 15 years. The Alkmaar region in Northern Holland covers about 300.000 inhabitants.

A full-time fellow was appointed to retrieve all data and evaluate patients at our clinic from January 2016 to September 2016.

Persons with a chronic HBV infection were defined as two positive Hepatitis B surface antigen (HBsAg) tests within 6 months. Chronic HCV infection was defined as two positive anti-HCV tests within 6 months confirmed with a positive HCV RNA test. Identified cases were compared with patients currently under follow-up in hospital or primary care. Persons without follow-up appointment were considered lost to follow up.

Due to Dutch privacy regulations, it was not allowed to directly contact identified persons since no active medical treatment agreement existed. Therefore, we informed the registered primary health care physician of identified persons and requested to refer them for evaluation at our clinic. Hence, only persons with updated contact details (registered primary health care physician, address) were eligible for retrieval. If persons moved to another area and no longer were registered at a primary health care physician in our region it was not possible for us to contact them. We were not allowed to use other databases, for instance municipality databases, to search for updated contact details.

Persons with severe comorbidity and an estimated survival of less than 1 year were excluded. If there was no referral within 2 months, we send a reminder to the primary health care physician.

Re-evaluation at our hospital included physical examination, blood examination for Alanine-aminotransferase (ALT), complete serology, HBV DNA load and genotype determination, and transient elastography of the liver. A management advice was proposed based on the outcome of evaluation in accordance to the Dutch guidelines on treatment of HBV and HCV infection [10].

The goal of the NHHRP was to retrieve patients lost to follow-up. In order to evaluate the feasibility of such a retrieval project, we aimed to evaluate the following outcomes:

- The number of persons with chronic HBV or HCV infection lost to follow-up
- The number of persons lost to follow-up we were able to retrieve and responded to our invitation for evaluation
- The number of persons for whom re-evaluation resulted in a change of management

Results were evaluated using descriptive statistics.

The Northern Holland Hepatitis Retrieval Project was approved by the local ethics committee.

Results

Chronic HBV

Concerning patients with chronic HBV we identified 552 cases and in our region.

In total, 356/552 (64.5%) HBV patients had no follow-up in primary or hospital care (see Fig. 1). Only 120/356 (33.7%) were eligible for retrieval and after consulting their primary care physician, 113/120 (94.1%) were invited for evaluation. The remaining 7 patients suffered from severe comorbidity. The majority of patients with HBV were not eligible for retrieval because of various reasons. In 97/236 (41.1%) patients the primary health care physician was unknown, 34/236 (14,4%) were imprisoned, 38/236 (16,1%) were asylum seekers with unknown address and 67/236 (28.4%) now resided in another region.

In total, 50 of the 113 (44.2%) responded to the invitation and were evaluated at our hospital. Patient characteristics and outcome of evaluation are described in Table 1.

All patients were hepatitis B e antigen (HBeAg) negative. Evaluation resulted in a change of management in 22/50 (44%) of patients. An additional indication for HCC-screening was recommended in 14/50 (28%), 5/50 (10%) had an indication for strict follow-up and 3/50 (6%) an indication to start antiviral therapy. The remaining 25/50 (50%) were advised to have a 6-12 monthly check of ALT levels and in 3/50 (6%) patients viral load was undetectable.

Chronic HCV

In total, 499 cases of chronic HCV were identified in our region (see Fig. 2).

In 150/499 (30.1%) persons, no follow-up was scheduled in primary or hospital care. Only 24/150 (16%) were eligible for retrieval and after consultation of their primary health care physician, 20/24 (83.3%) were invited for evaluation. Of the 126 persons not eligible for retrieval, in 45/126 (35.7%) their primary health care physician was unknown, 21/126 (16.7%) were asylum seekers with unknown address, 23/126 (18.3%) were imprisoned, 37/126 (29.4%) resided in another region.

Patient characteristics and outcome of evaluation are described in Table 2.

Only 4/20 (20%) of invited HCV patients responded to the invitation and were evaluated at our clinic and 3/4 (75%) started antiviral therapy.

Discussion

The NHHRP was initiated to retrieve chronic HBV and HCV patients without follow-up in primary or specialist care. We aimed to identify these patients and invite them for re-evaluation at our clinic.

The number of patients eligible for retrieval for both HBV and HCV was considerably lower than the total number of patients lost to follow-up. The major reason for this drawback was that updated contact details were lacking. About one-third of those identified to lost to

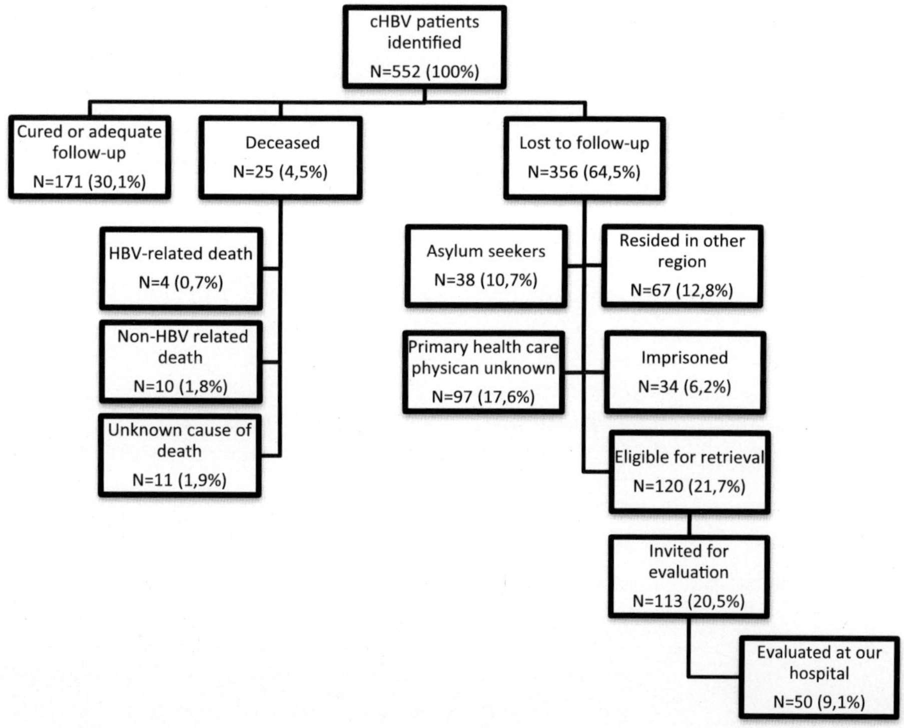

Fig. 1 Retrieval of chronic HBV patients, The flow-chart reflects the results of retrieval of 552 chronic HBV patients

Table 1 HBV patient characteristics and outcome of evaluation

	N = 50 (100%)
Sex	
Male	22 (44%)
Female	28 (56%)
Age (years) (mean ± SD)	48 ± 9.7
Migrational background	
Dutch / WE	4 (8%)
EE/EA	12 (24%)
NA	2 (4%)
SSA	7 (14%)
SEA	23 (46%)
LA	2 (4%)
ALT (U/l) (mean + SD) combined with HBV DNA levels (IU/mL)	
Normal (0-34 U/l) and HBV DNA < $2.0 \cdot 10^4$	44 (88%)
ALT >1xULN and HBV DNA < $2.0 \cdot 10^4$	3 (6%)
ALT >1xULN and HBV DNA > $2,0 \cdot 10^4$	3 (6%)
Fibrosis stage	
Unknown	2 (4%)
F0-F1	45 (90%)
F2-F3	3 (6%)
Management advice	
No Follow-up needed	3 (6%)
ALT levels every 6-12 months	25 (50%)
ALT levels and HCC screening every 6-12 months	14 (28%)
Strict follow-up every 3-6 months	5 (10%)
Antiviral therapy	3 (6%)

WE Western Europe, *EE* Eastern Europe, *EA* EuroAsia, *NA* North Africa, *SSA* Sub-Saharan Africa, *SEA* South East Asia, *LA* Latin America, *ALT* Alanine-aminotransferase, *ULN* Upper limit of normal, *HCC* Hepatocellular carcinoma

follow-up moved to another region and may have received adequate follow-up and care elsewhere. Due to national privacy regulations we were not allowed to search for updated data outside our own medical records, such as municipal databases. We expect this privacy regulation to be a major limitation in future retrieval projects. However, in Iceland, chronic HCV was defined as a public health threat and therefore a nationwide elimination programme, treatment as prevention for hepatitis C in Iceland (TRAP HEP C), was launched. Unlike our approach, in the context of this TRAP HEP C programme it was allowed to check updated contact details in the municipal database and to contact the patient directly [11].

Among the patients not eligible for retrieval we identified two important groups. The first group consisted of asylum seekers whose tests were performed in asylum seeker centers upon arrival. At the time of our retrieval project current address and legal status were unknown and therefore we were not able to retrieve and reevaluate this group. Our numbers suggest that this group could be a significant target group for retrieval and with better information and cooperation between asylum seeker centers and hepatitis treatment centers we could offer this group a chance of control or cure of their disease.

Second, prisoners tested positive during detention period are lost to follow-up after transferal to other detention centers or release to freedom without organizing follow-up in their place of residence. With close cooperation between prisons and hepatological centers this group is especially suitable for further evaluation and treatment of their chronic HBV or HCV. A large statewide programme in Australia showed that screening and treatment of prisoners can be very successful if it is done in a structured approach [12]. However, reimbursement of diagnostics and therapy within the detention period differs per country and could be a challenge.

Only 44% of chronic HBV patients eligible for retrieval was referred for re-evaluation. A lack of awareness of both patients and primary health care physician is a possible explanation. Awareness about chronic HBV and HCV can be created through education or media campaign. Increased awareness will contribute to the effect of a retrieval programme and may enhance the willingness of target groups to participate in these programmes.

The major change of management in chronic HBV patients was strict surveillance of the patient and to a lesser extent indication for antiviral therapy. Evaluation resulted in a major change of management in 44% of the patients. The remaining 50% had an indication for 6-12 monthly check of ALT levels and viral load. Patients were evaluated using the 2012 Dutch guideline on chronic HBV infection as standard. In 2017 the European Association of Studies of the Liver (EASL) released the updated guideline on HBV infection. This guideline sets a stricter cut-off point for indications for treatment with all patients with HBeAg-positive or –negative chronic hepatitis B, a viral load of $> 2.0 \cdot 10^3$ in combination with ALT greater than the upper limit of normal and/or at least moderate liver necroinflammation or fibrosis should be treated.

Three HBV patients started antiviral therapy based on viral loads in combination with elevated ALT levels. An additional 5 patients had an indication for strict follow-up because of elevated ALT levels or fibrosis stage F2-F3 despite viral load $< 2,0 \cdot 10^4$. These patients now may have an indication for therapy if HBV DNA levels are $> 2,0 \cdot 10^3$ according to the updated EASL guideline [7].

Concerning HCV patients, the results of retrieval were disappointing. We observed that two-third of patients had treatment or adequate follow-up, but the remaining one-third was hard to retrieve due to above-mentioned

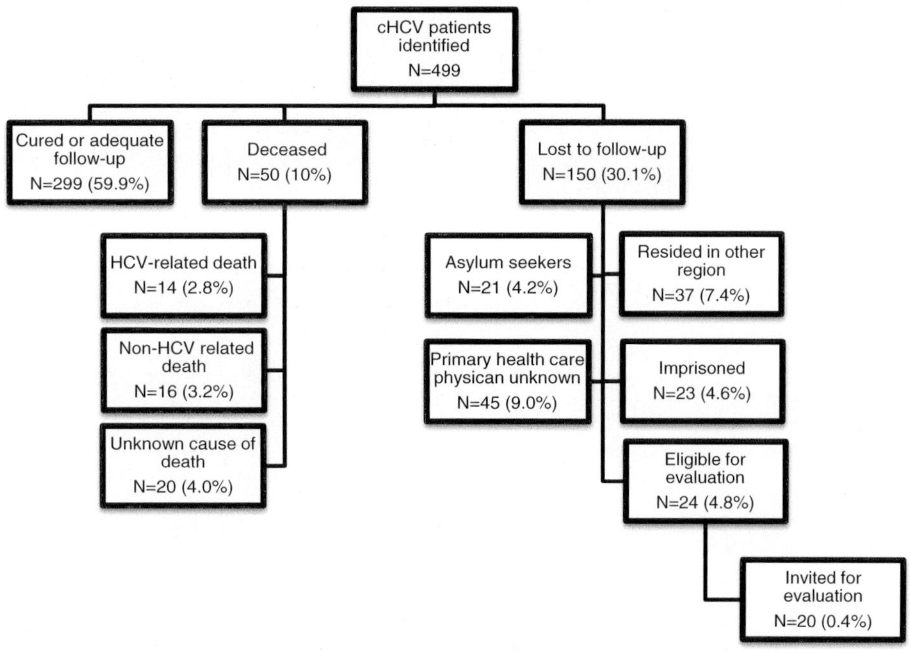

Fig. 2 Retrieval of chronic HCV patients, The flow-charts reflect the results of retrieval of 499 chronic HCV patients

reasons. Moreover, people who inject drugs (PWID) are an important target group as well. Because this group often has no permanent address, it is especially hard to reach them. However, treatment of PWID can be successfully in a multidisciplinary setting using strategies such as directly observed therapy and the involvement of nurse-practioners [13]. In close cooperation with addiction centers this group is particularly suitable for structured screening and therapy, for instance in conjunction with opioid substation therapy.

Table 2 HCV patient characteristics and outcome of evaluation

	N = 4 (100%)
Sex	
Male	2 (50%)
Female	2 (50%)
Age (years) (mean ± SD)	59 ± 21
Migrational background	
Dutch / WE	3 (75%)
EE/EA	1 (25%)
ALT (U/l) (mean + SD)	35 ± 18
Normal (0-34 U/l)	3 (75%)
> 1xULN	1 (25%)
Viral load (IU/mL) (median)	137,605
Fibrosis stage	
F0-F1	3 (75%)
F2-F3	1 (25%)
Management advice	
No therapy	1 (25%)
Antiviral therapy	3 (75%)

WE Western Europe, *EE* Eastern Europe, *EA* Euro Asia, *ALT* Alanine-aminotransferase, *ULN* Upper limit of normal

Despite difficulties with reaching above mentioned target groups, the effect of retrieval of chronic HCV patients will be significant. As of October 2015 direct antiviral agents for hepatitis C are approved for reimbursement of every basic health insurance in the Netherlands. Therefore, according to the Dutch guideline on hepatitis C, every patient with HCV infection has an indication for antiviral therapy. We started antiviral therapy in 3 of 4 patients, in one patient we did not start because of limited life expectancy.

A considerable larger number of HBV patients was lost to follow-up compared to HCV patients. The population of HBV patients predominantly consisted of migrants whereas the HCV population mainly consisted of PWID. It is possible that migrants have more difficulties with access to health care whilst PWID often have follow-up in addiction care and are easily referred to health care. Furthermore, in the past need for treatment and follow-up for chronic HBV infection was less strict compared to HCV patients and HBV patients therefore easily got lost to follow-up.

The most time-consuming element was the complicated construction to contact patients via their primary health care physician. Our region is a low-endemic region for HBV and HCV and most practices only have one or two HBV or HCV patients. Therefore, viral hepatitis is not a priority to most primary health care physicians. If it would be possible to approach the patients directly by using updated contact details, a retrieval project could be much more effective to perform. But we expect that, due to (inter) national privacy regulations, a direct approach will be hard to implement.

Our retrieval project is currently expanded to other regions in the Netherlands. The results of these projects will show us if large scale retrieval projects are worth the effort.

Conclusions

We conclude that a retrieval project comparing datafiles of the microbiological laboratory and medical records is time-consuming and will only lead to a limited percentage of patients lost to follow-up eligible for retrieval. Nonetheless it will lead to a change of management in a significant percentage of evaluated patients. Therefore, structured retrieval programmes of chronic HBV and HCV are an important element in the accomplishment of the WHO goal to eliminate HBV and HCV as public health care threat.

Abbreviations

ALT: Alanine-aminotransferase; EASL: European association of studies of the liver; HBeAg: Hepatitis B e antigen; HBsAg: Hepatitis B surface antigen; HBV: Hepatitis B virus; HCV: Hepatitis C virus; NHHRP: Northern Holland hepatitis retrieval project; PWID: People who inject drugs; WHO: World Health Organisation

Acknowledgements

not applicable

Funding

The Northern Holland Retrieval Project is funded by a grant from Gilead Sciences, grant number IN-NL-174-2008.

Authors' contributions

NB explored datafiles, NB and MK both analyzed and interpreted patient data. The manuscript was written by NB and MK. All authors read and approved the final manuscript.

Competing interests

N. Beekmans has received research funding from Gilead Sciences. M. Klemt-Kropp has served as a speaker, a consultant and advisory board member for AbbVie, Roche and Janssen, and has received research funding from Gilead Sciences.

References

1. Organization WH. Global hepatitis report 2017. Geneva; 2017.
2. Dienstag JL. Hepatitis B virus infection. New Engl J Med. 2008;359:1486–500.
3. Rosen HR. Clinical practice. Chronic hepatitis C infection. New Engl J Med. 2011;364(25):2429–38.
4. Westbrook RH, Dusheiko G. Natural history of hepatitis C. J Hepatol. 2014; 61(1 Suppl):S58–68.
5. van der Meer AJ, Veldt BJ, Feld JJ, Wedemeyer H, Dufour JF, Lammert F, et al. Association between sustained virological response and all-cause mortality among patients with chronic hepatitis C and advanced hepatic fibrosis. JAMA. 2012;308(24):2584–93.
6. Hsu YC, Ho HJ, Huang YT, Wang HH, Wu MS, Lin JT, et al. Association between antiviral treatment and extrahepatic outcomes in patients with hepatitis C virus infection. Gut. 2015;64(3):495–503.
7. European Association for the Study of the Liver. Electronic address eee, European Association for the Study of the L. EASL 2017 clinical practice guidelines on the management of hepatitis B virus infection. J Hepatol. 2017;67(2):370–98.
8. European Association for Study of L. EASL recommendations on treatment of hepatitis C 2015. J Hepatol. 2015;63:199–236.
9. NIV N, NVMDL, NVH, NVZA. HCV Richtsnoer. 2017.
10. NVMDL. Richtlijn Behandeling van een chronische Hepatitis-B-virusinfectie 2012. Available from: https://www.mdl.nl/sites/www.mdl.nl/files/richlijnen/Richtlijn_HBV_nieuwe_inzichten_2012.pdf
11. Olafsson S, Tyrfingsson T, Runarsdottir V, Bergmann OM, Björnsson ES, Johannsson B, et al. Treatment as prevention for hepatitis C in Iceland (TRAP HEP C). A real-world experience from a nationwide elimination program using direct acting antiviral agents. J Hepatol. 2017;66(1):S72.
12. McDonald L, Cragie A, Schulberg J, Scarmozzino J, Papaluca T, Stoove M, et al. Outcomes of treatment for hepatitis C virus infection in the prison setting. J Hepatol. 2017;66(1):S70-71.
13. Arain A, Robaeys G. Eligibility of persons who inject drugs for treatment of hepatitis C virus infection. World J Gastroenterol. 2014;20(36):12722–33.

21

Drug consumption rooms (DCRs) as a setting to address hepatitis C – findings from an international online survey

Vendula Belackova[1*], Allison M. Salmon[1], Eberhard Schatz[2] and Marianne Jauncey[1,3]

Abstract

Background: Prevalence of Hepatitis C Virus (HCV) among people who inject drugs (PWID) is high. Risky injecting behaviours have been found to decrease in drug consumption rooms (DCRs) and supervised injecting facilities (SIFs), yet HCV prevention and treatment in these settings have not been extensively explored.

Methods: To determine the range and scope of HCV prevention and treatment options in these services, we assessed DCR/SIF operational features, their clients' characteristics and the HCV-related services they provide. A comprehensive online survey was sent to the managers of the 91 DCRs/SIFs that were operating globally as of September 2016. A descriptive cross-country analysis of the main DCR/SIF characteristics was conducted and bivariate logistic models were used to assess factors associated with enhanced HCV service provision.

Results: Forty-nine valid responses were retrieved from DCRs/SIFs in all countries where they were established at the time of the survey (Australia, Canada, Denmark, France, Germany, Luxembourg, Netherlands, Norway, Spain and Switzerland). Internationally, the operational capacities of DCRs/SIFs varied in terms of funding, location, size and staffing, but their clients all shared common features of vulnerability and marginalisation. Estimated HCV prevalence rates were around 60%. Among a range of health and social services and referrals to other programs, most DCRs/SIFs provided HCV testing onsite (65%) and/or offered liver monitoring or disease management (54%). HCV treatment onsite was offered or was planned to be offered by 21% of DCRs/SIFs. HCV testing onsite was associated with provision of other services addressing blood-borne diseases and HCV treatment was linked to the provision of OST. HCV disease management was associated with employing a nurse at a DCR/SIF and HCV treatment was associated with employing a medical doctor.

Conclusions: DCRs/SIFs offer easy-to-access HCV-related services for PWID. The availability of onsite medical professionals and provision of support and education to non-medical staff are key to enhanced provision of HCV-related services in DCRs/SIFs. Funding and support for HCV treatment at the community level, via low-threshold services such as DCRs/SIFs, are worthy of action.

Keywords: Drug consumption rooms, Supervised injecting facilities, Hepatitis C testing, Hepatitis C support services, Hepatitis C treatment, People who inject drugs

* Correspondence: vbelackova@uniting.org
[1]Uniting Sydney Medically Supervised Injecting Centre (MSIC), Sydney, Australia
Full list of author information is available at the end of the article

Background

Drug consumption rooms (DCRs) / safe injecting facilities (SIFs) provide hygienic environments in which people who use/inject drugs (PWUD/PWID) can administer illegal drugs under the supervision of a health care professional, a trained allied service provider, or a peer (i.e., person who formerly used or currently uses illegal drugs), without the risk of arrest for drug possession [1]. DCRs/SIFs are evidence-based harm reduction interventions [2] with demonstrated effectiveness [3–11]. DCRs/SIFs generally target the most marginalised populations of people who use drugs (PWUD), people who inject drugs (PWID), and high-risk drug users (HRDU) [12, 13]. Studies among PWID have found that Hepatitis C Virus (HCV) prevalence at baseline is higher among DCR/SIF attendees than non-attendees [14], with daily attendees at greatest risk [15].

As such, DCRs/SIFs have the capacity to diagnose HCV among their clients in a timely way [16]. Several studies have documented the impact of DCRs/SIFs on HCV and HIV notifications [17–19], proving them cost-effective [20–22]. While decreases in risky injecting behaviour have been observed as an outcome of DCRs/SIFs attendance [23–26], HCV prevention and treatment in these settings has not been adequately explored in a cross-national context.

Recent research has demonstrated that high completion rates of HCV treatment among PWID [27], low rates of re-infection [28] and the provision of HCV treatment to active PWID are both effective and cost-effective [29, 30]. Adherence and response to the new, direct-acting antiviral agents (DAAs) therapy among PWID receiving opioid substitution treatment (OST) is comparable with people who never injected drugs [31], however numerous factors impede PWID participation in HCV treatment, including health system-related barriers, unstable housing or expectations of treatment side effects. Harm reduction services for PWID are an obvious avenue to circumventing some of these barriers [32] and can provide treatment-as-prevention [33], particularly to those clients attending on a daily basis or their "frequent attenders" [17, 34].

To date, surveys have not addressed HCV prevention and treatment among DCRs/SIFs clients [35, 36]. This study explored the range and scope of HCV-related services currently provided by DCRs/SIFs internationally, including HCV education, testing, disease management and treatment. We also explored their operational features and examined which factors were associated with the provision of enhanced HCV-related services at DCRs/SIFs.

Methods

To assess the range and scope of HCV-related services currently provided by the 91 DCRs/SIFs operating in 10 countries across the world at the time of this study (September – December 2016), an online survey was conducted. An invitation to participate in the study was sent to the mailing list of the International Network of Drug Consumption Rooms and of the Correlation Network (European Network for Social Inclusion and Health). The initial email requested a manager (or person in a similar position) completed the survey on behalf of the organisation. Managers were also asked to decline participation on behalf of their organization if they decided not to participate. Requests to participate were emailed three times to those who did not fill in the survey or did not respond (in October, November and early December 2016).

Survey questions focused on the DCRs/SIFs organisational structure and environment, staff composition and general client characteristics (18 items). Data on client characteristics were requested as an estimate in aggregated form. HCV-specific questions focused on (i) HCV-related onsite interventions and referrals (18 items), (ii) DCRs/SIFs client characteristics in relation to HCV (2 items), and (iii) barriers and facilitators to the expansion of HCV-related services (2 items). Open-ended questions like "other" or "please, specify" where included. The survey was distributed in English. German translation was available and when completed, answers were translated back to English and entered into the online tool by the study team.

The survey took approximately 45 min to complete. To facilitate survey completion, all answers were made non-compulsory, resulting in a different number of responses in each question. All participants provided consent and could withdraw from the study at any time. Ethics approval was granted by the South Eastern Sydney Local Health District Human Research Ethics Committee (16/258 LNR/16/POWH/482).

Study sample

The project used an exhaustive sampling method (i.e. approached all DCRs operating at the time of the survey). A total of 91 DCRs/SIFs from ten countries were invited to participate, namely from the Netherlands ($n = 30$ – number of DCRs in operation), Switzerland ($n = 13$), Germany ($n = 24$), Spain ($n = 13$), Norway ($n = 1$), Denmark ($n = 5$), Luxembourg ($n = 1$), Australia ($n = 1$), Canada ($n = 1$), and France ($n = 2$). In total, 86 survey responses were collected and from those, 37 were excluded from the analysis. Ten were excluded because they declined participation, nine due to duplicate responses, one response was from someone who wasn't eligible to take part in the study (not a DCR representative) and 17 were excluded as there was missing data for greater than 50% of answers. The remaining valid responses ($n = 49$) represented 54% of the DCRs/SIFs in operation at the time of the study.

Among the survey responses that were included in the analysis, each country was represented, i.e. the Netherlands ($n = 8$), Switzerland ($n = 7$), Germany ($n = 17$), Spain ($n = 9$), Norway ($n = 1$), Denmark ($n = 2$), Luxembourg ($n = 1$), Australia ($n = 1$), Canada ($n = 1$) and France ($n = 2$) (Table 1). Responses were grouped according to DCF/SIF country of operation. The countries where only a few DCRs/SIFs operated (< 5) were included in the "remaining countries" category ($n = 8$).

Data and analysis

Client characteristics and service provision data were analysed using descriptive analysis. T-test and chi2 test were used to assess the difference in the mean values (for continuous variables) and in proportions (for categorical variables) between each country of operation and all other countries.

To explore the factors associated with HCV service provision, three outcome variables were considered: (1) provision of HCV testing onsite – saliva, finger prick, both, or other test, (2) provision of liver health monitoring (e.g. via fibro-scanning) and/or provision of support for HCV disease management, (3) provision of HCV treatment onsite ("new" treatments, interferon, or both) and/or planning to provide HCV treatment in the future. Bivariate logistic regression models were fitted in order to explore the statistical significance and size/direction of the relationship between outcome variables and a set of variables pertaining to DCRs/SIFs operational characteristics (unadjusted odds ratios were calculated). A range of operational characteristics were included in the bivariate logistic models as independent factors (Table 2).

Table 1 DCRs/ SIFs operating internationally and those who responded to the survey

	No of DCRs operating (September 2016)	No of DCRs participating in the study	Participation rate
Netherlands	20	8	40%
Switzerland	18	7	39%
Germany	26	17	65%
Spain	15	9	60%
Remaining Countries	12	7	64%
Australia	1	1	100%
Canada*	1	1	100%
France	2	2	100%
Denmark	6	2	33%
Norway	1	1	100%
Luxembourg	1	1	100%
Total	91	49	54%

* For more recent developments in Canada, please see the Health Canada website dedicated to Supervised Consumption (https://www.canada.ca/en/health-canada/services/substance-abuse/supervised-consumption-sites)

Results

Descriptive Characteristics

DCRs/SIFs operational features

Most DCRs/SIFs were operated by a not-for-profit organisation (30/45, 67%). Other DCRs/SIFs providers included local, regional or national governments (18/45, 40%), private entities (3/45, 7%), or via contracts with a government (2/45, 4%) or religious organisation ($n = 1$). Services were funded from a variety of sources, often more than one. Funding was primarily provided by local (32/45, 71%), state/regional (16/45, 36%) or national (6/45, 13%) governments. Other funding sources included charities, drug service subsidies, donations or confiscated proceeds of crime.

The DCRs/SIFs were most commonly located in the centre of town (34/46, 74%), near a major travel hub (25/46, 54%) or within the boundaries of an established street-based drug scene (22/46, 48%). One fifth operated a mobile service (among those, two DCRs/SIFs operated a mobile service only). More than half were co-located with other services (26/46, 57%) and in four cases, these were shelters or overnight housing programs. About one third were stand-alone facilities, with other services used by their clients located nearby (14/46, 30%).

DCR/SIF capacities and services

The clinical staff at DCRs/SIFs included nurses (37/46, 80%), social workers (36/46, 78%), health educators/rescue workers (13/46, 35%) and medical doctors (20/46, 46%). Other professions employed by some DCRs/SIFs were psychiatrists, psychologists, case managers or researchers. Peers worked at one fifth and students / trainees in one sixth of the DCRs. About one third of DCRs/SIFs employed security personnel (15/46, 33%). Where estimated by the managers ($n = 42$), the average number of paid staff onsite on an average day was 7 (SD = 6.6, see Fig. 1 for details). A median of 10 spaces were offered for supervised drug consumption in DCRs/SIFs overall and the largest program had 63 spaces. See details of the operational capacities in Fig. 1.

Beyond the supervision of the drug administration, a range of services composed the "core business" of DCRs/SIFs and these were distribution of needles and syringes for onsite and offsite use, onsite overdose management and provision of referrals to health and social services. The majority of DCRs/SIFs also provided onsite HIV-related counselling (31/46, 67%) and HIV testing (25/46, 54%). A SIFs provided/SIFs provided medical treatments onsite:

Table 2 Per-country analysis of DCR/SIF characteristics (country vs. other; chi2 test, if not stated otherwise)

	Netherlands $n = 8$ proportion (%)	Switzerland $n = 7$ proportion (%)	Germany $n = 17$ proportion (%)	Spain $n = 9$ proportion (%)	Remaining countries $n = 8$ proportion (%)	Total $n = 49$ proportion (%)
Operational						
Operated by the government	4/8(50.0)	3/6(40.0)	*2/14(14.3*)*	4/9(44.4)	5/8(62.5)	18/45(40.0)
Funding from local government	*8/8(100.0*)*	3/5(60.0)	11/15(73.3)	6/9(66.7)	4/8(50.0)	32/45(71.1)
Co-located with another program	5/8(62.5)	4/6(66.7)	10/15(66.7)	3/9(33.3)	4/8(50.0)	26/46(56.5)
Stand-alone facility with other services nearby	*0/8(0.0*)*	2/6(33.3)	3/15(20.0)	4/9(44.4)	*5/8(62.5*)*	14/46(30.4)
Staff-Related						
Employing a nurse	*4/8(50.0*)*	6/6(100.0)	11/15(73.3)	8/9(88.9)	8/8(100.0)	37/46(80.4)
Employing a medical doctor	3/8(37.5)	*0/6(0.0*)*	7/15(46.7)	4/9(44.4)	*6/8(75.0*)*	20/46(43.5)
Employing peer workers	3/8(37.5)	2/6(33.3)	1/15(6.7)	1/9(11.1)	3/8(37.5)	10/46(21.7)
Number of paid staff on average day - n (mean country / other - t-test)	*6(3/8*)*	6(6/8)	13(8/7)	9(7/7)	*8(11/7*)*	42(7)
Client-Related						
Number of attendees per day - n (mean country / other - t-test)	*7(16/130*)*	5(158/100)	12(106/108)	8(109/107)	*4(206/95*)*	36(108)
% of clients tested for HCV - n (mean country / other - t-test)	5(59/72)	5(78/69)	14(77/67)	9(77/69)	8(54/75)	41(71)
% of clients estimated as HCV positive - n (mean country / other - t-test)	*5(33/61**)*	5(51/59)	15(57/58)	*8(69/55*)*	8(67/55)	41(58)
Service-Related						
Naloxone onsite	1/8(12.5)	1/6(16.7)	4/15(26.7)	*8/9(88.9***)*	3/8(37.5)	17/46(37.0)
HIV counselling onsite	*1/8(12.5***)*	3/6(50.0)	*14/15(93.3*)*	8/9(88.9)	6/8(75.0)	32/46(69.6)
HIV testing onsite	*0/8(0.0***)*	2/6(33.3)	9/15(60.0)	*8/9(88.9*)*	6/8(75.0)	25/46(54.4)
OST onsite	2/8(25.0)	0/6(0.0)	5/15(33.3)	3/9(33.3)	1/8(12.5)	11/46(23.9)
HBV vaccination onsite	1/8(12.5)	1/6(16.7)	7/15(46.7)	6/9(66.7)	4/8(50.0)	19/46(41.3)
Number of spaces for drug use - n (mean country / other - t-test)	7(10/12)	*5(26/10***)*	15(11/12)	*8(5/13*)*	6(13/12)	41(12)
HCV-Related services						
HCV testing onsite	*2/7(28.6*)*	4/7(57.1)	12/17(70.6)	8/9(88.9)	6/8(75.0)	32/48(66.7)
Liver monitoring or disease management onsite	2/7(28.6)	2/6(33.3)	11/17(64.7)	5/8(62.5)	5/8(62.5)	25/46(54.4)
HCV treatment onsite or plan to provide in the future	1/7(14.3)	0/6(0.0)	5/17(29.4)	1/9(11.1)	3/8(37.5)	10/47(21.3)

*statistically significant difference (country group vs. all other countries) on $p < 0.05$ level; **statistically significant difference on $p < 0.01$ level; ***statistically significant difference on $p = 0.00$ level

OST (11/46, 24%), abstinence-oriented treatment (5/46, 11%), or HIV treatment (2/46, 4%). The health and the social services provided at DCRs/SIFs are summarized in Figures 2 and 3 respectively. It was common to refer clients elsewhere when services were not provided onsite.

HCV rates and other characteristics among DCR clients

A median of 78 visits were made at a DCR each day (mean = 108, SD = 120, $n = 36$) and the largest number of visits made at a DCR on an average day was in Denmark (550).

Forty-one DCRs in the study provided estimates of the proportion of their clients who had been tested for HCV (median = 80%) and who were HCV positive (median = 60%). The highest rates of HCV positive clients (80% and more) were estimated in nine DCRs from across all European countries except for the Netherlands and France. The proportion of clients with HIV was 6% (estimated median).

The median age of DCR/SIF clients was approximately 40 years old and most were male (median = 80%, $n = 45$). Most DCR/SIF clients were estimated to have ever entered drug treatment (median = 70%, $n = 17$) and to be on OST at

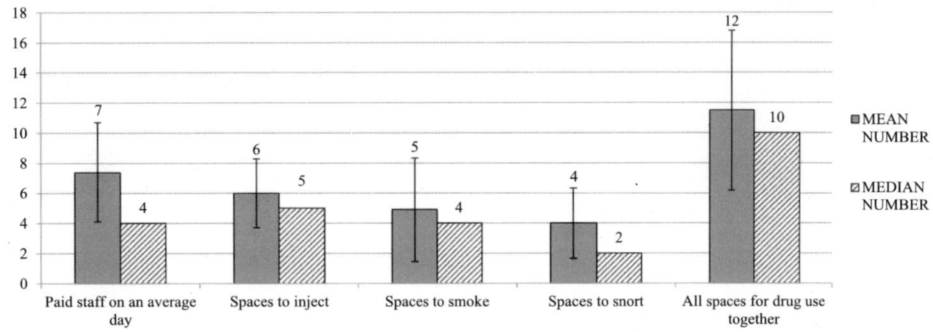

Fig. 1 Operational capacities of DCRs/SIFs

the time of the survey (median = 60%, $n = 27$). About one third of clients (median 34%, $n = 32$) were estimated to be homeless. All characteristics of DCRs/SIFs clients who participated in the survey are summarized in Fig. 4.

HCV-specific services provided at DCRs/SIFs

In response to the HCV rates reported above and as a prevention measure, almost all DCRs/SIFs in the study indicated that they provided HCV-related education (46/49, 94%). This took various forms (educational materials, consultations) and focused on providing information about transmission routes, infection symptoms, testing or treatment options (Table 3). The majority of the DCRs/SIFs also offered HCV testing onsite (32/49, 65%). The testing was most commonly done through a blood sample, but also saliva and/or finger prick tests were performed. From those facilities that were not providing HCV testing onsite ($n = 16$), eight were planning to do so in the future and nine currently referred clients elsewhere.

Almost all DCRs/SIFs referred their clients to HCV treatment programmes (Table 4). More than half (25/46, 54%) offered enhanced HCV services in the form of liver monitoring or disease management (Table 4). About half (24/47, 51%) of the DCRs/SIFs in the study planned to expand HCV referrals or the enhanced support services in the future. Only four DCRs/SIFs provided HCV treatment onsite at the time of the survey (8%), two of them in the form of DAAs. Six additional services were planning to provide HCV treatment in the near future: either new treatments ($n = 1$), interferon treatment ($n = 1$) or an unspecified type of treatment ($n = 4$).

Differences between countries

The Dutch DCRs/SIFs ($n = 8$ of the 49) differed from other countries in a number of ways: they were receiving funding from local government (chi2 = 3.95, $p = 0.047$), they did not offer stand-alone programs,

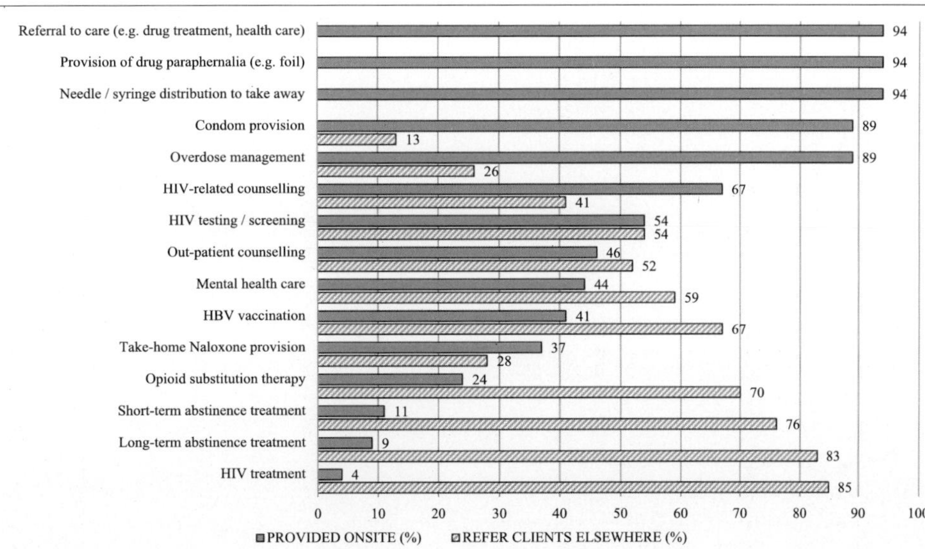

Fig. 2 Health services provided onsite and referred to offsite services by the DCRs/SIFs ($n = 46$)

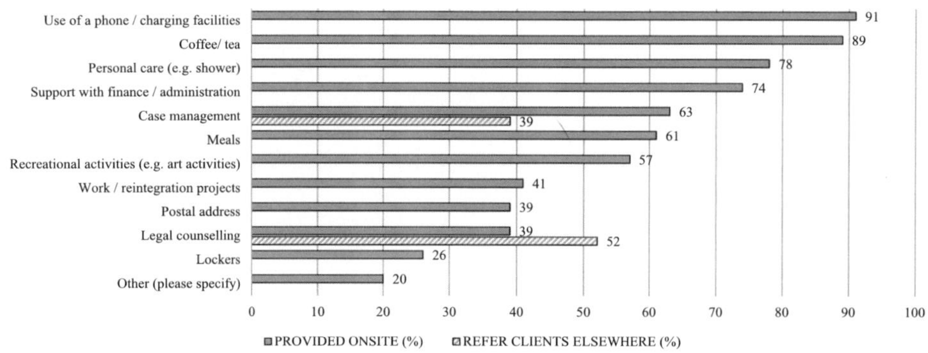

Fig. 3 Social services provided onsite and referred to offsite services by the DCRs/SIFs ($n = 46$)

and, they operated with fewer paid employees (chi2 = 6.36, $p = 0.012$) and fewer nurses (chi2 = 5.70, $p = 0.017$) than other services surveyed. They also reported a lower number of visitors per day ($t = 2.38$, $p = 0.01$), and provided a lower estimate of HCV-positive clients ($t = 3.03$, $p = 0.002$). The Dutch DCRs/SIFs were also less likely to provide onsite HIV services (chi2 = 11.53, $p = 0.00$) or HCV testing (chi2 = 5.35, $p = 0.02$) than those located elsewhere.

German DCRs/SIFs ($n = 17$) differed from those in other countries in that a lower proportion of them offered HIV counselling (chi2 = 5.94, $p = 0.015$). Also unique to German DCRs was that they were less likely to be operated by the government (chi2 = 5.60, $p = 0.018$).

The Spanish DCRs/SIFs offered onsite HIV testing more often than others (chi2 = 5.38, $p = 0.02$), and also over-performed with respect to providing Naloxone training onsite (chi2 = 12.95, $p = 0.00$). The Spanish DCRs/SIFs ($n = 9$) tended to have fewer drug consumption spaces ($t = 1.97$, $p = 0.03$) than other countries. Also, the Spanish DCRs/SIFs estimated a significantly higher proportion of HCV positive clients ($t = -1.80$, $p = 0.04$).

Contrastingly, a higher number of drug consumption spaces ($t = -3.46$, $p = 0.000$) was reported by the Swiss DCRs/SIFs ($n = 7$). At the same time, the Swiss programs were less likely to employ a medical doctor (chi2 = 5.31, $p = 0.021$).

In the group of "remaining countries" ($n = 8$), employing a medical doctor (chi2 = 3.95, $p = 0.048$) was more common than elsewhere, they employed a higher number of staff ($t = -1.83$, $p = 0.038$) and were more commonly operated as stand-alone facilities (chi2 = 4.70, $p = 0.030$). They also had a significantly higher number of attendees on an average day ($t = -1.79$, $p = 0.041$). See Table 2 for a more detailed cross-national comparison.

Factors associated with provision of HCV services at DCRs/SIFs

HCV testing was conducted more frequently in DCRs that provided HIV testing (OR = 44.6, $p = 0.00$) or HBV vaccination (OR = 7.3, $p = 0.01$). Factors positively associated with HCV support (defined as provision of liver monitoring or disease management) onsite at the DCR/SIF were: onsite HIV counselling (OR = 4.1, $p = 0.04$), testing (OR = 7.0, $p = 0.00$) and HBV vaccination (OR = 6.7, $p = 0.00$), onsite OST (OR = 5.4, $p = 0.03$), and employment of a nurse (OR = 12.4, $p = 0.01$) or a medical doctor (OR = 8.0, $p = 0.00$). Current or future provision of HCV treatment onsite was significantly associated with employing a

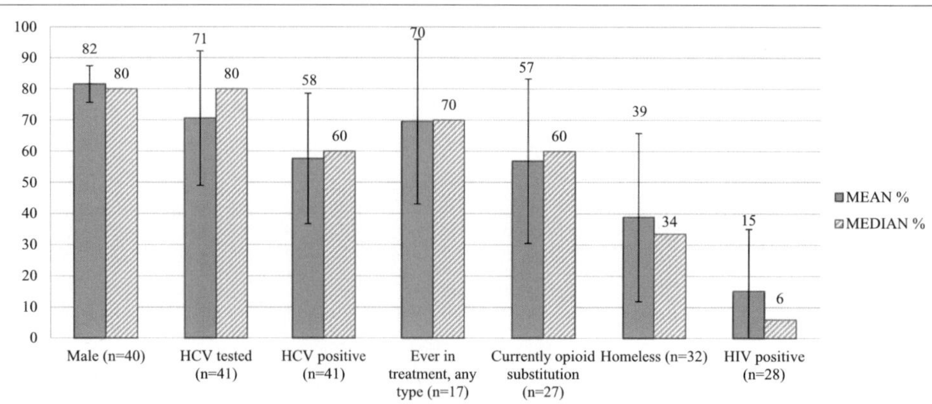

Fig. 4 DCR/SIF client characteristics, estimates reported by survey participants

Table 3 HCV education and testing provided onsite at DCRs/SIFs

Provided onsite		Form provided	
HCV education (multiple response)	$n = 49$	If HCV education provided onsite (multiple response)	$n = 46$
HCV prevention & transmission routes	94%	Brochures/pamphlets	90%
HCV testing	78%	Individual client consultations	88%
HCV infection symptoms	76%	Posters	69%
HCV treatment options	76%	Other (please specify)	20%
We don't provide any HCV information	6%	Digital resources (e.g., videos, quizzes)	20%
		Group education sessions	18%
HCV testing onsite	$n = 49$	If HCV testing provided onsite (multiple response)	$n = 32$
Yes	65%	BLOOD SAMPLE taken from a vein	68%
No	33%	SALIVA / oral fluid	39%
Don't know	2%	FINGER PRICK test	32%
		Other	10%

medical doctor (OR = 14.6, $p = 0.00$) and marginally associated (OR = 4.3, $p = 0.08$) with provision of OST onsite (Table 5).

When the managers were asked how they would spend any additional HCV-related funds, most said they would employ additional medical staff (24/46, 52%), develop client education around HCV (24/46, 52%) and/or provide additional staff training (21/46, 46%). Other responses included developing policies and procedures for staff, preparing educational material for clients or employing peer support workers. Conducting a needs assessment or developing referral pathways to a specialist were mentioned as well. Two organisations said that they would purchase a fibro-scan and one organisation mentioned that they would invest in advocacy to garner support to provide HCV treatment to "clandestine" persons.

When it comes to the reasons for not providing enhanced HCV-related services, some respondents indicated that HCV services were not part of the formal purpose of their facility (3/47, 6%). Other DCRs/SIFs mentioned that the site was already very busy or that the setting simply did not allow HCV services ($n = 2$), or that the DCRs/SIFs approach was non-medical and that current referral pathways worked well ($n = 1$). Other barriers included the high cost of rapid test kits ($n = 1$) or the fact that clients of the service were undocumented migrants who could not access treatment even if HCV positive.

Discussion

This study explored the range and scope of HCV-related services currently provided by DCRs/SIFs internationally and examined associated factors. We found that prevention and management of blood-borne infections is a priority for the vast majority of the DCRs/SIFs that responded to this online survey. Most of them reported that they provided HCV-related education in some form and referred their clients to HCV testing and treatment. Over two thirds provided onsite HCV testing. Over half of those surveyed offered enhanced HCV support services that

Table 4 HCV support services and treatment provided onsite at DCRs/SIFs and availability of HCV treatment to DCR clients

	Provide onsite	Plan to expand in future
HCV support (multiple responses possible)	$n = 46$	$n = 47$
Yes, referral to other services that can provide HCV treatment	96%	36%
Yes, disease self-management support (e.g. healthy diet, obesity)	50%	15%
Yes, liver health/cirrhosis monitoring (e.g. fibro-scan, blood test)	24%	11%
No	15%	49%
HCV treatment (one response only)	$n = 48$	$n = 39$
Yes, new HCV treatment forms (DAAs)	4%	3%
Yes, interferon-based treatment	0%	3%
Yes, both treatment options	4%	0%
Other (provided details)	–	10%
Don't know	8%	–
No	86%	84%

Table 5 Factors associated with HCV service provision at DCRs/SIFs - bi-variate logistic regression

	(1) Provide HCV testing onsite ($n = 32$; 665%) *OR (standard error), p-value*	(2) Provide liver monitoring or disease management onsite ($n = 25$; 51%) *OR (standard error), p-value*	(3) Provide HCV treatment onsite or planning to provide in near future ($n = 10$; 20%) *OR (standard error), p-value*
Operational			
Country (Netherlands)	*0.15* (0.13), 0.02*	1.48 (0.37), 0.11	1.39 (0.42), 0.26
Operated by the government	0.89 (0.58), 0.86	0.53 (0.33), 0.31	1.57 (1.23), 0.57
Funding from local government	0.55 (0.41), 0.41	0.76 (0.52), 0.69	0.64 (0.53), 0.59
Co-located with another program	1.38 (0.90), 0.61	1.67 (1.02), 0.40	2.84 (2.50), 0.21
Stand-alone facility with other services nearby	2.01 (1.51), 0.53	1.17 (0.76), 0.81	0.69 (0.62), 0.68
Staff-Related			
Employing a nurse	2.08 (1.60), 0.34	*12.38** (13.92), 0.01*	0.70 (0.64), 0.70
Employing a medical doctor	1.48 (0.98), 0.55	*8.00*** (5.66), 0.00*	*14.58*** (16.41), 0.00*
Employing peer workers	0.88 (0.70), 0.87	0.47 (0.34), 0.29	1.43 (1.31), 0.70
Higher than median number of paid staff on average day (> 4)	1.20 (0.80), 0.80	1.22 (0.77), 0.75	2.00 (1.62), 0.39
Client-Related			
Higher than median number of attendees per day (> 78)	1.42 (1.04), 0.63	0.62 (0.43), 0.49	2.14 (2.02), 0.41
Higher than median % of clients tested for HCV (> 80%)	1.98 (1.38), 0.32	0.38 (0.26), 0.15	0.51 (0.38), 0.36
Higher than median % of clients estimated as HCV positive (> 60%)	0.83 (0.57), 0.79	0.60 (0.40), 0.44	1.00 (0.75), 1.00
Service-Related			
Provide naloxone onsite	3.02 (2.25), 0.12	1.67 (1.07), 0.42	0.49 (0.43), 0.40
Provide HIV counselling onsite	2.57 (1.77), 0.17	*4.09* (2.90), 0.04*	3.36 (3.78), 0.23
Provide HIV testing onsite	*44.57*** (50.06), 0.00*	*7.00*** (4.75), 0.00*	2.84 (2.50), 0.21
Provide OST onsite	2.45 (2.11), 0.27	*5.40* (4.62), 0.03*	4.29 (3.52), 0.08
Provide HBV vaccination onsite	*7.29** (6.15), 0.01*	*6.67*** (4.67), 0.00*	1.47 (1.15), 0.62
Higher than median no of spaces for drug use (> 10)	0.63 (0.43), 0.49	0.62 (0.39), 0.44	2.97 (2.68), 0.21

*statistically significant difference (country group vs. all other countries) on $p < 0.05$ level; **statistically significant difference on $p < 0.01$ level; ***statistically significant difference on $p = 0.00$ level

included liver-health monitoring or disease management. One fifth of the DCRs/SIFs in the study offered or planned to offer HCV treatment in the near future.

Current provision of enhanced HCV-related services was (with one exception) independent of the DCR/SIF country of origin, the DCR/SIF source of funding, any co-location with other programs, the size of the DCRs/SIFs or the actual HCV prevalence rates among their clients. Factors positively associated with HCV service provision were the provision of services related to blood-borne disease prevention and care, the provision of OST and the staff health and medical qualifications.

Internationally, the operational capacities of DCRs/SIFs vary, but their clients all share common features of marginalisation, including estimated HCV prevalence rates of about 60%. DCRs/SIFs are well positioned to support PWUD to access HCV-related services, given the ease of access and the established relations between staff and clients which support uptake and adherence to HCV treatment [37]. The fact that HCV testing was significantly more likely to occur in DCRs/SIFs that offered HIV testing, or that provided vaccination for HBV onsite, is of high importance for PWUD who often live with hepatitis and HIV co-infections [38].

In HCV management, non-invasive liver disease assessment (e.g. fibro-scanning) is recommended as a feasible method in out-patient settings for PWUDs, alongside individualised disease management within a multidisciplinary team [39]. Treatment as prevention can significantly reduce HCV prevalence among PWUD and while DAAs make this approach more feasible [39], combining it with OST improves its effectiveness and can reduce population-level HCV rates [40].

In the Netherlands, HCV incidence and chronicity rates among PWUD have been the lowest in the European region [41] and have been decreasing for some time [42] in response to intensive prevention and treatment efforts. The decreasing rates of drug injection in the Netherlands have likely contributed to this trend [43, 44]. It was unsurprising then that the Dutch DCRs/SIFs were less likely to provide HCV testing and related services pertaining to blood-borne diseases.

There were other per-country differences in DCR operational characteristics. For instance, it has long been part of the Dutch DCR concept to run smaller facilities in multiple neighbourhoods and to co-locate them with other services, rather than one large stand-alone facility in a central area [45]. In contrast, our findings show countries with few DCRs/SIFs are more likely to operate as stand-alone services (for example, the Medically Supervised Injecting Centre in Sydney, Australia).

Between 2017 and 2018, about thirty new DCRs/SIFs were approved in Canada (in addition to Insite in Vancouver) [46]. The operational, financial and public health considerations of establishing additional DCRs/SIFs seem to favor smaller facilities which are well-integrated within existing agencies [47]. This study indicated that stand-alone facilities require larger investments in personnel, including medical staff. The advantage of the co-located services is that they can support PWUD/PWID directly with relevant care onsite.

When looking at the determinants of HCV service provision, these don't imply any causality and several other, unmeasured factors might play an important role. For instance, Australia has adopted universal access to HCV treatment, which is unprecedented internationally. Also, the Australian SIF employs a medical doctor. However, HCV treatment is not provided at the Sydney SIF, given the regulations around prescribing authority and it's close cooperation with a nearby health service. On the other hand, the local-level funding of DCRs in the Netherlands may have led to substantial local-level variability in operating procedures and funding priorities, including HCV provision. Local policies play an obvious role in the level of HCV service provision but this study wasn't designed to explore that in detail.

Low-threshold, harm reduction services such as DCRs/SIFs aim to "meet individuals where they are" in order to reduce individual and community-level harmful effects of drug use. Some clients might be systematically "falling through the net" of support services, leaving DCRs/SIFs the only programs they attend on a regular basis. This study found that HCV management and treatment were marginally more likely to be offered by DCRs/SIFs which also ran OST onsite. Unsurprisingly, the capacity to provide enhanced HCV care was closely related to the qualifications of DCRs/SIFs staff. Provision of liver monitoring or disease management were significantly associated with employing a nurse whereas HCV treatment was associated with employing a medical doctor. Enhancing staff qualifications via continuous education and greater engagement of health professionals in DCRs/SIFs operations will lead to more advanced HCV service provision and to continued engagement of the most vulnerable clients.

However, it needs to be acknowledged that hiring medical staff can represent a notable organisational and financial challenge for many DCRs/SIFs who are mostly funded outside of the general health funding schemes (e.g. local government budgets). Innovative protocols for the delivery of DAA treatments can include empowering existing staff via education and training to facilitate their cooperation with external medical professionals. In a recent Australian study, case managers who were supported by onsite nurses and medical doctors delivered DAA treatment in the community and achieved high completion rates [48]. This model can serve as an example for delivering flexible, patient-centred and cost-effective HCV treatment on community level. An additional barrier to implementing HCV treatments in DCRs might be the affordability of the medication. While the cost of medication is fully covered in Australia [49, 50], this has not been the situation in many low- and middle- income countries [51].

This study is limited by the relatively high non-response rate to the online survey (46%). Completing an online survey competes with other priorities and in some cases, filling in the survey was interrupted multiple times. In other instances, questions that required additional research into the DCR/SIF's internal resources were skipped.

The DCRs/SIFs that did not participate in the survey ($n = 52$) may offer different services to specific client groups, depending on their location and purpose, or have lower operational capacity. Some DCRs/SIFs in the study mentioned that enhanced provision of HCV-related services was not a key purpose of their operation. It is possible that DCRs/SIFs with greater affinity for HCV service provision chose to answer the survey. Beyond this survey, there is no official source of information that could be used to cross-validate the representativity of the sample. An important limitation to this study is that the survey wasn't available in all national languages (e.g. Spanish, Dutch, Danish or Norwegian) and misrepresentation of questions may have occurred.

Conclusions

The high infection rates of HCV among the DCRs/SIFs clients and the fact that HCV treatment as prevention can significantly reduce HCV rates among the population of PWUD warrant the attention for DCRs/SIFs to be seen as a potential space for the provision of HCV related services worldwide.

With their ease of access ('low threshold') and the regularity with which some clients attend them, DCRs/SIFs offer an important entry point to HCV treatment as well as a candidate program for the provision of new, DAA treatments. DCRs/SIFs can offer easy-to-access services and a trusted environment that is crucial in achieving HCV treatment adherence.

The main steps forward to enhance the onsite provision of HCV-related support in DCRs/SIFs are increasing their capacity to accommodate onsite medical professionals and educating existing staff. Funding and support for HCV treatment at the community level, via low-threshold services such as DCRs/SIFs, is worthy of action.

Abbreviations

DAA: Direct acting antivirals; DCR: Drug consumption room; HBV: Hepatitis B virus; HCV: Hepatitis C virus; HIV: Human immunodeficiency virus; OST: Opioid substitution treatment; PWID: People who inject drugs; PWUD: People who use drugs; SIF: Supervised injecting facility

Acknowledgements

The authors would like to thank all DCR/SIF managers who participated in the study. They would also like to thank Associate Professor Carolyn Day and Dr. Edmund Silins for providing comments to the manuscript, to Dr Libby Topp for reviewing the study questionnaire and protocol.

Funding

No specific funding was obtained to conduct this study.

Authors' contributions

AS and ES designed the study. All the authors (VB, AS, ES, MJ) contributed to developing the study tools and protocols. VB conducted data analysis and prepared the draft manuscript. All authors (VB, AS, ES, MJ) contributed to interpretation of the findings and to the writing of the manuscript. All authors read and approved the final manuscript.

Competing interests

The authors declare that they have no competing interests.

Author details

[1]Uniting Sydney Medically Supervised Injecting Centre (MSIC), Sydney, Australia. [2]Correlation network, Foundation De Regenboog Groep, Amsterdam, The Netherlands. [3]School of Public Health and Community Medicine, University of New South Wales, Sydney, NSW, Australia.

References

1. BCCS. Supervised consumption services: operational guidance. In: Edited by the steering Committee for the Supervised Consumption Services Guidelines. British Columbia: British Columbia Centre on Substance Use, Ministry of Health; 2018.
2. EMCDDA. Drug consumption rooms: an overview of provision and evidence. In: Perspectives on drugs. Lisbon: European Monitoring Centre for Drugs and Drug Addiction; 2016.
3. Hedrich D, Hartnoll R. Harm reduction interventions. Textbook of Addiction Treatment: International Perspectives. 2015:1291–313.
4. Hedrich D, Kerr T, Dubois-Arber F. Drug consumption facilities in Europe and beyond. In: Rhodes T, Hedrich D, editors. EMCDDA Scientific Monograph Series No 10- Harm Reduction: Evidence, Impacts and Challenges. Lisbon: The European Monitoring Centre for Drugs and Drug Addiction (EMCDDA); 2010.
5. Kerr T, Kimber J, DeBeck K, Wood E. The role of safer injection facilities in the response to HIV/AIDS among injection drug users. Current HIV/AIDS Reports. 2007;4(4):158–64.
6. Kimber J, Dolan K, Van Beek I, Hedrich D, Zurhold H. Drug consumption facilities: an update since 2000. Drug and Alcohol Review. 2003;22(2):227–33.
7. Kimber J, Palmateer N, Hutchinson S, Hickman M, Goldberg D, Rhodes T. Harm reduction among injecting drug users-evidence of effectiveness. In: Rhodes T, Hedrich D, editors. Harm Reduction: evidence, impacts and challenges. Lisbon: EMCDDA; 2010. p. 115–63.
8. Milloy MJ, Wood E. Emerging role of supervised injecting facilities in human immunodeficiency virus prevention. Addiction. 2009;104(4):620–1.
9. Monico D. Out of the alley: lessons from safe injecting facilities (SIF). Graduate Annual. 2015;3(1):12.
10. Potier C, Laprévote V, Dubois-Arber F, Cottencin O, Rolland B. Supervised injection services: what has been demonstrated? A systematic literature review. Drug Alcohol Depend. 2014;145:48–68.
11. Semaan S, Fleming P, Worrell C, Stolp H, Baack B, Miller M. Potential role of safer injection facilities in reducing HIV and hepatitis C infections and overdose mortality in the United States. Drug Alcohol Depend. 2011;118:11.
12. Wood E, Tyndall MW, Li K, Lloyd-Smith E, Small W, Montaner JSG, Kerr T. Do supervised injecting facilities attract higher-risk injection drug users? Am J Prev Med. 2005;29(2):126–30.
13. van Beek I, Kimber J, Dakin A, Gilmour S. The Sydney medically supervised injecting Centre: reducing harm associated with heroin overdose. Crit Public Health. 2004;14(4):391–406.
14. Bravo MJ, Royuela L, De la Fuente L, Brugal MT, Barrio G, Domingo-Salvany A, Itínere project group. Use of supervised injection facilities and injection risk behaviours among young drug injectors. Addiction. 2009;104(4):614–9.
15. Wood E, Tyndall MW, Qui Z, Zhang R, Montaner JSG, Kerr T. Service uptake and characteristics of injection drug users utilizing north Americas first medically supervised safer injecting facility. Am J Public Health. 2006;96(5):770–3.
16. Parés-Badell O, Espelt A, Folch C, Majó X, González V, Casabona J, Brugal MT. Undiagnosed HIV and hepatitis C infection in people who inject drugs: from new evidence to better practice. J Subst Abus Treat. 2017;77:13–20.
17. KPMG. Further evaluation of the Medically Supervised Injecting Centre during its extended trial period (2007-2011): Final report. Sydney: KPMG. p. 2010.
18. MSIC Evaluation committee. Final report of the evaluation of the Sydney medically supervised injecting Centre. Sydney: Authors; 2003.
19. Salmon AM, van Beek I, Amin J, Grulich A, Maher L. High HIV testing and low HIV prevalence among injecting drug users attending the Sydney medically supervised injecting Centre. Aust N Z J Public Health. 2009;33(3):280–3.
20. Andresen MA, Boyd N. A cost-benefit and cost-effectiveness analysis of Vancouver's supervised injection facility. International Journal of Drug Policy. 2010;21(1):70–6.
21. Bayoumi AM, Zaric GS. The cost-effectiveness of Vancouver's supervised injection facility. Can Med Assoc J. 2008;179(11):1143–51.
22. Pinkerton SD. Is Vancouver Canada's supervised injection facility cost-saving? Addiction. 2010;105(8):1429–36.
23. Stoltz J-A, Wood E, Small W, Li K, Tyndall M, Montaner J, Kerr T. Changes in injecting practices associated with the use of a medically supervised safer injection facility. Journal of Public Health. 2007;29(1):35–9.
24. Wood E, Tyndall MW, Stoltz J-A, Small W, Lloyd-Smith E, Zhang R, Montaner JSG, Kerr T. Factors Associated with Syringe Sharing Among Users of a Medically Supervised Safer Injecting Facility. American Jounral of Infectious Diseases. 2005:1(1).
25. Kinnard EN, Howe CJ, Kerr T, Hass VS, Marshall BD. Self-reported changes in drug use behaviors and syringe disposal methods following the opening of a supervised injecting facility in Copenhagen Denmark. Harm Reduct J. 2014;11(1):1.
26. Zurhold H, Degkwitz P, Verthein U, Haasen C. Drug consumption rooms in Hamburg, Germany: evaluation of the effects on harm reduction and the reduction of public nuisance. J Drug Issues. 2003;33(3):663–88.

27. Dimova RB, Zeremski M, Jacobson IM, Hagan H, Des Jarlais DC, Talal AH. Determinants of hepatitis C virus treatment completion and efficacy in drug users assessed by meta-analysis. Clin Infect Dis. 2013;56(6):806–16.
28. Grady BP, Schinkel J, Thomas XV, Dalgard O. Hepatitis C virus reinfection following treatment among people who use drugs. Clin Infect Dis. 2013; 57(suppl 2):S105–10.
29. Martin NK, Vickerman P, Miners A, Foster GR, Hutchinson SJ, Goldberg DJ, Hickman M. Cost-effectiveness of hepatitis C virus antiviral treatment for injection drug user populations. Hepatology. 2012;55(1):49–57.
30. Visconti AJ, Doyle JS, Weir A, Shiell AM, Hellard ME. Assessing the cost-effectiveness of treating chronic hepatitis C virus in people who inject drugs in Australia. J Gastroenterol Hepatol. 2013;28(4):707–16.
31. Grebely J, Hajarizadeh B, Dore GJ. Direct-acting antiviral agents for HCV infection affecting people who inject drugs. Gastoenterology & Hepatology. 2017;1:1–11.
32. McGowan CE, Fried MW. Barriers to hepatitis C treatment. Liver Int. 2012;32(s1):151–6.
33. Dillon JF, Lazarus JV, Razavi HA. Urgent action to fight hepatitis C in people who inject drugs in Europe. Hepatology, Medicine and Policy. 2016;1(2):1–10.
34. Dubois-Arber F, Benninghoff F, Jeannin A. Typology of injection profiles of clients of a supervised drug consumption facility in Geneva Switzerland. European Addiction Research. 2008;14(1):1–10.
35. Woods S. Organisational overview of drug consumption rooms in Europe. Amsterdam: European Harm Reduction Network – Regenboog Groep; 2014.
36. Kimber JO, Dolan K, Wodak A. Survey of drug consumption rooms: service delivery and perceived public health and amenity impact. Drug and Alcohol Review. 2005;24(1):21–4.
37. Rich ZC, Chu C, Mao J, Zhou K, Cai W, Ma Q, Volberding P, Tucker JD. Facilitators of HCV treatment adherence among people who inject drugs: a systematic qualitative review and implications for scale up of direct acting antivirals. BMC Public Health. 2016;16(1):994.
38. Nielsen S, Gassowski M, Wenz B, Bannert N, Bock C-T, Kücherer C, Ross RS, Bremer V, Marcus U, Zimmermann R. Concordance between self-reported and measured HIV and hepatitis C virus infection status among people who inject drugs in Germany. Hepatology, Medicine and Policy. 2016;1(1):8.
39. Grebely J, Robaeys G, Bruggmann P, Aghemo A, Backmund M, Bruneau J, Byrne J, Dalgard O, Feld JJ, Hellard M. Recommendations for the management of hepatitis C virus infection among people who inject drugs. International Journal of Drug Policy. 2015;26(10):1028–38.
40. Martin NK, Hickman M, Hutchinson SJ, Goldberg DJ, Vickerman P. Combination interventions to prevent HCV transmission among people who inject drugs: modeling the impact of antiviral treatment, needle and syringe programs, and opiate substitution therapy. Clinical Infectious Diseases. 2013;57(suppl_2):S39–45.
41. Wiessing L, Ferri M, Grady B, Kantzanou M, Sperle I, Cullen KJ, Hatzakis A, Prins M, Vickerman P, Lazarus JV. Hepatitis C virus infection epidemiology among people who inject drugs in Europe: a systematic review of data for scaling up treatment and prevention. PLoS One. 2014;9(7):e103345.
42. van de Laar TJ, Molenkamp R, van den Berg C, Schinkel J, Beld MG, Prins M, Coutinho RA, Bruisten SM. Frequent HCV reinfection and superinfection in a cohort of injecting drug users in Amsterdam. J Hepatol. 2009;51(4):667–74.
43. Van Ameijden E, Coutinho R. Large decline in injecting drug use in Amsterdam, 1986–1998: explanatory mechanisms and determinants of injecting transitions. J Epidemiol Community Health. 2001;55(5):356–63.
44. van de Laar TJ, Langendam MW, Bruisten SM, Welp EA, Verhaest I, van Ameijden EJ, Coutinho RA, Prins M. Changes in risk behavior and dynamics of hepatitis C virus infections among young drug users in Amsterdam, the Netherlands. J Med Virol. 2005;77(4):509–18.
45. Dolan K, Kimber J, Fry C, McDonald D, Fitzgerald J, Trautmann F. Drug consumption facilities in Europe and the establishment of supervised injecting centres in Australia. Drug and Alcohol Review. 2000;19(3):337–46.
46. Health Canada. Supervised consumption sites: status of applications. Vancouver: Government of Canada; 2018.
47. Williams S: Opinion: Safe injection sites a small step but big milestone in saving lives. In: Edmonton Journal. vol. 25th October, 2017. Edmonton; 2017. https://edmontonjournal.com/opinion/columnists/opinion-safe-injection-sites-a-small-step-but-big-milestone-in-saving-lives, Retrieved on 30th July, 2018.
48. Morris L, Smirnov A, Kvassay A, Leslie E, Kavanagh R, Alexander N, Davey G, Williams O, Gilks C, Najman J. Initial outcomes of integrated community-based hepatitis C treatment for people who inject drugs: findings from the Queensland injectors' health network. Int J Drug Policy. 2017;47:216–20.
49. Lazarus JV. Edito-in-Chief's welcome to Hepatology, medicine and policy. BMJ Hepatology, Medicine and Policy. 2016;1(1):1–3.
50. Iyengar S, Tay-Teo K, Vogler S, Beyer P, Wiktor S, de Joncheere K, Hill S. Prices, costs, and affordability of new medicines for hepatitis C in 30 countries: an economic analysis. PLoS Med. 2016;13(5):e1002032.
51. FitzSimons D, Hendrickx G, Hallauer J, Larson H, Lavanchy D, Lodewyckx I, Shouval D, Ward J, Van Damme P. Innovative sources for funding of viral hepatitis prevention and treatment in low-and middle-income countries: a roundtable meeting report. Hepatology, Medicine and Policy. 2016;1(1):16.

22

Design of the Prospective Real-world Outcomes Study of hepatic encephalopathy Patients' Experience on Rifaximin-α (PROSPER)

Aleksander Krag[1*], Marcus Schuchmann[2], Hanna Sodatonou[3], Jeff Pilot[3], James Whitehouse[4], Simone I. Strasser[5] and Mark Hudson[6]

Abstract

Background: Hepatic encephalopathy (HE) is one of the most important severe complications of liver cirrhosis. Thought to be caused by elevated blood levels of gut-derived neurotoxins (particularly ammonia) entering the brain, HE manifests as a wide range of neurological or psychiatric abnormalities, which increase the risk of mortality, result in substantial morbidity and negatively affect the quality of life (QoL) of both patients and their caregivers. HE is also associated with a substantial economic burden. Rifaximin-α 550 mg is a locally acting oral antibiotic that reduces the effects of ammonia-producing intestinal flora, and which is used to help reduce the recurrence of overt HE. The efficacy of rifaximin-α 550 mg was established in a randomised controlled trial and long-term extension study. However, 'real-world' evidence is also required to assess how this efficacy may translate into effectiveness in clinical practice, including the potential impact of treatment on healthcare resource utilisation.

Methods: The Prospective Real-world Outcomes Study of HE Patients' Experience on Rifaximin-α 550 mg (PROSPER) is a multinational, multicentre, observational study that will be conducted under real-world clinical practice conditions. Comprising a retrospective phase (up to 12 months) and a prospective phase (up to 24 months), and employing a robust statistical methodology, PROSPER has been specifically designed to minimise the bias associated with observational studies. The primary endpoint will be the effect of rifaximin-α 550 mg treatment on HE- and liver-related hospitalisation rate and duration of hospitalisation. Secondary endpoints will include comprehensive assessments of the impact of treatment on the QoL and workplace productivity of patients and caregivers, a global assessment of treatment effectiveness and safety/tolerability. Approximately 550 patients will be enrolled.

Conclusions: PROSPER will provide valuable real-world information on the effectiveness of rifaximin-α 550 mg in reducing the recurrence of HE, and its impact on the QoL and work productivity of patients and their caregivers. By providing data on both the direct costs (e.g., hospitalisation rate, duration of hospitalisation) and indirect costs (such as work productivity) of HE, PROSPER should help confirm whether rifaximin-α 550 mg treatment represents a good use of economic resources.

Keywords: Cirrhosis, Health economics, Hepatic encephalopathy, Hospitalisation, Liver disease, Patient-reported outcomes, Quality of life, Real-world, Rifaximin-α 550 mg, Work productivity

* Correspondence: aleksanderkrag@hotmail.com
[1]Department of Gastroenterology and Hepatology, Odense University Hospital, University of Southern Denmark, Odense, Denmark
Full list of author information is available at the end of the article

Introduction

Hepatic encephalopathy (HE) is a brain dysfunction caused by liver insufficiency and/or portosystemic shunting, which manifests as a wide spectrum of neurological or psychiatric abnormalities [1]. It is now widely recognised as one of the most important severe complications of liver cirrhosis, along with conditions such as ascites and variceal bleeding [1]. HE severity is categorised using West Haven criteria from 'minimal' through grade 1 to 4 [1]. 'Covert HE' is defined as West Haven minimal and grade 1, and 'overt HE' is defined as West Haven grades 2 to 4 [1]. Overt HE occurs in 30–40% of patients with cirrhosis at some time during their clinical course [1]. HE increases the risk of mortality [2] and is one of the most debilitating complications of liver disease [1], negatively affecting the lives of both patients and caregivers [1, 3].

HE is also associated with a substantial economic burden, in terms of direct healthcare costs resulting from, for example, emergency room visits and hospitalisation [1, 4–11]. Although difficult to accurately determine, the indirect costs of HE (e.g., loss of work productivity, car accidents) also represent a substantial economic burden, which is likely to be further increased when the impact on caregivers is taken into account [3, 7, 12].

The neuropsychiatric symptoms of HE are thought to result from elevated blood levels of gut-derived neurotoxins (particularly ammonia), which enter the brain due to the inability of the cirrhotic liver to remove them from the blood [13]. Rifaximin-α 550 mg is a locally acting oral antibiotic that is minimally absorbed in the gut to reduce the effects of intestinal flora, including ammonia-producing species [14]. Its clinical activity may be due to its effects on the metabolic function of gut microbiota, rather than a change in relative bacterial abundance [15]. Rifaximin-α 550 mg is indicated in Europe for the reduction in recurrence of episodes of overt HE in patients aged ≥18 years [16]. In Australia, it has the same indication, but is restricted to where other treatments have failed or are contraindicated [17]. The efficacy of rifaximin-α 550 mg has been confirmed in a randomised controlled trial (RCT), in which rifaximin-α 550 mg twice daily (administered concomitantly with lactulose therapy in approximately 91% of patients) reduced the relative risks of recurrence of overt HE and HE-related hospitalisation by 58% and 50%, respectively, compared with placebo (absolute risk reductions: 24% and 9%, respectively) [18]. In a subsequent 2-year extension study, long-term treatment with rifaximin-α 550 mg (with concomitant lactulose in approximately 90% of patients) provided a continued reduction in the rate of HE-related and all-cause hospitalisation, without an increased rate of adverse events [19].

Although RCTs are essential in the clinical development of new treatments, they do not necessarily reflect clinical practice conditions. Typically, they are conducted in carefully defined patient populations using specific inclusion and exclusion criteria. By contrast, in clinical practice, patients are more diverse in terms of clinical characteristics than those recruited for RCTs. In addition, whereas RCTs employ rigid treatment protocols, in clinical practice treatment is tailored on a patient-by-patient basis. Consequently, 'real-world' studies are required to complement evidence from RCTs by determining how the efficacy of an agent translates into effectiveness in clinical practice. Since real-world studies have a higher likelihood of inherent bias than RCTs, it is important when designing a real-world study to eliminate as much bias as possible and minimise the impact of any remaining bias in the statistical analysis methodology employed. Real-world data are particularly useful for hard-to-reach patient populations (such as HE patients), for which clinical trial recruitment is challenging. Moreover, national reimbursement authorities are increasingly requesting real-world data to support evidence from clinical trials when examining the economic rationale for supporting new treatments [20, 21]. Real-world studies are therefore important both clinically and from a patient access perspective.

An important aspect of real-world studies is to assess patient- and caregiver-reported outcomes, since the effectiveness of a treatment is not only dependent on its efficacy and safety/tolerability, but also on its effects on the patient's quality of life (QoL) and ability to function, and the associated impact on those who care for them. This is particularly true for chronic conditions, such as HE, where an agent's effectiveness relies primarily on the patient being willing and able to be compliant with the treatment over the long term.

We here describe the design of the Prospective Real-world Outcomes Study of HE Patients' Experience on Rifaximin-α 550 mg (PROSPER), which will evaluate the clinical effectiveness of rifaximin-α 550 mg and its impact on healthcare resources when used for the management of HE in routine clinical practice.

Methods/design

PROSPER is a multinational, multicentre, observational study that will be conducted in secondary/tertiary care centres across Europe and Australia (ClinicalTrials.gov identifier: NCT02488993). Study site selection will be based on an initial feasibility assessment to evaluate the volume of patients seen and local expertise in HE at potential centres. The principal country for patient recruitment will be Denmark, where no ethical approval is required for observational studies.

Ethical approval in other individual countries will be sought, where appropriate.

Study design

PROSPER will be conducted under 'real-world' clinical practice conditions. Consequently, no changes to the management of HE patients will be made for the purposes of the study.

Once eligible patients have been recruited and consented to participate in the study, two data collection phases will be undertaken (Fig. 1). The first will be a retrospective phase, involving the review of the patients' medical records and electronic hospital admissions data. Up to 12 months of data prior to study entry will be reviewed and collected. The level and nature of missing data will be assessed and accounted for in the statistical analysis plan, if necessary. The retrospective phase will be followed by a prospective phase, during which data will be collected from all patients either receiving rifaximin-α 550 mg (rifaximin-α 550 mg cohort) or not receiving rifaximin-α 550 mg (control cohort) from the point of study entry. Up to 24 months of data following study entry will be collected and analysed.

In order to minimise bias and the influence of confounding factors, the study outcomes will be compared between the treatment cohorts in three ways (Fig. 1). The first approach will initially involve the clinical characterisation of the study population, based on retrospective chart review (Fig. 1, comparison 1a), following which outcomes between the cohorts will be compared after adjustment of statistical methods on the basis of the findings from comparison 1a (Fig. 1, comparison 1b). Secondly, for each cohort individually, outcomes pre and post baseline will be compared (Fig. 1, comparisons 2a and 2b). Thirdly, the difference between the two cohorts in pre/post changes will be compared (Fig. 1, comparison 3).

Patients will be eligible to enrol during or following hospitalisation for the qualifying episode of overt HE (Fig. 2; timepoint 1). Patients will also be eligible to enter the study at the time of resolution of the qualifying episode of overt HE (Fig. 2; timepoint 2) or at a follow-up appointment, providing this is within 12 weeks of resolution of the qualifying episode of overt HE (Fig. 2; timepoint 3).

Study population

Patients with cirrhosis and HE will be enrolled into PROSPER. The study will employ a limited number of inclusion and exclusion criteria in order to reflect the diversity of patients encountered in clinical practice (Table 1).

Study assessments

The study's primary endpoint will be the HE- and liver-related hospitalisation rate and the resulting duration of hospitalisation (number of bed-days). Secondary endpoints will include the rate of all-cause hospitalisation and the resulting duration of hospitalisation (number of bed-days), mortality rate, and the number, duration and severity of HE episodes. Effects of treatment on the underlying liver disease will also be assessed as secondary endpoints using the Child-Turcotte-Pugh score, Model for End-stage Liver Disease (MELD) score or MELD-Na score (a modified MELD score including serum sodium [22]). In addition, the effectiveness of treatment will be assessed by the patient, caregiver and physician, using the Global Evaluation of Treatment Effectiveness (GETE) questionnaire. This consists of the single question *'How effective has [your treatment/the treatment] been in controlling [your/the patient's] HE?'*, which is answered by choosing one of five responses: *'Complete control of HE'*, *'Marked improvement in HE'*, *'Limited improvement in HE'*, *'No appreciable change in HE'* or *'Worsening of HE'*.

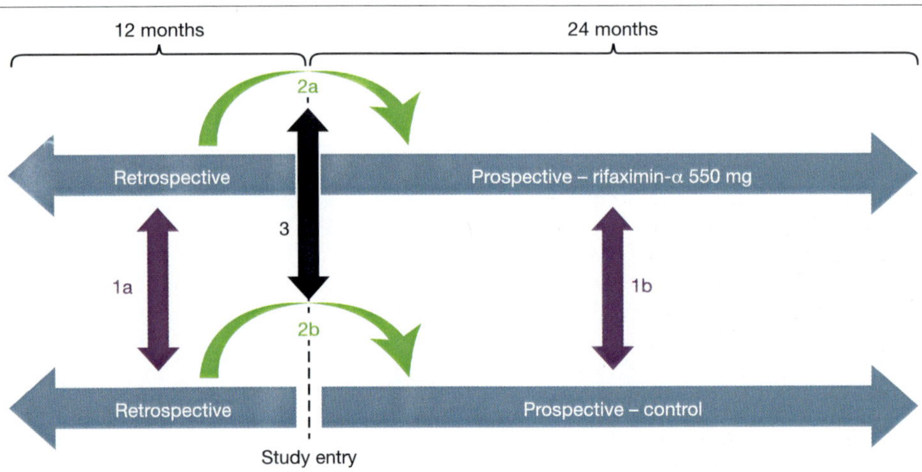

Fig. 1 Study design

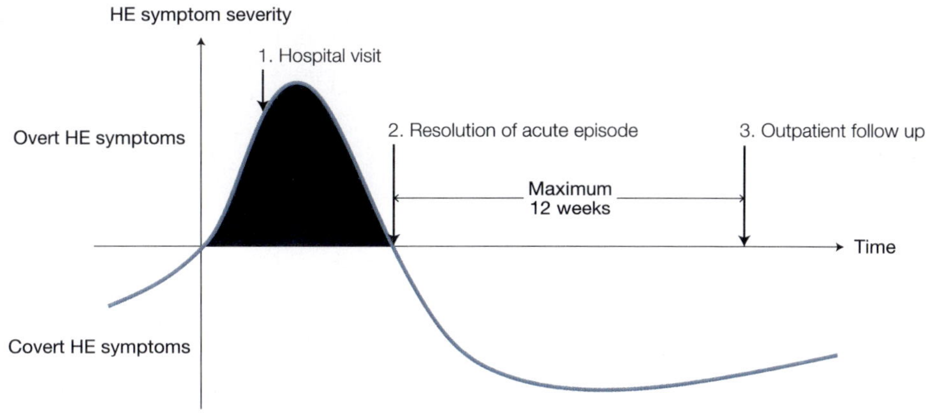

Fig. 2 Timing of entry into study, relative to overt HE episode. HE, hepatic encephalopathy

The safety of treatment with rifaximin-α 550 mg will be evaluated by assessing the frequency and nature of adverse events (AEs) and serious AEs. This will include classification of the severity of AEs and their relationship/causality in relation to medical treatment of HE.

The effects of treatment on health-related QoL will be assessed using the patient-reported Chronic Liver Disease Questionnaire (CLDQ) [23], the patient-reported Euroqol-5 Dimension-5 level (EQ-5D-5L) measure and the caregiver-reported proxy EQ-5D-5L:1 measure [24]. The CLDQ is a 29-item questionnaire assessing a wide range of physical, emotional and psychosocial QoL-related factors during the previous 2 weeks [23]. The EQ-5D-5L and proxy EQ-5D-5L are six-item questionnaires assessing the patient's mobility, ability to self-care, ability to undertake usual activities, pain/discomfort, anxiety/depression and overall health status on the particular day in question [24].

Workplace productivity impairment will be assessed in patients using the Work Productivity and Activity Impairment Questionnaire: General Health V2.0 (WPAI:GH) and in caregivers using the Work Productivity and Activity Impairment Questionnaire: General Health Care Giving V2.0 (WPAI:GH-CG) [25]. These are six-item questionnaires assessing the effects of the patient's health problems (WPAI:GH), or the effects of caregiving for the patient's health problems (WPAI:GH-CG), on the individual's ability to work and perform daily activities. A schedule for these assessments is shown in Table 2.

Sample size calculation

In observational studies where multivariable modelling is expected to be performed, the study should have at least 10 events for every variable included in the model. Therefore, in order to consider approximately 10 variables, 100 events would need to be observed in each of the study cohorts (patients receiving and not receiving rifaximin-α 550 mg). On the basis of an open-label maintenance study of rifaximin-α 550 mg in patients with HE [19], approximately 45% of patients would be expected to have experienced a hospitalisation within the first 12 months of follow-up. Assuming a dropout rate of 10%, approximately 247 patients would be required for each of the two cohorts, or 494 patients overall. Thus, a total study population of 550 would be sufficient to assess the primary endpoint of the study at

Table 1 Inclusion and exclusion criteria

Inclusion criteria	Exclusion criteria
• Diagnosis of cirrhosis	• West Haven score of ≥2 at study entry
• Age ≥ 18 years	• A mental health disorder that makes HE diagnosis questionable (e.g., dementia, psychosis)
• Enrolment within 12 weeks of resolution of an episode of overt HE associated with a hospital visit	• Prior treatment with rifaximin[a] within 12 months prior to the qualifying overt HE episode
• Ability to provide informed consent	• Contraindications to the use of rifaximin-α 550 mg, as per the local Summary of Product Characteristics [16, 17]
• Clinical eligibility to receive rifaximin-α 550 mg, in the opinion of the participating physician, regardless of HE treatment actually received	

HE hepatic encephalopathy
[a]All types and dose strengths of rifaximin

Table 2 Schedule of assessments

	Enrolment	1 month[a]	3 months[a]	6 months[a]	12 months[a]	18 months[a]	24 months[a]
Informed consent provided by patient and caregiver (note that caregiver consent is optional for patient study inclusion)	X						
Retrospective chart review (collection of demographic and medical history data)	X						
Ongoing clinical data, including clinical outcomes, laboratory measures, medication dose/schedule, resource utilisation, medication adherence[b]		X	X	X	X	X	X
GETE[c]		X		X			
CLDQ[b]	X				X		X
EQ-5D-5L (patient)[d]	X		X	X	X	X	X
EQ-5D-5L Proxy (caregiver)[d,e]	X		X	X	X	X	X
WPAI (patient)[c]	X		X	X	X	X	X
WPAI (caregiver)[c]	X		X	X	X	X	X

CLDQ Chronic Liver Disease Questionnaire, *EQ-5D-5 L* Euroqol-5 Dimension-5 level measure, *GETE* Global Evaluation of Treatment Effectiveness questionnaire, *WPAI* Work Productivity and Activity Impairment questionnaire

[a]Target dates only; flexible depending on patient response

[b]To be collected at all clinic visits but not at fixed time intervals; clinic visits will be scheduled by investigator and patient according to normal management and not defined by study protocol

[c]To be collected at the clinic visit closest to the indicated study date; no additional clinic visits to be scheduled for study participation

[d]To be requested for patient completion via paper submission or online portal or at clinic visit closest to the indicated date; clinic visit may not be required

[e]Australia, UK, Ireland, France and Germany, where the proxy response has been validated

an interim follow-up of 12 months, with additional precision following the full 24-month follow-up period.

Statistical analysis

A primary aim of PROSPER will be to minimise any bias typically associated with observational studies. This will be achieved by the three-step comparative structure incorporated into the study's design (as described above) and the associated statistical methodology. An overview of the statistical considerations is presented here.

The primary outcome of HE- and liver-associated hospitalisation rate will be analysed as a count, using either Poisson or negative binomial regression, depending on the level of observed dispersion. An offset term will be included to account for length of time eligible to experience a hospitalisation, accounting for mortality or other competing risk events. The primary outcome of duration of HE- and liver-associated hospitalisation (number of bed-days) will be analysed either as a continuous variable or a count, depending on the observed distribution. Methodologies such as median regression may be employed to account for the likelihood of right skew resulting from a small proportion of extended hospital stays. Comparison of the primary outcomes between treatment cohorts will adjust for key covariates using either multivariable regression analysis or a propensity score analysis (to be confirmed based on an exploratory review of the data). Due to the observational nature of the study, it is expected that some patients could change, discontinue or be non-compliant with therapy during the course of follow-up. These scenarios will be considered during statistical analysis and techniques that account for exposure to therapy will be applied, if applicable.

The rate of all-cause hospitalisation and the resulting duration of hospitalisation will be analysed in the same way as the primary endpoints. Numeric measures (e.g., CLDQ, EQ-5D-5L and GETE scores) will be analysed using a linear regression model, with longitudinal methodology to account for repeated measures, if applicable. Event-based variables and count data (e.g., AEs, HE episodes, mortality) will be analysed using Poisson or negative binomial regression, with offset terms to account for exposure time, length of time eligible to receive hospitalisation and competing risks (e.g., death); analyses will also adjust for underlying differences between cohorts (i.e., confounding factors). Time-to-event methods (e.g., Kaplan Meier analysis) will be used for variables such as time until death. Categorical demographic and clinical characteristics will be presented descriptively as frequency/percentage distribution and compared using a chi-squared test. Continuous demographic and clinical characteristics will be presented descriptively as means with 95% confidence intervals and compared using a Student's *t*-test.

It is anticipated that additional analyses will include treatment adherence and switching, and the integration of survival data with QoL data, to assess quality-adjusted life-years (QALYs). Other exploratory analyses may also be conducted.

Current status

PROSPER aims to enrol approximately 550 patients. Patient recruitment commenced in June 2015. An interim analysis will be performed after 12 months of data collection. Additional *ad hoc* and exploratory analyses may also occur during the course of data collection. The full dataset should be available for analysis by January 2020.

Discussion

Data on the real-world effectiveness of secondary prophylaxis with rifaximin-α 550 mg and its impact on healthcare resource utilisation are currently limited. Although several studies have been conducted in the USA [7, 26–29], studies in Europe are scarce and none have yet been published in Australia. In the UK retrospective observational IMPRESS study, details of inpatient hospitalisations and hospital visits in the 12 months prior to and following initiation of rifaximin-α 550 mg treatment for HE were extracted from 11 NHS Trust electronic databases [4]. A total of 145 patients were evaluated (mean age 61 years; 61% male), 82% of whom were being treated with lactulose. A comparison of resource use in the 12 months pre- and post-initiation of rifaximin-α 550 mg revealed that there were significant reductions in the number of hospitalisations with overnight stay per patient (mean 2.7 vs. 1.7; $p = 0.002$), total number of bed days per inpatient (mean 31.7 vs. 16.4; $p < 0.001$) and number of critical care bed days per inpatient (mean 11.3 vs. 2.4; $p = 0.017$). The number of emergency room visits per patient also decreased but the difference was not statistically significant (mean 2.4 vs. 1.8; $p = 0.099$). Treatment with rifaximin-α 550 mg was generally well tolerated: three patients (2%) had adverse drug reactions and four (3%) developed *C. difficile* infection, but none of these patients discontinued treatment [4].

Another UK study specifically assessed the impact of rifaximin-α 550 mg treatment on healthcare resource utilisation using data from seven liver treatment centres [30]. Clinical, demographic and hospital admissions data from 326 patients were collected retrospectively for the time-periods 3, 6 and 12 months before and following initiation of rifaximin-α 550 mg treatment, and admission rates and hospital length of stay before and during therapy were compared. Rifaximin-α 550 mg treatment reduced the total length of stay in hospital by an estimated 31–53%, decreasing inpatient costs by £4858–6607 per patient per year. When the cost of treatment was taken into account (£3379 per patient per year), the estimated annual mean saving was £1480–3228 per patient [30].

Other data from Europe on the impact on healthcare resource utilisation are the results of cost-effectiveness modelling analyses conducted for the UK, Belgium, Sweden and the Netherlands [8–11], which applied country-specific costings to data derived from the original rifaximin-α 550 mg RCT [18] and open-label extension study [19]. The UK analysis found that the 5-year average cost of care for HE with rifaximin-α 550 mg plus lactulose was £22,971, a saving of £573 compared with the 5-year average cost of standard care (placebo plus lactulose) [8]. The corresponding values for benefit were 2.4 and 1.8 QALYs, respectively, representing a dominant base-case incremental cost-effectiveness ratio (ICER) over a 5-year horizon for rifaximin-α 550 mg. The positive impact of rifaximin-α 550 mg on healthcare costs was due to its reducing the rate of overt HE episodes, the likelihood of hospitalisation and hospital length of stay [8]. Similarly, beneficial cost-effectiveness results for rifaximin-α 550 mg treatment were demonstrated in modelling analyses conducted for Belgium and Sweden [9, 10]. The analysis conducted for the Netherlands incorporated indirect costs into the model, in terms of loss of work productivity and the costs of travelling to attend outpatient visits [11]. The time horizon was again 5 years, and costs and benefits were discounted at 4.0% and 1.5%, respectively. The total discounted and undiscounted 5-year costs for a patient treated with rifaximin-α 550 mg plus lactulose were €67,018 and €87,154, respectively, compared with €37,365 and €45,755, respectively, for a patient treated with placebo plus lactulose. Although the cost of lost productivity was higher for placebo plus lactulose than for rifaximin-α 550 mg plus lactulose (because of more frequent overt HE events), travel and informal costs were higher for rifaximin-α 550 mg plus lactulose than for placebo plus lactulose due to increased survival. The incremental health benefits for rifaximin-α 550 mg over a lifetime scenario were 0.93 QALYs (discounted) and 1.09 (undiscounted). Although the ICER amounted to €31,897 per QALY (discounted) and €38,027 per QALY (undiscounted), these values were well below the threshold recommended by the country's Scientific Council for Government Policy (€80,000 per QALY) [11].

Although encouraging, these cost-effectiveness analyses were modelled using RCT data and their results therefore need to be confirmed with real-world evidence. PROSPER will address this need by providing valuable real-world information on the impact of rifaximin-α 550 mg treatment in Europe and Australia on both the direct costs (e.g., hospitalisation rate, duration of hospitalisation) and indirect costs (e.g., work productivity) of HE. PROSPER could also afford a better understanding of the burden and natural history of HE, and of variability in disease management between different countries and regions. Additionally, PROSPER is likely to provide the type of evidence required by payors and decision bodies to confirm whether rifaximin-α 550 mg treatment represents a good use of economic resources (as indicated by cost-effectiveness models), thereby ultimately allowing access to the right treatment for the right patients.

Since the findings and implications of real-world studies are often limited by bias, PROSPER has been specifically developed to minimise bias, in terms of both its design and the robust statistical methodology it employs. As such, it is broadly in line with the International Society for Pharmacoeconomics and Outcomes Research (ISPOR) Good Research Practices Taskforce guidelines, which state that the choice of study design may strengthen the ability to address potential biases and confounding in prospective observational studies, separately from the analytic and statistical approaches employed [20]. The details provided in the present article also address the guidelines' recommendation that the reasoning behind all study design and analytic choices should be transparent and explained in the study protocol [20].

The ISPOR guidelines acknowledge the increasing importance of real-world studies in informing health policy decisions and highlight the consequent necessity for rigour and transparency when conducting such studies [20]. In addressing these concerns, it is anticipated that the findings of PROSPER will be widely applicable to clinical practice and may help inform future approaches to HE management.

Conclusions

PROSPER will provide valuable real-world information on the effectiveness of rifaximin-α 550 mg in reducing the recurrence of HE, and its impact on the QoL and work productivity of patients and their caregivers. PROSPER will also help to confirm whether rifaximin-α 550 mg treatment is cost effective, by providing real-world information on its impact on both the direct and indirect costs of HE.

Abbreviations

AE: Adverse event; CLDQ: Chronic Liver Disease Questionnaire; EQ-5D-5L: Euroqol-5 Dimension-5 level; GETE: Global Evaluation of Treatment Effectiveness; HE: Hepatic encephalopathy; ICER: Incremental cost-effectiveness ratio; ISPOR: International Society for Pharmacoeconomics and Outcomes Research; MELD: Model for End-stage Liver Disease; NHS: National Health Service; PROSPER: Prospective Real-world Outcomes Study of HE Patients' Experience on Rifaximin-α 550 mg; QALY: Quality-adjusted life-year; QoL: Quality of life; RCT: Randomised controlled trial; WPAI:GH: Work Productivity and Activity Impairment Questionnaire: General Health V2.0; WPAI:GH-CG: Work Productivity and Activity Impairment Questionnaire: General Health Care Giving V2.0

Acknowledgements

Medical writing support was provided by John Scopes of m*X*m Medical Communications.

Funding

This study is sponsored by Norgine. Medical writing support for the preparation of this manuscript was funded by Norgine.

Authors' contributions

All authors were involved in the development and preparation of this manuscript, and take full responsibility for its content. All authors read and approved the final manuscript.

Competing interests

AK: Norgine advisory board, speaker and investigator.
MS: Lecture and travel fees from AbbVie, Gilead, Falk and Norgine; in addition, advisory board honoraria from AbbVie and Norgine.
HS, JP and JW: Employees of Norgine Ltd.
SIS: Advisory board membership/speaker fees from Norgine, Gilead Sciences, AbbVie, Bristol Myers Squibb, MSD, Bayer Healthcare and Astellas.
MH: Speaker fees and travel expenses from Norgine, Astellas, Janssen and AbbVie.

Author details

[1]Department of Gastroenterology and Hepatology, Odense University Hospital, University of Southern Denmark, Odense, Denmark. [2]Department of Internal Medicine, Constance Medical Centre, Constance, Germany. [3]Norgine Ltd Clinical Development & Medical Affairs, Harefield, UK. [4]Norgine Global Health Outcomes, Norgine Ltd, Uxbridge, UK. [5]AW Morrow Gastroenterology and Liver Centre, Royal Prince Alfred Hospital and University of Sydney, Sydney, Australia. [6]Liver Unit, Freeman Hospital, Newcastle upon Tyne Hospitals NHS Trust and Institute of Cellular Medicine, Newcastle University, Newcastle upon Tyne, UK.

References

1. American Association for the Study of Liver Diseases; European Association for the Study of the Liver. Hepatic encephalopathy in chronic liver disease: 2014 practice guideline by the European Association for the Study of the Liver and the American Association for the Study of Liver Diseases. J Hepatol. 2014;61:642–59.
2. Cordoba J, Ventura-Cots M, Simón-Talero M, Amorós À, Pavesi M, Vilstrup H, Angeli P, Domenicali M, Ginés P, Bernardi M, Arroyo V, CANONIC Study Investigators of EASL-CLIF consortium. Characteristics, risk factors, and mortality of cirrhotic patients hospitalized for hepatic encephalopathy with and without acute-on-chronic liver failure (ACLF). J Hepatol. 2014;60:275–81.
3. Bajaj JS, Wade JB, Gibson DP, Heuman DM, Thacker LR, Sterling RK, Stravitz RT, Luketic V, Fuchs M, White MB, Bell DE, Gilles H, Morton K, Noble N, Puri P, Sanyal AJ. The multi-dimensional burden of cirrhosis and hepatic encephalopathy on patients and caregivers. Am J Gastroenterol. 2011;106: 1646–53.
4. Aspinall R, Radwan A, Shaya G, Sodatonou H, Cipelli R, Hudson M. The impact of rifaximin-alpha on NHS hospital resource use in UK patients with hepatic encephalopathy: a retrospective observational study (IMPRESS). J Hepatol. 2016;64(Suppl 2):S283 (abstract THU-376).
5. Bajaj JS, Reddy KR, Tandon P, Wong F, Kamath PS, Garcia-Tsao G, Maliakkal B, Biggins SW, Thuluvath PJ, Fallon MB, Subramanian RM, Vargas H, Thacker LR, O'Leary JG. North American Consortium for the Study of End-Stage Liver Disease. The 3-month readmission rate remains unacceptably high in a large North American cohort of cirrhotic patients. Hepatology. 2016;64:200–8.
6. Montagnese S, Bajaj JS, Angeli P, Krag A. Real-world evidence: does it really change clinical practice? Treatment strategies. Hepatology. 2015;2:35–42.
7. Neff GW, Kemmer N, Duncan C, Alsina A. Update on the management of cirrhosis - focus on cost-effective preventative strategies. Clinicoecon Outcomes Res. 2013;5:143–52.
8. Berni E, Poole CD, Conway P, Radwan A, Currie CJ. Cost effectiveness of rifaximin-α 550mg in the reduction of recurrence of overt hepatic encephalopathy in United Kingdom. Value Health. 2015;18:A626 [abstract].
9. Berni E, Connolly M, Conway P, Radwan A, Currie CJ. Evaluation of the cost effectiveness of rifaximin-α in the reduction of recurrence of overt hepatic encephalopathy in Belgium. Value Health. 2015;18:A628 [abstract].
10. Poole CD, Berni E, Conway P, Radwan A, Currie CJ. Evaluation of the cost effectiveness of rifaximin-α 550mg in the reduction of recurrence of overt hepatic encephalopathy in Sweden. Value Health. 2015;18:A626 [abstract].

11. Whitehouse JT, Berni E, Conway P, Radwan A, Henrar R, Currie CJ. Evaluation of the cost effectiveness and societal impact of rifaximin-α 550mg in the reduction of recurrence of overt hepatic encephalopathy in The Netherlands. Value Health. 2015;18:A629 [abstract].
12. Grover VP, Tognarelli JM, Massie N, Crossey MM, Cook NA, Taylor-Robinson SD. The why and wherefore of hepatic encephalopathy. Int J Gen Med. 2015;8:381–90.
13. Williams R. Review article: bacterial flora and pathogenesis in hepatic encephalopathy. Aliment Pharmacol Ther. 2007;25(Suppl 1):17–22.
14. Scott LJ. Rifaximin: a review of its use in reducing recurrence of overt hepatic encephalopathy episodes. Drugs. 2014;74:2153–60.
15. Bajaj JS. Review article: potential mechanisms of action of rifaximin in the management of hepatic encephalopathy and other complications of cirrhosis. Aliment Pharmacol Ther. 2016;43(Suppl 1):11–26.
16. TARGAXAN® Summary of Product Characteristics. http://www.medicines.org.uk/emc/medicine/27427/SPC/TARGAXAN+550+mg+film-coated+tablets/. Accessed 15 March 2017.
17. XIFAXAN® Product Information. https://www.ebs.tga.gov.au/ebs/picmi/picmirepository.nsf/pdf?OpenAgent&id=CP-2012-PI-02052-3. Accessed 15 March 2017.
18. Bass NM, Mullen KD, Sanyal A, Poordad F, Neff G, Leevy CB, Sigal S, Sheikh MY, Beavers K, Frederick T, Teperman L, Hillebrand D, Huang S, Merchant K, Shaw A, Bortey E, Forbes WP. Rifaximin treatment in hepatic encephalopathy. N Engl J Med. 2010;362:1071–81.
19. Mullen KD, Sanyal AJ, Bass NM, Poordad FF, Sheikh MY, Frederick RT, Bortey E, Forbes WP. Rifaximin is safe and well tolerated for long-term maintenance of remission from overt hepatic encephalopathy. Clin Gastroenterol Hepatol. 2014;12:1390–7.
20. Berger ML, Dreyer N, Anderson F, Towse A, Sedrakyan A, Normand SL. Prospective observational studies to assess comparative effectiveness: the ISPOR good research practices task force report. Value Health. 2012; 15:217–30.
21. NHS England. Commissioning through Evaluation. https://www.england.nhs.uk/commissioning/spec-services/npc-crg/comm-eval/#. Accessed 15 March 2017.
22. Biggins SW, Kim WR, Terrault NA, Saab S, Balan V, Schiano T, Benson J, Therneau T, Kremers W, Wiesner R, Kamath P, Klintmalm G. Evidence-based incorporation of serum sodium concentration into MELD. Gastroenterology. 2006;130:1652–60.
23. Younossi ZM, Guyatt G, Kiwi M, Boparai N, King D. Development of a disease specific questionnaire to measure health related quality of life in patients with chronic liver disease. Gut. 1999;45:295–300.
24. Herdman M, Gudex C, Lloyd A, Janssen M, Kind P, Parkin D, Bonsel G, Badia X. Development and preliminary testing of the new five-level version of EQ-5D (EQ-5D-5L). Qual Life Res. 2011;20:1727–36.
25. Reilly MC, Zbrozek AS, Dukes EM. The validity and reproducibility of a work productivity and activity impairment instrument. PharmacoEconomics. 1993; 4:353–65.
26. Neff GW, Kemmer N, Zacharias VC, Kaiser T, Duncan C, McHenry R, Jonas M, Novick D, Williamson C, Hess K, Thomas M, Buell J. Analysis of hospitalizations comparing rifaximin versus lactulose in the management of hepatic encephalopathy. Transplant Proc. 2006;38:3552–5.
27. Leevy CB, Phillips JA. Hospitalizations during the use of rifaximin versus lactulose for the treatment of hepatic encephalopathy. Dig Dis Sci. 2007;52:737–41.
28. Leevy CB. Economic impact of treatment options for hepatic encephalopathy. Semin Liver Dis. 2007;27:26–31.
29. Huang E, Esrailian E, Spiegel BM. The cost-effectiveness and budget impact of competing therapies in hepatic encephalopathy - a decision analysis. Aliment Pharmacol Ther. 2007;26:1147–61.
30. Orr JG, Currie CJ, Berni E, Goel A, Moriarty KJ, Sinha A, Gordon F, Dethier A, Dillon J, Clark K, Richardson P, Middleton P, Patel V, Shawcross D, Preedy H, Aspinall RJ, Hudson M. The impact on hospital resource utilisation of treatment of hepatic encephalopathy with rifaximin-α. Liver Int. 2016;36: 1295–303.

23

Seroprevalence of hepatitis B and C

Marcelo Contardo Moscoso Naveira*, Komal Badal*, Jagadish Dhakal, Neichu Angami Mayer, Bina Pokharel and Ruben Frank Del Prado

Abstract

Introduction: Hepatitis B and C represent an important co-infection for people living with HIV worldwide. Nepal wants to be part of the international mobilization for viral hepatitis elimination, and has pursued better understanding of the epidemic in its territory through scientific research.

Methods: We performed a systematic review of seroprevalence studies hepatitis B and C in Nepal following the PRISMA 2009 Flow Diagram.

Results: Fifty-four scientific publications and reports were selected for this review. Nearly a quarter of these documents have been issued in recent years and many are authored by non-governmental organizations in Nepal. The collective of information displays a wide range of alarming prevalence rates, particularly for girls and women survivors of human trafficking and a progressive participation of civil society in viral hepatitis epidemiology research in the country.

Conclusion: This paper presents a most complete review of hepatitis B and C and HIV co-infection prevalence studies in different population groups from 1973 to 2016. A comprehensive analysis of the epidemiology and apparent trends in public health research and policy making in Nepal are also addressed in this document. We expect this to be a most important tool for improvements in future interventions for both epidemics in the country.

Keywords: Viral hepatitis, Hepatitis B, Hepatitis C, Systematic review, Epidemiology, Nepal

Background

Viral hepatitis has become a leading cause of death and disability worldwide - estimated to be responsible for over 1.4 million deaths every year. Chronic viral hepatitis, mostly represented by the hepatitis B and C viruses infections (HBV and HCV, respectively), is a major cause of increasing events of high morbidity and mortality such as cirrhosis, end-stage liver disease and hepatocellular carcinoma. Both viruses are more easily transmissible than HIV [1].

The Sustainable Development Goals (SDG) establishes the year of 2030 as a desirable deadline for the end of many epidemics, including viral hepatitis. Nepal, a landlocked central Himalayan country in South Asia, has committed to the seventeen ambitious goals of SDG, and pursues to graduate from the least developed country rank by 2022. Nepal already presented remarkable achievements in infectious diseases, particularly the HIV response [2–4]. However, the understanding of viral hepatitis impacts to the country is limited. There is no national plan devised for the elimination of viral hepatitis and hepatitis C has only been briefly mentioned in the National HIV Strategic Plan 2016–2021 (Nepal HIVision 2020) [5].

Multiple community- and facility-based seroepidemiological surveys for viral hepatitis and co-infections have taken place in Nepal since 1973 [6–8]. Studies have assessed different population groups mostly in urban areas of Kathmandu Valley and to a lesser extent in other development regions.

As new National Guidelines for Viral Hepatitis are being developed, the Joint United Nations Programme on HIV/AIDS in Nepal (UNAIDS Nepal) understands this comprehensive review is a most welcome tool for future research. We expect this document to be useful for mathematical

* Correspondence: mnaveir1@alumni.jh.edu; talktobadal@gmail.com; badalk@unaids.org
UNAIDS Nepal, UN House, Pulchowk, Lalitpur GPO 107, Nepal

models, advocacy for key populations, improvements in public health policy, and setting priorities for successful elimination of hepatitis B and C.

Methods

We conducted a systematic review of seroprevalence studies of hepatitis B and C following the PRISMA 2009 Flow Diagram [9]. Our main sources of data for this research were: 1) PubMed (Medline), through the following search expression "((("Hepatitis B"[Mesh] OR "Hepatitis B, Chronic"[Mesh] OR "Hepatitis B virus"[Mesh] OR "Hepatitis B Surface Antigens"[Mesh] OR "Hepatitis B Antibodies"[-Mesh] OR "Hepatitis B"[Text] OR "Hepatitis C"[Mesh] OR "Hepatitis C, Chronic"[Mesh] OR "Hepatitis C Antibodies"[Mesh] OR "Hepatitis C"[Text]) AND ("Nepal"[Mesh] OR "Nepal"[Text]))"; 2) reports provided by the Government of Nepal (GoN); 3) reports authored by international agencies and non-governamental organizations (NGOs); and 4) personal correspondence to authors.

Study selection

Two researchers took part in all steps of the reviewing process. We assessed our initial search results for eligibility through title, abstract and full-text analysis. Duplicates were not identified, but two publications were found to be supplemental to previously evaluated studies. One review obtained during the search presented additional data for three studies unavailable in digital media. Personal correspondences were sent to authors to obtain additional information. We could not identify any repetition of datasets.

Publications were considered eligible for inclusion if they presented own and original data (absolute numbers or percentage) for any population group, Nepalese or residing in Nepal, at any given site and time for at least one of the following outcomes of interest: 1) hepatitis B seroprevalence, active infection or exposure; and 2) hepatitis C seroprevalence as detected by anti-HCV tests.

Selected publications were excluded if full-text material could not be retrieved, if published before 1981 and if abstract could not provide sufficient information for any of the three outcomes of interest.

Data extraction

The following data were then extracted from each eligible study included in this review: year of publication, population group, site, month and/or year of data collection, sample size, numbers/percentage of positive results for hepatitis B, C, HIV and syphilis; and authors' name.

Seven studies did not provide details of which tests were used to define active HBV infection [7, 10–15]. One study identified did not provide details about which tests were used to define seroprevalence of exposition to HBV [16].

We chose to display results for every study total population and for as many subgroups as possible. Figures were obtained through full-text analysis and personal correspondence with authors. All numbers were thoroughly revised.

Results

This review selection process is depicted in Fig. 1, as adapted from the PRISMA 2009 Flow Diagram [9]. Initial search expression resulted in ninety different records with no duplicates. Forty-two citations were excluded after title, abstract and full-text screening and one citation was found to be supplemental. One report from Asian Network of People Who Use Drugs (ANPUD), one from HEPA Foundation/United Nations Office on Drugs and Crime (UNODC), one from United Nations Development Program (UNPD), two from Nepal Red Cross Society (NRCS) and six from Ministry of Health of Nepal (MoH), including the Global AIDS Response Progress Report 2015 (GARRP), were added to the group of forty-eight eligible citations, resulting in fifty-nine documents.

Five records were excluded because full-text could not be retrieved and their abstracts did not have data on any of the three outcomes of interest. Three additional documents from 1987 to 1990, which were not listed in PubMed, were identified from a review and later included in the collective. Fifty-seven documents relevant to fifty-five relevant prevalence studies were selected for this review.

Table 1 presents the collective of viral hepatitis prevalence studies with stratified population groups according to WHO key terms.

Table 2 presents an analysis of the reviewed data and Cochran's Q tests performed by Weill Cornell Medical College in Qatar. Estimated prevalence and heterogeneity has been presented for five population groups: PWID, populations at intermediate risk, populations at low risk (general population), populations with liver-related conditions and special clinical populations [17].

Population groups

Candidates for blood donation account for just seven prevalence studies and yet represent approximately 90 % of the population evaluated for viral hepatitis in Nepal since 1973. This overwhelming presence of candidates for blood donation in seroprevalence studies does not contribute to the understanding of populations at increased risk of HBV, HCV and HIV co-infection in Nepal as they rarely present seroprevalence rates higher than 1 % [12, 13, 18–22].

It is understood that people at increased risk of HBV, HCV and HIV co-infections should be properly represented in our review. We have succeeded to identify studies for most groups of interest: general population, children, adults, pregnant women, people who inject drugs

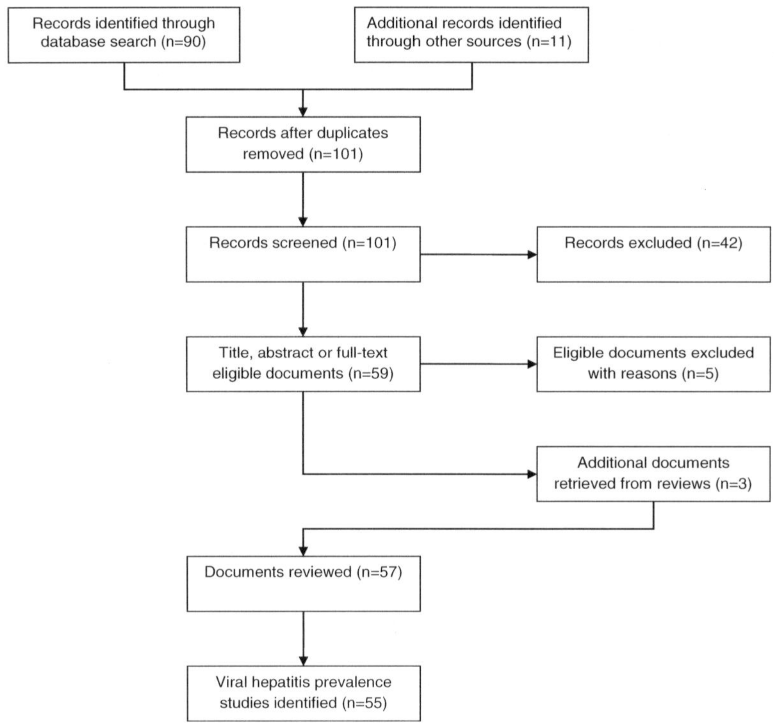

Fig. 1 Flow of article selection for the viral hepatitis B and C prevalence studies in Nepal

(PWID), patients attending healthcare services, sexual and household contacts of people chronically infected by HBV, sex workers (SW), healthcare workers (HCW), migrant workers, refugees/displaced persons and survivors of human trafficking.

We found only one survey of viral hepatitis in lesbian, gay, bisexual or transgender population (LGBT), including men who have sex with other men (MSM); and another in people with history of incarceration. All collected documents only referred to drug use as injection and did not acknowledge people who use drugs (PWUD) or different methods of drug administration (e.g. smoking heroin). [23, 24].

Hepatitis B

A disease preventable by vaccination, hepatitis B has been identified in our review in forty-six studies. HBsAg (surface antigen) positive tests had highest values in PWID (1.3–81.9%), [8, 25] patients with jaundice, chronic liver disease, cirrhosis or hepatocellular carcinoma (7.5–60%); [16, 26–28] sexual and household contacts of people chronically infected by HBV (6.6–31), [29] girls and women survivors of sex trafficking (30%), [7] Tibetan population living in Kathmandu Valley (10–20%) [30] and Nepalese people outside Nepal (2.7–19.3) [31, 32]. On the other hand, the overall prevalence of hepatitis B in Nepal is estimated at 0.9%, [33].

Children, adults and general population cohorts also present interesting ranges for figures of hepatitis B seroprevalence. Older age groups present higher values for HBsAg [20, 34] and children born after vaccine implementation display reduced disease prevalence. [35].

Unfortunately, only one document presents viral hepatitis prevalence in LGBT population (MSM included), but it lacks important information on sample size and number of positive tests.

Exposure to hepatitis B virus, defined by anti-HBc (antibody against core antigen), has been assessed only in one key population - PWID, in two studies nearly twenty years apart. In 1996, more than 80 % of PWID had positive results for anti-HBc [25] and in 2015, when less than 45 % had positive results for the same marker [8].

Hepatitis C

One of the most important causes of morbidity [36] and mortality, particularly for people living with HIV (PLWH), [37] hepatitis C seroprevalence has been featured in thirty-one studies, in a total of approximately one million people in Nepal. Prevalence rates range from zero to more than 80%, with highest figures found in PWID (85.5 in males; 24.6 in females), [38] PLHIV (43.3) and patients with hepatocellular carcinoma (17.6). [27, 38, 39].

Regardless of key population status, different prevalence rates have been observed in males and females [40]. Statistically significant differences according to gender can be verified in studies by Shrestha AC et al., between male and female candidates for blood donation in 2009 (0.69 vs.

Table 1 Studies reporting hepatitis B and C in Nepal

SN	YEAR	POPULATION, SITE, TIME	SAMPLE SIZE, N	ANTI-HIV(%)	HBV			ANTI-HCV	NOTES	AUTHOR(S)
					HBSAG(%)	**ANTI-HBC(%)**	**ANTI-HBS(%)**			
1	1973	Patients attending hospitals in Kathmandu during infectious hepatitis outbreak, January 1973 to October 1973	53 sera samples	–	0 (0.00)	–	–	–	–	Hillis A et al. [6]
2	1984	Hospitalized patients with jaundice referred to Shree Tribhubn Chandra Military Hospital, Kathmandu and Infectious Disease Hospital, Teku, 1981 to 1982	41 patients	–	6 (7.50)	–	–	–	–	Kane MA et al. [28]
		Outpatients referred to Shree Tribhubn Chandra Military Hospital, Kathmandu and Infectious Disease Hospital, Teku, 1981 to 1982	39 patients	–		–	–	–	–	
3	1987	Children age 0–10 years, Surkhet Valley	45 children[a]	–	(6.6)	–	(22.2)	–	–	Shreshta SM. [72]
		Children, teenagers and adults age 11–20 years, Surkhet Valley	65 children, teenager and adults[a]	–	(3.0)	–	(46.6)	–	–	
		Adults age 21–40 years, Surkhet Valley	82 adults[a]	–	(9.7)	–	(44.0)	–	–	
		Adults 41+ years, Surkhet Valley	33 adults[a]	–	(6.0)	–	(25.0)	–	–	
		Girls and women, 0–41+ years, Surkhet Valley	–	–	(9.8)		–	–	–	
		Boys and men, 0–41+ years, Surkhet Valley	–	–	(4.4)	–	–	–	–	
		General population age 0–41+, Surkhet Valley	225 people[a]	–	(6.6)	–	(35.0)	–	–	
4	1987	Tibetan children age 0–9 years, Hemza, Tashi Ling, Pokhara; Jawalkhel, Kathmandu Valley	34 children	–	(20.0)	(32.0)[a]	–	–	–	Shrestha SM. [30]
		Tibetan children, teenagers and adults age 10–19 years, Hemza, Tashi Ling, Pokhara; Jawalkhel, Kathmandu Valley	79 children, teenagers and adults	–	(10.0)	(39.0)[a]	–	–	–	
		Tibetan adults age 20–29 years, Hemza, Tashi Ling, Pokhara; Jawalkhel, Kathmandu Valley	106 adults	–	(18.0)	(55.0)[a]	–	–	–	
		Tibetan adults age 30–39 years, Hemza, Tashi Ling, Pokhara; Jawalkhel, Kathmandu Valley	61 adults	–	(20.0)	(46.0)[a]	–	–	–	
		Tibetans age 40–49 years, Hemza, Tashi Ling, Pokhara; Jawalkhel, Kathmandu Valley	95 adults	–	(15.0)	(36.0)[a]	–	–	–	
		Tibetans age 0–49 years, Hemza, Tashi Ling, Pokhara; Jawalkhel, Kathmandu Valley	375 people	–	(16.0)	(45.0)[a]	–	–	–	
		Nepalese children age 0–9 years, Hemza, Tashi Ling, Pokhara; Jawalkhel, Kathmandu Valley	113 children	–	(0.0)	(3.5)[a]	–	–	–	
		Nepalese children, teenagers and adults age 10–19 years, Hemza, Tashi Ling, Pokhara; Jawalkhel, Kathmandu Valley	198 children, teenagers and adults	–	(0.5)	(5.0)[a]	–	–	–	
		Nepalese adults age 20–29 years, Hemza, Tashi Ling, Pokhara; Jawalkhel, Kathmandu Valley	110 adults	–	(1.8)	(5.4)[a]	–	–	–	
		Nepalese adults age 30–39 years, Hemza, Tashi Ling, Pokhara; Jawalkhel, Kathmandu Valley	49 adults	–	(0.0)	(32.6)[a]	–	–	–	
		Nepalese adults age 40–49 years, Hemza, Tashi Ling, Pokhara; Jawalkhel, Kathmandu Valley	25 adults	–	(0.0)	(16.0)[a]	–	–	–	
		Nepalese adults age 50+ years, Hemza,	45 adults	–	(2.2)	(7.8)[a]	–	–	–	

Table 1 Studies reporting hepatitis B and C in Nepal *(Continued)*

SN	YEAR	POPULATION, SITE, TIME	SAMPLE SIZE, N	ANTI-HIV(%)	HBV			ANTI-HCV	NOTES	AUTHOR(S)
					HBSAG(%)	**ANTI-HBC(%)**	**ANTI-HBS(%)**			
		Tashi Ling, Pokhara; Jawalkhel, Kathmandu Valley								
		Nepalese age 11–41+ years, Hemza, Tashi Ling, Pokhara; Jawalkhel, Kathmandu Valley	540 people	–	(0.7)	(36.0)[a]			–	
5	1988	Patients during 1983 enterically transmitted non A–non B hepatitis outbreak, Kathmandu Valley	150 patients	–	34 (13.60)[a]			–	–	Nuti M [10]
		Controls during 1983 non A–non B hepatitis outbreak, Kathmandu Valley	100 people	–				–	–	
6	1988	Lactating women from six villages of Kathmandu Valley	26 women	–	0 (0.00)	4 (15.38)	8 (30.77)	–	–	Reynolds RD et al. [73]
		Breastfed infants age 2–6 months from six villages of Kathmandu Valley	26 infants	–	–			–	–	
7	1989	Patients age 20–40 years attending four Kathmandu hospitals, Kathmandu, 1985	460 sera samples	0 (0.00)	5 (1.09)	64 (13.91)	–	–	–	Mertens T et al. [74]
8	1990	Children age 0–5 years	57 healthy children	–	0 (0.00)	–	5 (8.77)	–	–	Shrestha SM [75]
		Children and teenagers age 6–15 years	359 healthy children ad teenagers	–	8 (2.23)	–	15 (4.18)	–	–	
		Teenagers and adults age 16–41 years	1788 healthy teenagers and adults	–	16 (0.89)	–	158 (8.84)	–	–	
		Adults, 41+ years	351 healthy adults	–	2 (0.57)	–	35 (9.97)	–	–	
		Girls and women, 0–41+ years	1529 healthy women	–	9 (0.59)	–	76 (7.40)	–	–	
		Boys and men, 0–41+ years	1026 healthy men	–	17 (1.65)	–	138 (9.02)	–	–	
		General population, 0–41+ years	2555 healthy individuals	–	26 (1.02)	23 (0.90)	214 (8.4)	–	–	
9	1991	Spouses of HBsAg chronic carriers	34 people	–	6 (17.65)	–	15 (44.12)	–	–	Shrestha SM et al. [29]
		Offspring of HBsAg chronic carriers	73 people	–	15 (20.55)	–	17 (23.29)	–	–	
		Siblings of HBsAg chronic carriers	29 people	–	9 (31.03)	–	11 (37.93)	–	–	
10	1993	Children age 0–4 years, Gurkha Contingent, Singapore	177 children	–	64 (19.28)	161 (17.05)	213 (22.56)	–	–	Goh et al. [32]
		Children age 5–14 years, Gurkha Contingent, Singapore	155 children	–				–	–	
		Children and adults age 15–24 years, Gurkha Contingent, Singapore	227 children and adults	–	–			–	–	
		Adults age 25–34 years, Gurkha Contingent, Singapore	289 people	–	–			–	–	
		Adults 35+ years, Gurkha Contingent, Singapore	96 people	–	–			–	–	
		Gurkha Community members, Gurkha Contingent, Singapore	944 people	–	26 (2.75)			–	–	
11	1994	Patients with chronic hepatitis attending Bir Hospital, Kathmandu	20 patients	–	12 (60.00)	–	–	5 (25.00)	–	Shreshta SM et al. [26]
		Patients with cirrhosis attending Bir Hospital,	63 patients	–	25 (39.68)	–	–	9	–	

Table 1 Studies reporting hepatitis B and C in Nepal *(Continued)*

SN	YEAR	POPULATION, SITE, TIME	SAMPLE SIZE, N	ANTI-HIV(%)	HBV			ANTI-HCV	NOTES	AUTHOR(S)
					HBSAG(%)	**ANTI-HBC(%)**	**ANTI-HBS(%)**			
		Kathmandu						(14.28)		
		Patients with hepatocellular carcinoma attending Bir Hospital, Kathmandu	62 patients	–	20 (29.41)	–	–	6 (9.68)	–	
		Patients with chronic hepatitis, cirrhosis or hepatocellular carcinoma attending Bir Hospital, Kathmandu	145 patients	–	57 (39.31)	–	–	20 (13.79)	–	
		Pregnant women attending Bir Hospital, Kathmandu	83 women	–	0 (0.00)	–	–	3 (3.61)	–	
		Medical or paramedical personnel serving at Bir Hospital, Kathmandu	296 people	–	5 (1.69)	–	–	10 (3.38)	–	
12	1994	Female sex workers, Kathmandu Valley	341 women	3 (0.88)	37 (10.85)[a]			–	Syphilis: 73 (21.41)	Bhatta P et al. [76]
13	1994	Villagers, Dharan, Sunsari; Pancha Kanya Village Development Committee, Ilam; Dhankuta Hile, Dhankuta; Basantapur Village Development Committee, Tehrathm	303 serum samples	–	0 (0.00)	–	6 (1.98)	–	–	Rai SK et al. [77]
14	1995	Villagers, Bhadrakali and Kotyang villages, 1987	676 blood samples	–	2 (0.29)	52 (7.69)	–	1 (0.15)	–	Nakashima K et al. [78]
15	1996	People who inject drugs	72 people	–	4 (5.55)	59 (81.94)	–	58 (80.55)	–	Shrestha SM et al. [25]
16	1997	People who use drugs	72 people	–	2 (2.78)	44 (61.11)[b]		43 (59,72)	–	Shrestha SM et al. [16]
		People with chronic kidney disease	41 people	–	1 (2.44)	6 (14.63)[b]		1 (2.44)	–	
		People with chronic liver disease	145 people	–	57 (39.31)	74 (51.03)[b]		12 (8.27)	–	
		HBsAg carriers	49 people	–	49 (100.00)	49 (100.00)[b]		0 (0.00)	–	
		Healthy individuals undergoing routine check-ups	181 people	–	9 (4.97)	46 (25.41)[b]		0 (0.00)	–	
17	1998	Patients age ≤ 15 years attending Amp Pipal Hospital, Gorkha district, 1993	101 children and adults	–	–	0/9 (0.00)	1/9 (11.11)	0/9 (0.00)	–	De Bruyn et al. [44]
		Patients age 16–25 years attending Amp Pipal Hospital, Gorkha district, 1993		–	–	0/34 (0.00)	0/34 (0.00)	4/34 (11.76)	–	
		Patients age 26–35 years attending Amp Pipal Hospital, Gorkha district, 1993		–	–	1/20 (5.00)	0/21 (0.00)	0/21 (0.00)	–	
		Patients age 36–45 years attending Amp Pipal Hospital, Gorkha district, 1993		–	–	2/14 (14.28)	2/13 (15.38)	0/13 (0.00)	–	
		Patients age 46–55 years attending Amp Pipal Hospital, Gorkha district, 1993		–	–	1/8 (12.50)	1/8 (12.50)	0/8 (0.00)	–	
		Patients age ≥ 56 years attending Amp Pipal Hospital, Gorkha district, 1993		–	–	3/10 (30.00)	4/10 (40.00)	0/10 (0.00)	–	
18	1999	Male villagers age ≤ 24 years from Bhadrakali and Kotyang villages, August 1996 to September 1996	44 boys and men	–	0 (0.00)	1 (2.27)	–	1 (2.27)	–	Sawayama Y et al. [40]
		Female villagers age ≤ 24 years from Bhadrakali and Kotyang villages, August 1996 to September 1996	43 girls and women	–	1 (2.32)	1 (2.32)	–	0 (0.00)	–	
		Villagers age ≤ 24 years from Bhadrakali and Kotyang villages, August 1996 to September 1996	87 people	–	1 (1.15)	2 (2.30)	–	1 (1.15)	–	
		Male villagers 25–34 years from Bhadrakali and Kotyang villages, August 1996 to	40 men	–	0 (0.00)	2 (5.00)	–	2 (5.00)	–	

Table 1 Studies reporting hepatitis B and C in Nepal *(Continued)*

SN	YEAR	POPULATION, SITE, TIME	SAMPLE SIZE, N	ANTI-HIV(%)	HBV			ANTI-HCV	NOTES	AUTHOR(S)
					HBSAG(%)	**ANTI-HBC(%)**	**ANTI-HBS(%)**			
		September 1996								
		Female villagers 25–34 years from Bhadrakali and Kotyang villages, August 1996 to September 1996	37 women	–	1 (2.70)	2 (5.40)	–	0 (0.00)	–	
		Villagers 25–34 years from Bhadrakali and Kotyang villages, August 1996 to September 1996	77 people	–	1 (1.30)	4 (5.19)	–	2 (2.60)	–	
		Male villagers 35–44 years from Bhadrakali and Kotyang villages, August 1996 to September 1996	49 men	–	0 (0.00)	1 (2.04)	–	1 (2.04)	–	
		Female villagers 35–44 years from Bhadrakali and Kotyang villages, August 1996 to September 1996	41 women	–	0 (0.00)	1 (2.44)	–	0 (0.00)	–	
		Villagers 35–44 years from Bhadrakali and Kotyang villages, August 1996 to September 1996	90 people	–	0 (0.00)	2 (2.22)	–	1 (1.11)	–	
		Male villagers 45–54 years from Bhadrakali and Kotyang villages, August 1996 to September 1996	29 men	–	0 (0.00)	1 (3.45)	–	2 (6.90)	–	
		Female villagers 45–54 years from Bhadrakali and Kotyang villages, August 1996 to September 1996	44 women	–	0 (0.00)	2 (4.54)	–	1 (2.27)	–	
		Villagers 45–54 years from Bhadrakali and Kotyang villages, August 1996 to September 1996	73 people	–	0 (0.00)	3 (4.11)	–	3 (4.11)	–	
		Male villagers 55–64 years from Bhadrakali and Kotyang villages, August 1996 to September 1996	29 men	–	1 (3.45)	5 (17.24)	–	0 (0.00)	–	
		Female villagers 55–64 years from Bhadrakali and Kotyang villages, August 1996 to September 1996	39 women	–	2 (5.13)	6 (15.38)	–	1 (2.56)	–	
		Villagers 55–64 years from Bhadrakali and Kotyang villages, August 1996 to September 1996	68 people	–	3 (4.41)	11 (16.18)	–	1 (1.47)	–	
		Male villagers ≥65 years from Bhadrakali and Kotyang villages, August 1996 to September 1996	38 men	–	0 (0.00)	7 (18.42)	–	0 (0.00)	–	
		Female villagers ≥65 years from Bhadrakali and Kotyang villages, August 1996 to September 1996	25 women	–	0 (0.00)	4 (16.00)	–	0 (0.00)	–	
		Villagers ≥65 years from Bhadrakali and Kotyang villages, August 1996 to September 1996	63 people	–	0 (0.00)	11 (17.46)	–	0 (0.00)	–	
		Female villagers age 15–90 years from Bhadrakali and Kotyang villages, August 1996 to September 1996	229 women	–	4 (1.75)	16 (6.97)	–	2 (0.87)	–	
		Male villagers age 15–90 years from Bhadrakali and Kotyang villages, August 1996 to September 1996	229 men	–	1 (0.44)	17 (7.42)	–	6 (2.62)	–	
		Villagers age 15–90 years from Bhadrakali and Kotyang villages, August 1996 to September 1996	458 people	–	5 (1.09)	33 (7.20)	–	8 (1.75)	–	
19	2000	Healthy Nepalese Men from Eastern development region, October 1996 to March 1997	100 men	–	2 (2.00)	–	–	–	–	Manandhar K et al. [79, 80]

Table 1 Studies reporting hepatitis B and C in Nepal *(Continued)*

SN	YEAR	POPULATION, SITE, TIME	SAMPLE SIZE, N	ANTI-HIV(%)	HBV			ANTI-HCV	NOTES	AUTHOR(S)
					HBSAG(%)	**ANTI-HBC(%)**	**ANTI-HBS(%)**			
		Healthy Nepalese Men from Central development region, October 1996 to March 1997	100 men	–	3 (3.00)	–	–	–	–	
		Healthy Nepalese Men from Western development region, October 1996 to March 1997	100 men	–	4 (4.00)	–	–	–	–	
		Healthy Nepalese Men from Mid Western development region, October 1996 to March 1997	97 men	–	4 (4.12)	–	–	–	–	
		Healthy Nepalese Men from Far Western development region, October 1996 to March 1997	81 men	–	5 (6.17)	–	–	–	–	
		Healthy Nepalese Men from five different development regions, October 1996 to March 1997	478 men	–	18 (3.76)	–	–	–	17 < 40 yrs. old -	
20	2002	Nepalese men age 16–50 years who required medical check-ups for employment abroad, July 1999 to September 1999	2585 men	–	24 (0.93)	–	–	–	–	Bidya S [81]
21	2003	Boys and men < 19 years, Baba Medical Center, Kathmandu, September 2003 to June 2004	52 boys and men	0 (0.00)	0 (0.00)	–	–	–	–	Joshi SK et al. [34]
		Men age 20–29 years, Baba Medical Center, Kathmandu, September 2003 to June 2004	375 men	5 (1.33)	9 (2.40)	–	–	–	Syphilis: 4/545	
		Men age 30–39 years, Baba Medical Center, Kathmandu, September 2003 to June 2004	170 men	5 (2.94)	7 (4.11)	–	–	–		
		Men age 40+ years, Baba Medical Center, Kathmandu, September 2003 to June 2004	30 men	–	1 (3.33)	–	–	–	–	
22	2003	People who inject drugs, Siddhi Polyclinic, Dillibazaar, Kathmandu	400 people	–	–	–	–	342 (85.5)	–	Shrestha IL [38]
		Adults without history of injection drug use, Siddhi Polyclinic, Dillibazaar, Kathmandu	400 people	–	–	–	–	3 (0.75)	–	
23	2003	Candidates for blood donation at Blood Bank Centre, NRCS, Teaching Hospital, Bhairahawa, February 2001 to April 2003	1548 samples	2 (0.13)	7 (0.45)	–	–	2 (0.13)	–	Chander A et al. [18]
24	2004	Sherpa people age 15–66 years, Lukla, Solukhumbu district, 2004	103 people	–	2 (1.94)	25 (24.27)	23 (22.33)	–	–	Chiba H et al. [82]
25	2005	Bhutanese refugees, Beldangi 2 Extension Camp, March 1998 to July 1998	467 people	–	4 (0.86)	–	–	–	–	Shah BK et al. [83]
26	2006	Healthcare workers of Bir Hospital, Kathmandu, December 2001 to February 2002	145 people	–	2 (1.38)	21 (14.48)	–	–	–	Shrestha SK et al. [68]
27	2006	Male villagers, migrant-returnes from India and non-migrants, from five village development committees, Doti District, April 2001	149 people	1 (0.67)	16 (10.74)	–	–	–	–	Poudel K et al. [31]
28	2007	Patients with liver cirrhosis or hepatocellular carcinoma attending Liver Foundation Nepal clinic, January 1998 to January 2004	121 patients	–	48 (39.67)	85 (70.25)	–	15 (12.40)	–	Shrestha SM et al. [27]
		Patients with liver cirrhosis attending Liver Foundation Nepal clinic, January 1998 to January 2004	70 patients	–	20 (28.57)	47 (67.14)	–	6 (8.57)	–	
		Patients with hepatocellular carcinoma attending Liver Foundation Nepal clinic, January 1998 to January 2004	51 patients	–	28 (54.90)	38 (74.51)	–	9 (17.65)	–	
29	2008	Symptomatic people living with HIV/AIDS at Manipal Teaching Hospital, Pokhara, March	54 patients	PLWH	1 (1.85)[a]			1 (1.85)	–	Dhungel BA et al. [11]

Table 1 Studies reporting hepatitis B and C in Nepal *(Continued)*

SN	YEAR	POPULATION, SITE, TIME	SAMPLE SIZE, N	ANTI-HIV(%)	HBV			ANTI-HCV	NOTES	AUTHOR(S)
					HBSAG(%)	**ANTI-HBC(%)**	**ANTI-HBS(%)**			
		2004 to September 2005								
30	2008	Candidates for blood donation, NRSC, CBTS, hospital units/mobile camps all over Nepal, 2001 to 2002	72,459 blood samples	–	627 (0.86)	–	–	384 (0.52)	–	Karki S et al. [19]
		Candidates for blood donation, NRSC, CBTS, hospital units/mobile camps all over Nepal, 2002 to 2003	73,758 blood samples	–	911 (1.23)	–	–	417 (0.56)	–	
		Candidates for blood donation, NRSC, CBTS, hospital units/mobile camps all over Nepal, 2003 to 2004	76,647 blood samples	–	663 (0.86)	–	–	321 (0.41)	–	
		Candidates for blood donation, NRSC, CBTS, hospital units/mobile camps all over Nepal, 2004 to 2005	82,677 blood samples	–	644 (0.77)	–	–	373 (0.45)	–	
		Candidates for blood donation, NRSC, CBTS, hospital units/mobile camps all over Nepal, 2005 to 2006	103,067 blood samples	–	887 (0.86)	–	–	366 (0.35)	–	
		Candidates for blood donation, NRSC, CBTS, hospital units/mobile camps all over Nepal, 2006 to 2007	115,720 blood samples	–	430 (0.37)	–	–	628 (0.54)	–	
		Candidates for blood donation, NRSC, CBTS, hospital units/mobile camps all over Nepal, 2001 to 2007	524,328 blood samples	–	4162 (0.82)	–	–	2489 (0.47)	–	
31	2008	Sex trafficked women and girls assisted by Maiti Nepal, Kathmandu	246 women and girls	74 (30.08)	66/210 (31.43)[a]			–	Syphilis: 48%	Silverman J et al. [7]
32	2009	Candidates for blood donation at the Central Blood Transfusion Service, Nepal Red Cross Society (NRCS), Kathmandu, December 2006 to September 2007	33,255 individual samples	65 (0.19)	–			–	–	Karki S et al. [12]
		People living with HIV/AIDS diagnosed during blood donation at the Central Blood Transfusion Service, NRCS, Kathmandu, December 2006 to September 2007	65 individual samples tested positive for anti-HIV	PLWH	–			7 (10.76)	–	
33	2009	Pregnant women admitted in the ward of NMCTH, Kathmandu, 2001 to 2007	5602	–	18 (0.32)[a]			–	–	Shreshta P et al. [84]
34	2009	People who inject drugs on Oral Substitution Therapy (OST), Kathmandu Valley, June 2009	118 people	–	–	–	–	95 (80.50)	–	HEPA Foundation [85]
		People who inject drugs, Kathmandu Valley, June 2009	82 people	–	–	–	–	47 (57.32)	–	
35	2009	Male candidates for blood donation, NRCS, Central Blood Transfusion Service (CBTS), Kathmandu, March 2008 to September 2008	18,434 blood samples of male candidates	25 (0.13)	92 (0.50)	–	–	128 (0.69)	Coinfection HIV/HCV: 8/ 128	Shrestha AC et al. [20]
		Female candidates for blood donation, NRCS, Central Blood Transfusion Service (CBTS), Kathmandu, March 2008 to September 2008	3282 blood samples of female candidates	2 (0.06)	10 (0.30)	–	–	11 (0.33)	–	
		Candidates for blood donation age ≤ 20 years, NRCS, Central Blood Transfusion Service (CBTS), Kathmandu, March 2008 to September 2008	3310 blood samples	2 (0.06)	7 (0.21)	–	–	7 (0.21)	–	
		Candidates for blood donation age 31–30 years, NRCS, Central Blood Transfusion Service (CBTS), Kathmandu, March 2008 to September 2008	9818 blood samples	12 (0.12)	45 (0.45)	–	–	75 (0.76)	–	
		Candidates for blood donation age 31–	5763 blood	10	29 (0.50)	–	–	42	–	

Table 1 Studies reporting hepatitis B and C in Nepal *(Continued)*

SN	YEAR	POPULATION, SITE, TIME	SAMPLE SIZE, N	ANTI-HIV(%)	HBV			ANTI-HCV	NOTES	AUTHOR(S)
					HBSAG(%)	**ANTI-HBC(%)**	**ANTI-HBS(%)**			
		40 years, NRCS, Central Blood Transfusion Service (CBTS), Kathmandu, March 2008 to September 2008	samples	(0.17)				(0.72)		
		Candidates for blood donation age 41–50 years, NRCS, Central Blood Transfusion Service (CBTS), Kathmandu, March 2008 to September 2008	2433 blood sample	3 (0.12)	19 (0.78)	–	–	13 (0.53)	–	
		Candidates for blood donation age 51–60 years, NRCS, Central Blood Transfusion Service (CBTS), Kathmandu, March 2008 to September 2008	392 blood samples	0 (0.00)	3 (0.51)	–	–	2 (0.51)	–	
		Candidates for blood donation, NRCS, Central Blood Transfusion Service (CBTS), Kathmandu, March 2008 to September 2008	21,716 blood samples	27 (0.12)	102 (0.46)	–	–	139 (0.64)	–	
36	2010	Candidates for blood donation in Banke blood transfusion service, July 2006 to June 2007	5211	–	63 (1.21)[a]			6 (0.11)	–	Tiwari BR et al. [13]
		Candidates for blood donation in Kaski blood transfusion service, July 2006 to June 2007	5995	–	21 (0.35)[a]			10 (0.17)	–	
		Candidates for blood donation in Morang blood transfusion service, July 2006 to June 2007	5351	–	47 (0.88)[a]			14 (0.26)	–	
		Candidates for blood donation in Banke, Kaski and Morang blood transfusion services, July 2006 to June 2007	16,557	–	131 (0.79)[a]			32 (0.19)	–	
37	2011	People who inject drugs, age 18–40 years, 2011	40 people	–	–	–	–	7 (17.50)	–	ANPUD. [86]
38	2012	Children age 10–12 years born from April 2000 to April 2002, before hepatitis B vaccine introduction, Kathmandu, April 2012	1200 children	–	3 (0.25)	–	–	–	–	Upreti SR et al. [35]
		Children age 5–6 years born from April 2006 to April 2007, after hepatitis B vaccine introduction, Kathmandu, April 2012	2187 children	–	3 (0.14)	–	–	–	–	
39	2012	Patients with ascites attending Nepal Medical College Hospital (NMCTH), Kathmandu, September 2011 to February 2012	43 patients	–	–	–	–	2 (4.65)	–	Adhikari P et al. [87]
40	2013	People with one or more risk behaviors attending National Public Health Laboratory (NPHL), Kathmandu, November 2011 to May 2012	678 people	105 (15.49)	–	–	–	–	–	Ojha CR et al. [88]
		People living with HIV/AIDS diagnosed among study population, November 2011 to May 2012	105 people	PLWH	–	–	14 (13.33)	–	–	
41	2014	People living with HIV/AIDS attending B P Koirala Institute of Health Sciences (BPKIHS), Dharan; Society for Positive Atmosphere and Related Support to HIV and IDS (SPARSHA), Kathmandu; Sukhra Raj Tropical and Infectious Disease Hospital, Teku, Kathmandu, April 2010 to March 2011	108 patients	PLWH	4 (3.70)[a]			3 (2.78)	HBV/HCV: 0 (0.00)	Barnawal SP et al. [15]
		People who inject drugs living with HIV/AIDS attending BPKIHS, Dharan; SPARSHA, Kathmandu; Sukhra Raj Tropical and Infectious Disease Hospital, Teku, Kathmandu, April 2010 to March 2011	205 patients	PLWH	24 (11.71)[a]			137 (66.83)	HBV/HCV: 10 (4.88)	

Table 1 Studies reporting hepatitis B and C in Nepal *(Continued)*

SN	YEAR	POPULATION, SITE, TIME	SAMPLE SIZE, N	ANTI-HIV(%)	HBV			ANTI-HCV	NOTES	AUTHOR(S)
					HBSAG(%)	**ANTI-HBC(%)**	**ANTI-HBS(%)**			
42	2014	Women living with HIV/AIDS, 18 years or older, February to March 2010	136 women	PLWH	–	–	–	9 (6.61)	–	Poudel KC et al. [39]
		Men living with HIV/AIDS, 18 years or older, February to March 2010	183 men	PLWH	–	–	–	129 (70,49)	–	
		People who do not inject drugs living with HIV/AIDS, 18 years or older, February to March 2010	189 people	PLWH	–	–	–	13 (6.88)	–	
		People who inject drugs living with HIV/AIDS, 18 years or older, February to March 2010	130 people	PLWH	–	–	–	125 (95.15)	–	
		People living with HIV/AIDS, 18 years or older, February to March 2010	319 people	PLWH	–	–	–	138 (43.26)	–	
43	2014	Central Blood Transfusion Centre, 2012–2013	67,644 blood samples	45 (0.07)	150 (0.22)	–	–	317 (0.47)	Syphilis: 394 (0.58)	NRCS [21]
		Regional Blood Transfusion Centre, 2012–2013	47,733 blood samples	40 (0.08)	188 (0.39)	–	–	126 (0.26)	Syphilis: 284 (0.59)	
		District/Emergency Blood Transfusion Centre, 2012–2013	61,624 blood samples	35 (0.06)	195 (0.32)	–	–	121 (0.20)	Syphilis: 118 (0.19)	
		Hospital Blood Transfusion Unit, 2012–2013	12,320 blood samples	3 (0.02)	32 (0.26)	–	–	21 (0.17)	Syphilis: 8 (0.06)	
		Total, 2012–2013	189,321 blood samples	123 (0.06)	565 (0.30)	–	–	585 (0.31)	Syphilis: 804 (0.42)	
44	2014	Children age 0–15 years with acute hepatitis attending the liver clinic of Bir Hospital and Norvic International Hospital of Kathmandu, Kathmandu, January 2006 to December 2010	312 children	–	15 (4.81)[a]			–	–	Sudhamshu KC et al. [14]
45	2015	Women who inject drugs attending Recovering Nepal services submitted to HIV testing, Nepalgunj	3 women	0 (0.00)	–	–	–	0 (0.00)	–	Kinkel HT et al. [8]
		Men who inject drugs attending Recovering Nepal services submitted to HIV testing, Nepalgunj	76 men	6 (7.89)	–	–	–	18 (23.68)	–	
		People who inject drugs attending Recovering Nepal services submitted to HIV testing, Nepalgunj	79 people	6 (7.59)	–	–	–	18 (22.78)	–	
		Women who inject drugs attending Recovering Nepal services, Dharan; Biratnagar	69 women	9 (13.04)	3 (4.35)	–	–	17 (24.64)	–	
		Men who inject drugs attending Recovering Nepal services, Dharan; Biratnagar	72 men	12/70 (17.14)	5 (6.94)	–	–	50 (69.44)	–	
		People who inject drugs attending Recovering Nepal services, Dharan; Biratnagar	141 people	21/139 (15.11)	8 (5.67)	–	–	67 (47.52)	–	
		Women who inject drugs attending Recovering Nepal services submitted to HIV testing, Kathmandu; Lalitpur; Chitwan	28 women	0 (0.00)	1 (3.57)	–	–	2 (7.14)	–	
		Men who inject drugs attending Recovering Nepal services submitted to HIV testing, Kathmandu; Lalitpur; Chitwan	153 men	22/108 (20.37)	2 (1.31)	–	–	113 (73.86)	–	
		People who inject drugs attending Recovering Nepal services submitted to HIV testing, Kathmandu; Lalitpur; Chitwan	181 people	22/136 (16.18)	3 (1.66)	–	–	115 (63.53)	–	
		Women who inject drugs attending Recovering Nepal services, Nepalgunj;	100 women	9 (9.00)	4 (4.00)	–	–	19 (19.00)	–	

Table 1 Studies reporting hepatitis B and C in Nepal *(Continued)*

SN	YEAR	POPULATION, SITE, TIME	SAMPLE SIZE, N	ANTI-HIV(%)	HBV			ANTI-HCV	NOTES	AUTHOR(S)
					HBSAG(%)	**ANTI-HBC(%)**	**ANTI-HBS(%)**			
		Dharan; Biratnagar; Kathmandu; Lalitpur; Chitwan,								
		Men who inject drugs attending Recovering Nepal services submitted to HIV testing, Nepalgunj; Dharan; Biratnagar; Kathmandu; Lalitpur; Chitwan,	301 men	40/ 254 (15.75)	10 (3.32)	–	–	181 (60.13)	–	
		People who inject drugs attending Recovering Nepal services submitted to HIV testing, Nepalgunj; Dharan; Biratnagar; Kathmandu; Lalitpur; Chitwan,	354 people	49 (13.84)	–	–	–	–	–	
		People who inject drugs attending Recovering Nepal services, Nepalgunj; Dharan; Biratnagar; Kathmandu; Lalitpur; Chitwan,	401 people	92/ 397 (23.17)	14 (3.49)	146 (43.89)	–	200 (49.87)	–	
46	2015	Patients attending Manipal Teaching Hospital, Pokhara, 2008 to 2013	25,708 individual blood samples	218 (0.85)	–	–	–	–	–	Supram HS et al. [89]
		People living with HIV/AIDS at Manipal Teaching Hospital, Pokhara, 2008 to 2013	218 individual blood samples	PLWH	7 (3.21)	–	–	9 (4.13)	–	
47	2015	Boys and men 15+ years who inject drugs, Sunsari, Morang and Jhapa districts, July 2015	360 boys and men	30 (8.33)	3 (0.83)	–	–	171 (47.50)	Syphilis: 4 (1.11); Syphilis History: 8 (2.22)	MoH/ NCASC [90]
48	2015	Boys and men 16+ years who inject drugs, Kathmandu, Lalitpur and Bhaktapur districts, Kathmandu Valley, June 2015 to July 2015	340 boys and men	22 (6.47)	0 (0.00)	–	–	75 (22.06)	Syphilis: 0 (0.00); Syphilis History: 0 (0.00)	MoH/ NCASC [91]
49	2015	Boys and men 16+ years who inject drugs, Pokhara Valley, June 2015 to July 2015	345 boys and men	10 (2.90)	6 (1.74)	–	–	45 (13.04)	-STI: 4 (1.16)	MoH/ NCASC [92]
50	2015	People living with HIV/AIDS in Eastern Development Region,	140 people	PLWH	5 (3.57)	–	–	67 (47.86)	–	UNDP/ DFID/CMDN [2, 93]
		People living with HIV/AIDS in Central Development Region,	137 people	PLWH	7 (5.11)	–	–	30 (21.90)	–	
		People living with HIV/AIDS in West Development Region,	203 people	PLWH	13 (6.40)	–	–	20 (9.85)	–	
		People living with HIV/AIDS in Midwest Development Region,	51 people	PLWH	0 (0.00)	–	–	12 (23.53)	–	
		People living with HIV/AIDS in Far West Development Region,	146 people	PLWH	5 (3.42)	–	–	3 (2.05)	–	
		People living with HIV/AIDS in all Development Regions,	677 people	PLWH	30 (4.43)	–	–	132 (19.50)	–	
		People who inject drugs living with HIV/ AIDS in all Development Regions,	562 people	PLWH	8 (1.42)	–	–	91 (16.19)	–	
		Sex workers living with HIV/AIDS in all Development Regions,	–	PLWH	(0.1)	–	–	0 (0.00)	–	
		Migrant workers living with HIV/AIDS in all Development Regions,	–	PLWH	(1.0)	–	–	(1.8)	–	
		Gay, Lesbian and Transgender people living with HIV/AIDS in all Development Regions,	–	PLWH	(0.4)	–	–	(0.4)	–	
		Non most at risk population living with HIV/ AIDS in all Development Regions,	–	PLWH	(1.3)	–	–	(1.0)	–	

Table 1 Studies reporting hepatitis B and C in Nepal *(Continued)*

SN	YEAR	POPULATION, SITE, TIME	SAMPLE SIZE, N	ANTI-HIV(%)	HBV			ANTI-HCV	NOTES	AUTHOR(S)
					HBSAG(%)	**ANTI-HBC(%)**	**ANTI-HBS(%)**			
51	2016	People who inject drugs with last 30-day frequent injection drug use attending re-habilitation centers, Kathmandu; Bhaktapur; Lalitupur; Sindupalchowk	167 people	–	–	–	–	20/87 (22.99)	–	Loewinger G et al. [94]
52	2016	Girls and women 16+ years who inject drugs, Kathmandu, Lalitpur and Bhaktapur districts, Kathmandu Valley, April 2016 to July 2016	160 girls and women	14 (8.75)	3 (1.87)	–	–	34 (21.25)	12 (7.50)	MoH/ NCASC [95]
53	2016	Boys and men 15+ years who inject drugs, Rupandehi, Kapilvastu, Dang, Banke, Kailali and Kanchanpur districts	300 boys and men	7 (2.33)	5 (1.67)	–	–	24 (8.00)	Syphilis: 1 (0.33); Syphilis History: 5 (1.67)	MoH/ NCASC [96]
54	2016	Patients who came in contact with HIV or other chronic liver disease and jaundice attending Teku Hospital, Tribhuvan University Teaching Hospital, NRCS	2700 patients	–	–	–	–	100 (3.70)	–	Nepal A et al. [97]
55	2016	Central Blood Transfusion Centre, 2014–2015	69,303 blood samples	21 (0.03)	192 (0.28)	–	–	224 (0.32)	Syphilis: 360 (0.52)	NRCS [22]
		Regional Blood Transfusion Centre, 2014–2015	42,511 blood samples	13 (0.03)	151 (0.35)	–	–	56 (0.23)	Syphilis: 115 (0.27)	
		District/Emergency Blood Transfusion Centre, 2014–2015	77,016 blood samples	27 (0.03)	227 (0.29)	–	–	119 (0.15)	Syphilis: 260 (0.34)	
		Hospital Blood Transfusion unit, 2014–2015	28,324 blood samples	7 (0.02)	47 (0.16)	–	–	23 (0.08)	Syphilis: 25 (0.09)	
		Total, 2014–2015	217,154 blood samples	68 (0.03)	617 (0.28)	–	–	422 (0.19)	Syphilis: 760 (0.35)	

[a]: Study describes seroprevalence of active HBV infection. Test(s) used in the survey is(are) not specified
[b]: Study describes seroprevalence of exposure to HBV. Test(s) used in the survey is (are) not specified

0.33, respectively), [20] and Kinkel HT et a, between male and female PWID attending Recovering Nepal services in 2015 (19.00 vs. 60.13).

Age has been fundamental to the design of hepatitis C public health policies in many countries. It is known that age can relate to many factors in the epidemic: year of introduction of the virus, availability of tests and distribution of contaminated blood products, cumulative exposure (such as injection drug use, unprotected sexual activity across adult life), and status of harm reduction

Table 2 Findings of the meta-analyses for hepatitis C virus (HCV) prevalence measures

Populations at risk	Studies	Samples	HCV prevalence estimates		Heterogeneity measures			
	Total N	Total N	Mean (%)	95% CI	Q (*p*-value)[a]	τ^{2b}	I^2 (confidence limits-%)[c]	Prediction interval (%)[d]
People who inject drugs	15	3140	45.17	26.34–64.73	1714.1 (< 0.0001)	0.1487	99.2 (99.0–99.3)	0–100
Populations at intermediate risk	12	4998	12.76	5.44–22.47	668.83 (< 0.0001)	0.0486	98.4 (97.9–98.7)	0–59.58
Populations at low risk (general population)	28	972,123	0.68	0.54–0.86	683.44 (< 0.0001)	0.2027	96.0 (95.1–96.8)	0.26–1.75
Populations with liver-related conditions	6	411	11.51	7.73–15.87	7.40 (0.1926)	0.0018	32.4 (0–72.7)	3.48–22.89
Special clinical populations	3	133	1.67	0–5.81	2.79 (0.2473)	0.0022	28.4 (0–92.6)	0–75.38

[a]Q: the Cochran's Q statistic is a measure assessing the existence of heterogeneity in HCV prevalence estimates
[b]τ^2: the estimated between-study variance in the double arcsine transformed proportions of the true HCV prevalence estimates. The back-transformed τ^2 was not calculated as the methodology to do so is not currently available
[c]I^2: a measure assessing the magnitude of between-study variation that is due to differences in HCV prevalence estimates across studies rather than chance
[d]Prediction interval: estimates the 95% interval in which the true HCV prevalence in a new HCV study will lie

strategies [41–43]. In Nepal, age and hepatitis C have only been featured in two studies. De Bruyn et al. found anti-HCV to be positive in 11.8% of patients age 16–65 years attending Amp Pipal Hospital at Gorkha district in 1993; and Sawayama Y et al. found 2.27% in female villagers 45–54 years from Bhadrakali and Kotyang villages in 1996 [40, 44].

HIV co-infection prevalence

The first HIV prevalence study in Nepal dates 1989, [44] 1 year after the first case of HIV was detected in the country [45]. So far, eighteen prevalence studies also assessed at some time the HIV infection in their population, almost half a million people and roughly half of the population evaluated for HBV or HCV infection since 1985, the year of debut of anti-HIV ELISA tests.

As stated previously for overall population, candidates for blood donation represent the majority of the population tested for HIV co-infection in Nepal in the fifty-five viral hepatitis prevalence studies of this review. Yet, regardless of age and/or gender subgroups, candidates for blood donation have failed to present HIV seropositivity rates above 0.2% [20, 12, 18], constituting themselves a population of low prevalence for HIV co-infection. This data must not considered a proxy for general population, as candidates for blood donation have shown to be a "poor control group for non-genetic studies of diseases related to environmentally, behaviourally, or socially patterned exposures", [46] but a reason to pursue further detection of viral hepatitis in priority populations.

As we evaluate the remaining studied population, we find that the highest rates of HIV infection found in this review do not belong to PWID, but sex trafficked girls and women, at an approximate 30% rate of infection in 2008 (74/246) [7]. This is closely followed by PWID attending Recovering Nepal services, if accounted the participation of those with previously defined HIV status, with rates as high as 23.17% in 2015. Such findings are consonant with latest numbers of Family Health International data for HIV prevalence in PWID in Kathmandu (21% in 2009) [3] and increase of HIV and sexually transmitted infections in survivors of sex traffic, particularly for Nepalese girls and women [47–49].

Discussion

This review collects all available surveys performed in Nepal or with Nepalese population. It provides relevant information to policy makers, researchers and activists.

Developments of improved strategic information

It has been 44 years since the first viral hepatitis prevalence study took place in Nepal. Since then, sixty different publications, of which fifty-five are available in this review, have dedicated themselves to the better understanding of these epidemics.

Almost a quarter of these scientific publications and reports have been issued in the last 3 years. While there is still much to investigate, it is undeniable that Nepal's civil society organizations and academia have been successful in their struggle to improve the reactive approach to viral hepatitis and HIV, shaping public health policy and visibility of key populations.

Superior strategic information and overall engagement to the epidemics lead to additional victories: the inclusion of LGBT issues in government policies, the return of harm reductions strategy in 2007, increase in donor funding for the response to HIV, and stronger ties between emerging and existing networks of key populations and representatives, healthcare professionals, academia, UNAIDS and GoN [50–55]. Such echoing common voice for change lead to the preliminary discussion of National Viral Hepatitis Guidelines and negotiation of licensed generic drugs for hepatitis C treatment at a fraction of prices offered to other developing countries [41, 56–59]. This recent collective represents a cornerstone for viral hepatitis in Nepal.

Gaps and key populations

It would seem to be that the shared modes of transmission of viral hepatitis and HIV, and the resulting similar epidemiological profiles, could translate into one equally successful public health intervention for both epidemics.

This is hardly the truth. Regardless of improvements in blood safety, availability of harm reduction services and assistance to sexually transmitted and reproductive tract infections, with significant drops in HIV prevalence since the last decade, many key populations sustain subpar decrease in hepatitis C numbers. Such is the case of PWID in Nepal: hepatitis C exceeds three times the HIV prevalence in several cohorts.

Since 2000, PWID, PLHIV, sex workers and LGBT have figured in no less than seventeen different viral hepatitis prevalence studies, almost a third of studies collected in this review, contributing without precedents to the national strategic information and deeper understanding of the response to public health interventions. Additional publications also developed initial data for other population groups such as refugees/misplaced persons and survivors of sex traffic.

Our research could not retrieve any studies regarding transgender population, male sex workers or incarcerated persons in Nepal.

Hepatitis B vaccine coverage and elimination of vertical transmission (EVT)

Hepatitis B is a highly contagious, yet preventable disease [60, 61]. In recent years, many countries have chosen to scale up maternal and newborn care in order to secure a generation 'free of hepatitis B'.

Our review provided two studies depicting hepatitis B in infancy in Nepal. The first study states hepatitis B is responsible for approximately 5 % of the cases of acute hepatitis in children 0–15 years [14]. The second study describes observed benefits of hepatitis B vaccine introduction to children in Nepal in 2002.

While no routine for hepatitis B immunoglobulin in prevention of vertical transmission has been implemented in Nepal, the rates of acute hepatitis related to HBV infection in children are quite different than the prevalence values of HBV in pregnant women (0.32%), an indicator that perhaps household exposure during infancy, and not mother-to-child transmission, is the reason for new but likely overlooked exposure during infancy (households).

Commercial vaccines for hepatitis B have been available worldwide since 1981 [62]. In Nepal, however, it has only been introduced in 2002. After fifteen years and despite recommendations issued by GoN, the country still struggles to provide appropriate vaccine coverage [35, 63].

Official government reports state that from 2002 until 2009, third-dose hepatitis B vaccine coverage for children 12–23 months stood at approximately 80%. [63, 64] World Health Organization (WHO) and United Nations Children's Fund (UNICEF) estimate improved coverage in 20,012 and 2013, slightly above 95%. [65] Such higher vaccine coverage numbers are not homogenous in Nepal - not all municipalities have immunization plans or appropriate structure at their disposal [63, 64]. Moreover, the intervention requires timely birth-dose vaccination for a most successful response, [66] and faces many other obstacles [67].

Hepatitis B vaccine is available to healthcare workers (HCW) in many countries. In Nepal, HCW are featured in two studies as an alternative to controls, with HBsAg seropositivity rates of 1.38 and 1.69% [26, 68]. These figures are lower than the ones presented by key populations, but still higher than those of candidates for blood donation. Further investigation reveals that HCW and students in Nepal have largely mishandled biosafety procedures while at high risk of exposure to the infective agent. Studies in tertiary care centers have shown frequent needle-stick and sharps-related injuries, and incomplete or fully ignored vaccination and post prophylaxis procedures [69–71].

Nevertheless, UNAIDS understands that the strengthening of the immunization plan and maternal health must be accompanied of a nationwide awareness campaign for HCW and future health professionals.

Community and the strengthening of health systems

Communities were the first responders to the HIV epidemic, nearly thirty years ago. They have continuously played an essential role in development of research, health services and shaping of public health policy worldwide, expanding their activities to sustainable and affordable vaccines and medicines for viral hepatitis.

Moreover, these collectives of advocates, researchers, clients or providers have the ability to work unisonous with marginalized populations, increasing the reach and quality of health systems and health services, often detecting overlooked issues such as stigma and discrimination. Whether leading research or promoting health services, civil society engagement improves awareness, prevention, diagnosis and retention in care. This has been the case of both viral hepatitis and HIV epidemic.

In Nepal, these initiatives are considered to be just as important as developments provided by academia, government and international agencies. It is clear that these endeavors provide a unique opportunity to fill critical gaps such as strategic information, low immunization coverage rates and elimination of mother-to-child and household transmission.

Conclusion

The present review illustrates different turning points in viral hepatitis and HIV co-infection epidemiology in Nepal. Since 1973, when the first study on viral hepatitis in the country was published, there have been many changes in the understanding of these epidemics.

These include the indirect effects of successful public health policies aimed towards HIV, such as the decrease of viral hepatitis prevalence in PWID, and their limitations, revealing overlooked population groups and issues in viral hepatitis that require public health policies of their own.

The review also allows one to witness the progressive scientific development by Nepalese researchers and institutions, and civil society representatives' participation. Such collaboration correlates with increased number of studies and sample sizes in recent years including the survey of key populations, and will be fundamental for the success of the National HIV Strategic Plan 2016–2021 and achieving the SDG by 2030.

Acknowledgements

We are grateful for the support provided by the Biostatistics, Epidemiology, and Biomathematics Research Core at the Weill Cornell Medical College in Qatar. The authors are also grateful for the valuable suggestions and comments by the reviewers of this article.

Authors' contributions

MCMN and KB performed the systematic review. KB supervised the research and provided inputs for discussion. All authors contributed equally to the discussion, conclusion and review of this manuscript. All authors read and approved the final manuscript.

Competing interests

The authors declare that they have no competing interests.

References

1. Kleinman S, Busch M. The risk of transfusion-transmitted infection: direct estimation and mathematical modelling. Ballière's Clinical Haematology. 2000;13(4):631–49.
2. Government of Nepal. Ministry of Health and Population. National Centre for AIDS and STD Control. Country Progress Report Nepal. 2015.
3. Narain JP. Three decades of HIV/AIDS in Asia. New Delhi: Vivek Mehra for SAGE Publications India Pvt Ltd; 2012.
4. Government of Nepal. National Planning Comission. Sustainable development goals 2016–2030. Kathmandu: National Preliminary Report; 2015.
5. Government of Nepal. Ministry of Health. National Centre for AIDS and STD Control. Kathmandu: Nepal HIVision 2020 - Ending the AIDS epidemic as a public health threat, by 2030; 2016.
6. Hillis A, Shrestha S, Saha N. An epidemic of infectious hepatitis in the Kathmandu Valley. J Nepal Med Assoc. 1973;11(5):145–53.
7. Silverman JG, Decker MR, Gupta J, Dharmadhikari A, Seage G, Raj A. Syphilis and hepatitis co-infection among HIV-infected, sex-trafficked women and girls, Nepal. Emerg Infect Dis. 2008;14(6):932–4.
8. Kinkel HT, Karmacharya D, Shakya J, Manandhar S, Panthi S, Karmacharya P, et al. Prevalence of HIV, hepatitis B and C infections and an assessment of HCV-genotypes and two IL28B SNPs among people who inject drugs in three regions of Nepal. PLOS One. 2015;10(8):1–18.
9. Moher D, Liberati A, Tetzlaff J, Altman DG, PRISMA Group. Preferred reporting items for systematic reviews and meta-analyses: the PRISMA statement. PLoS Med. 2009;6(7):e1000097.
10. Nuti M. The low prevalence of HBV markers in Nepal. Transact R Soc Trop Med Hyg. 1988;82:144.
11. Dhungel B, Dhungel K, Easow J, Singh Y. Opportunistic infection among HIV seropositive cases in Manipal Teaching Hospital, Pokhara, Nepal. Kathmandu Univ Med J. 2008;6(3):335–9.
12. Karki S, Ghimire P, Tiwari BR, Shrestha AC, Gautam A, Rajkarnikar M. Seroprevalence of HIV and hepatitis C co-infection among blood donors in Kathmandu Valley, Nepal. Southeast Asian J Trop Med Public Health. 2009;40(1):67–70.
13. Tiwari B, Ghimire P, Kandel S, Rajkarnikar M. Seroprevalence of HBV and HCV in blood donors: a study from regional blood transfusion services of Nepal. Asian J Transfus Sci. 2010;4(2):91–3.
14. Sudhamshu K, Sharma D, Poudyal N, Basnet BK. Acute viral hepatitis in pediatric age groups. J Nepal Med Assoc. 2014;52(193):687–91.
15. Barnawal SP, Niraula SR, Agrahari AK, Bista N, Jha N, Pokharel PK. Human immunodeficiency virus and hepatitis C virus coinfection in Nepal. Indian J Gastroenterol. 2014;33(2):141–5.
16. Shrestha SM, Shrestha S, Tsuda F, Sawada N, Tanaka T, Okamoto H, et al. Infection with GB virus C and hepatitis C virus in drug addicts, patients on maintenance hemodialysis, or with chronic liver disease in Nepal. J Med Virol. 1997;53:157–61.
17. Mohamoud YA, Mumtaz GR, Riome S, Miller D, Abu-Raddad LJ. The epidemiology of hepatitis C virus in Egypt: a systematic review and data synthesis. BMC Infectious Diseases. 2013;13:288. https://doi.org/10.1186/1471-2334-13-288.
18. Chander A, Pahwa V. Status of infectious disease markers among blood donors in a teaching hospital, Bhairahawa, western Nepal. J Commun Dis. 2003;35(3):188–97.
19. Karki S, Ghimire P, Tiwari BR, Maharjan A, Rajkarnikar M. Trends in hepatitis B and hepatitis C seroprevalence among Nepalese blood donors. Jpn J Infect Dis. 2008;61:324–6.
20. Shrestha AC, Ghimre P, Tiwari BR, Rajkarnikar M. Transfusion-transmissible infections among blood donors in Kathmandu, Nepal. J Infect Dev Ctries. 2009;3(10):794–7.
21. Nepal Red Cross Society National Blood Transfusion Service. Annual Progress Report 2069/070 (2012/13).
22. Nepal Red Cross Society. Annual Progress Report 2071/072 (2014/15).
23. Chatterjee A, Uprety L, Chapagain M, Kafle K. Drug abuse in Nepal: a rapid assessment study. Bull Narc. 1996;48(1):11–33.
24. Lam L. Comments on Strang et al.'s "Heroin smoking by 'chasing the dragon': origins and history". Addiction. 1997;92(6):685–95. https://onlinelibrary.wiley.com/doi/pdf/10.1080/09652149737665.
25. Shrestha S, Shrestha D, Gafney T, Maharjan K, Tsuda F, Okamoto H. Hepatitis B and C infection among drug abusers in Nepal. Trop Gastroenterol. 1996;17(4):212–3.
26. Shrestha SM, Tsuda F, Okamoto H, Tokita H, Horikita M, Tanaka T, et al. Hepatitis B virus subtypes and hepatitis C virus genotypes in patients with chronic liver disease in Nepal. Hepatol. 1994;19(4):805–9.
27. Shrestha SM, Shrestha S, Shreshta A, Tsuda F, Endo K, Takahashi M, et al. High prevalence of hepatitis B virus infection and inferior vena cava obstruction among patients with liver cirrhosis or hepatocellular carcinoma in Nepal. Hepatol. 2007;22:1921–8.
28. Kane MA, Bradley DW, Shrestha SM, Maynard J, Cook EH, Mishra RP, et al. Recovery of a possible etiologic agent and transmission studies in marmosets. JAMA. 1984;252(22):3140–5.
29. Shrestha SM, Shrestha I, Maharjan K. Family clustering of HBV infection in the household of persistent HBsAg carriers: spread of HBV by horizontal transmission. J Inst Med. 1991;13:319–26.
30. Shrestha SM. Seroepidemiology of viral hepatitis in Surkhet, Nepal. J Inst Med. 1987;9:1–10.
31. Poudel KC, Jimba M, Okumura J, Wakai S. Emerging co-infection of HIV and hepatitis B virus in far western Nepal. Trop Doct. 2006;36:186–7.
32. Goh K, Kong K, Heng B, Oon C. Seroepidemiology of hepatitis A and hepatitis B virus infection in a Gurkha Community in Singapore. J Med Virol. 1993;41:146–9.
33. Shrestha SM, Shrestha S. Chronic hepatitis B in Nepal: an Asian country with low prevalence of HBV infection. Trop Gastroenterol. 2012;33(2):95–101.
34. Joshi S, Ghimire G. Serological prevalence of antibodies to Human Immunodeficiency Virus (HIV) and hepatitis B virus (HBV) among healthy Nepalese males - a retrospective study. Kathmandu Univ Med J. 2003;1(4):251–5.
35. Upreti SR, Gurung S, Patel M, Dixit S, Krause K, Shakya G, et al. Prevalence of chronic hepatitis B virus infection before and after implementation of a hepatitis B vaccination program among children in Nepal. Vaccine. 2014; 32(34):4304–9.
36. Lavanchy D. The global burden of hepatitis C. Liver Int. 2009;29(Suppl 1):74–81.
37. Sulkowski M, Thomas DL. Hepatitis in the HIV-infected person. Ann Intern Med. 2003;138(3):197–208.
38. Shrestha IL. Seroprevalence of antibodies to hepatitis C virus among injecting drug users from Kathmandu. Kathmandu Univ Med J. 2003;1(2):101–3.
39. Poudel KC, Palmer PH, Jimba M, Mizoue T, Kobayashi J, Poudel-Tandukar K. Coinfection with hepatitis C virus among HIV-positive people in Kathmandu Valley, Nepal. J Int Assoc Provid AIDS Care. 2014;13(3):277–83.
40. Sawayama Y, Hayashi J, Ariyama I, Furusyo N, Kawasaki T, Kawasaki M, et al. A ten year serological survey of hepatitis A, B and C viruses infections in Nepal. J Epidemiol. 1999;9(5):350–4.
41. Mesquita F, Santos MÉ, Benzaken A, Corrêa R, Cattapan E, Sereno L, et al. The Brazilian comprehensive response to hepatitis C: from strategic thinking to access to interferon-free therapy. BMC Public Health. 2016;16(1132)
42. European Centre fr Disease Prevention and Control. Hepatitis C surveillance in Europe 2013. Stockholm: ECDC; 2015.
43. U.S. Department of Health and Human Services. Centers for Disease Control and Prevention. Hepatitis C - why people born from 1945–1965 should get tested. United States: CDC; 2016.
44. de Bruyn G, Song E. Seroepidemiology of hepatotropic viral infections in Amp Pipal, Nepal. Trop Doct. 1998;28:173–4.
45. Hannun J. AIDS in Nepal: communities confronting an emerging epidemic. New York: AmFAR in Association with Seven Stories Press; 1997.
46. Golding J, Northstone K, Miller L, Davey Smith G, Pembrey M. Differences between blood donors and a population sample: implications for case-control studies. Int J Epidemiol. 2013;42(4):1145–56.
47. Joffres C, Mills E, Joffres M, Khanna T, Walia H, Grund D. Sexual slavery without borders: trafficking for commercial sexual exploitation in India. Int J Equity Health. 2008;7(22)
48. Sarkar K, Bal B, Mukherjee R, Chakraborty S, Saha S, Ghosh A, et al. Sex-trafficking, violence, negotiating skill, and HIV infection in brother-based sex workers of Eastern India, adjoining Nepal, Bhutan, and Bangladesh. J Health Popul Nutr. 2008;26(2):223–31.
49. Silverman J, Decker M, Gupta J, Maheshwari A, Willis B, Raj A. HIV prevalence and predictors of infection in sex-trafficked Nepalese girls and women. JAMA. 2007;298(5):536–42.
50. UNDP, USAID. Being LGBT in Asia. Bangkok: Nepal Country Report; 2014.
51. Federal Ministry for Economic Cooperation and Development. Division for Health and Population. Opioid substitution therapy in Nepal. Bonn: Deutsche Gesellschaft für Internationale Zusammenarbeit (GIZ) GmbH; 2016.
52. UNDP, Williams Institute. Surveying Nepal's sexual and gender minorities: an inclusive approach. Bangkok: UNDP; 2014.

53. UNDP. Lost in transition: transgender people, rights and HIV vulnerability in the Asia-Pacific Region. Bangkok: UNDP; 2012.
54. Ministry of Health and Population. National Centre for AIDS and STI Control. National targeted intervention operational guidelines - injecting drug users. 2010.
55. Thomson N. Harm reduction history, response, and current trends in Asia. J Food Drug Anal. 2013;21(Suppl 4):113–6.
56. Natco Pharma. News & Announcements. 2017. http://natcopharma.co.in/about/news/. Accessed 21 Feb 2017.
57. Gilead Sciences, Inc. Chronic hepatitis C treatment expansion - generic manufacturing for developing countries. 2015.
58. Bristol-Myers Squibb Company, Medicines Patent Pool. Medicines Patent Pool. 2015. https://medicinespatentpool.org/uploads/2015/11/MPP-HCV-License-Agreement-BMS-FINAL-Web-00000002.pdf. Accessed 21 Feb 2017.
59. Iyengar S, Tay-Teo K, Vogler S, Beyer P, Wiktor S, de Joncheere K, et al. Prices, costs, and affordability of new medicines for hepatitis C in 30 countries: an economic analysis. PLOS Med. 2016;13(5):e1002032.
60. Lavanchy D. Chronic viral hepatitis as a public health issue in the world. Best Pract Res Clin Gastroenterol. 2008;22(6):991–1008.
61. Mandell G, Bennett J, Mandell DR. In: Mandell JEBRD GL, editor. Douglas, and Bennett's Principles and Practice of Infectious Diseases. 7th ed. Philadelphia: Elsevier; 2010.
62. Blumberg BS. The discovery of the hepatitis B virus and the invention of the vaccine: a scientific memoir. J Gastroenterol Hepatol. 2002;17(Suppl):502–3.
63. Ministry of Health & Population. Department of Health Services. Child Health Division. National immunization program - reaching every child - comprehensive multi-year plan 2068/2072 (2011–2016). Kathmandu: Government of Nepal; 2011.
64. Ministry of Health. Department of Health Services. Child Health Division. National immunization program of Nepal - reaching every village - multi-year plan of action 2007–2011. Kathmandu: Government of Nepal; 2007.
65. Berger S. Hepatitis B: global status: GIDEON Informatics Inc; 2016.
66. World Health Organization. Global health sector strategy on viral hepatitis, 2016–2021. Geneva: World Health Organization; 2016.
67. Tajiri K, Shimizu Y. Unsolved problems and future perspectives of hepatitis B virus vaccination. World J Gastroenterol. 2015;21(23):7074–83.
68. Shrestha S, Bhattarai M. Study of hepatitis B among different categories of health care workers. J Coll Physicians Surg Pak. 2006;16(2):108–11.
69. Bhattarai S, Smriti K, Pradhan PM, Lama S, Rijal S. Hepatitis B vaccination status and needle-stick and sharps-related injuries among medical school students in Nepal: a cross-sectional study. BMC Res Notes. 2014;7(774)
70. Gurubacharya D, Mathura K, Karki D. Knowledge, attitude and practices among health care workers on needle-stick injuries. Kathmandu Univ Med J. 2003;1(2):91–4.
71. Singh B, Paudel B, KC S. Knowledge and practice of health care workers regarding needle stick injuries in a tertiary care center of Nepal. Kathmandu Univ Med J. 2015;13:230–3.
72. Shrestha SM. Acute sporadic viral hepatitis in Nepal. Trop Gastroenterol. 1987;8:99–105.
73. Reynolds RD, Moser P, Acharya S, McConnell W, Andon M, Howard MP. Nutritional and medical status of lactating women and their infants in the Kathmandu valley of Nepal. Am J Clin Nutr. 1988;47:722–8.
74. Mertens T, Tondorf G, Siebolds M, Kruppenbacher J, Shrestha S, Mauff G, et al. Epidemiology of HIV and hepatitis B virus (HBV) in selected African and Asian populations. Infection. 1989;17(1):4–7.
75. Shrestha SM. Seroepidemiology of hepatitis B in Nepal. J Commun Dis. 1990;22:27–32.
76. Bhatta P, Thapa S, Neupane S, Baker J, Friedman M. Commercial sex workers in Kathmandu Valley: profile and prevalence of sexually transmitted diseases. J Nepal Med Assoc. 1994;32(111):191–203.
77. Rai SK, Shibata H, Satoh M, Murakoso K, Sumi K, Kubo T, et al. Seroprevalence of hepatitis B and C viruses in Eastern Nepal. Kansenshogaku Zasshi. 1994;68(12):1492–7.
78. Nakashima K, Kashiwagi S, Noguchi A, Hirata M, Hayashi J, Kawasaki T, et al. Human T-lymphotropic virus type-I, and hepatitis A, B and C viruses in Nepal: a serological survey. J Trop Med Hyg. 1995;98(5):347–50.
79. Manandhar K, Shrestha B. Prevalence of HBV infection among the healthy Nepalese males: a serological survey. J Epidemiol. 2000;10(6):410–3.
80. Manandhar K, Shrestha B. Prevalence of hepatitis B virus infection amongst healthy Nepalese males. Trop Gastroenterol. 1998;19(4):145–7.
81. Bidya S. HBsAg carriers among healthy Nepalese men: a serological survey. J Health Popul Nutr. 2002;20(3):235–8. http://www.recoveringnepal.org.np/image/info_materials/20111103081156838553767.pdf.
82. Chiba H, Takezaki T, Neupani D, Kim J, Yoshida S, Mizoguchi E, et al. An epidemiological study of HBV, HCV and HTLV-1 in Sherpas of Nepal. Asian Pac J Cancer Prev. 2004;5:370–3.
83. Shah B, Bhattacharya S, Parija S. Seroprevalence of hepatitis B virus among Bhutanese refugees residing in Nepal. Kathmandu Univ Med J. 2005;3(3):239–42.
84. Shrestha P, Bhandari D, Sharma D, Bhandari B. A study of viral hepatitis during pregnancy in Nepal Medical College Teaching Hospital. Nepal Med Coll J. 2009;11(3):192–4.
85. HEPA Foundation, United Nations Office on Drugs and Crime (UNODC). Prevalence of hepatitis C in OST client.
86. Asian Network of People Who Use Drugs. Barriers to hepatitis C diagnosis, management and treatment among people who inject drugs in 4 Asian countries: a community led study in India, Indonesia, Malaysia & Nepal. Bangkok: Asian Network of People who Use Drugs (ANPUD); 2011.
87. Adhikari P, Pathak U, Uprety D, Sapkota S. Profile of ascites patients admitted in Nepal Medical College Teaching Hospital. Nepal Med Coll J. 2012;14(2):111–3.
88. Ojha CR, Khagendra K, Shakya G. Co-infection of hepatitis C among HIV-infected population with different risk groups in Kathmandu, Nepal. Biomed Res. 2013;24(4):441–4.
89. Supram HS, Gokhale S, Sathian B, Bhatta DR. Hepatitis B virus (HBV) and hepatitis C virus (HCV) co-infection among HIV infected individuals at tertiary care hospital in Western Nepal. Nepal J Epidemiol. 2015;5(2):488–93.
90. Ministry of Health and Population. National Centre for AIDS and STD Control. Integrated biological and behavioral surveillance (IBBS) survey among people who inject drugs (PWID-male) in the Eastern Terai Highway Districts (Jhapa, Morang and Sunsari) of Nepal, 2015. Teku, Kathmandu: Government of Nepal; 2015.
91. Ministry of Health and Population. National Centre for AIDS and STD Control. Integrated biological and behavioral surveillance (IBBS) survey among people who inject drugs (PWID) in Kathmandu Valley, 2015. Teku, Kathmandu: Government of Nepal; 2015.
92. Ministry of Health and Population. National Centre for AIDS and STD Control. Integrated biological and behavioral surveillance (IBBS) survey among people who inject drugs (PWIDs) in Pokhara Valley, 2015. Kathmandu: Government of Nepal; 2015.
93. United Nations Development Program/Department for International Development/Center for Molecular Dynamics Nepal. Draft report of four PLHIV surveys. 2012.
94. Loewinger G, Sharma B, Karki DK, Khatiwoda P, Kainee S, Poudel K. Low knowledge and perceived hepatitis C risk despite high risk behaviour among injection drug users in Kathmandu, Nepal. Int J Drug Policy. 2016;33:75–82.
95. Ministry of Health. National Centre for AIDS and STD Control. Integrated biological and behavioral surveillance (IBBS) survey among female injecting drug users in Kathmandu Valley. Teku, Kathmandu: Government of Nepal; 2016.
96. Ministry of Health. National Centre for AIDS and STD Control. Integrated biological and behavioral surveillance (IBBS) survey among people who inject drugs (PWID-male) in Western to Far Western Terai Highway Districts of Nepal. Kathmandu: Government of Nepal; 2016.
97. Nepal A, Kunwar B. Evidence of hepatitis C virus infection and associated treatment in Nepal. J Mol Biomark Diagn. 2016;7(2):270.

Racial/ethnic- and county-specific prevalence of chronic hepatitis B and its burden

Mehlika Toy[1*], Bin Wei[1], Tejpal S. Virdi[1], An Le[2], Huy Trinh[3], Jiayi Li[4], Jian Zhang[5], Ann W. Hsing[6], Samuel K. So[1] and Mindie H. Nguyen[2]

Abstract

Background: In the United States, the highest burden of chronic hepatitis B (CHB) and CHB-related liver cancer is in the state of California, primarily in the San Francisco (SF) Bay and Los Angeles (LA) areas. The aim of this study was to estimate county-specific hepatitis B surface antigen (HBsAg) prevalence and quantify CHB cases by age, race/ethnicity, nativity, and disease activity status.

Methods: Twelve counties in SF Bay Area and three large counties in LA area were included for this analysis. Race/ethnicity-specific prevalence of HBsAg for each county and the state of California as a whole, was estimated by including prevalence data from the National Health and Nutrition Examination Survey and various studies that estimated HBsAg prevalence in US and foreign-born Asian Pacific Islanders, Hispanic, and Black populations. In addition, clinical data of 2000 consecutive CHB patients (collected between 2009 and 2014) from a large clinical consortium in the SF Bay area were used to calculate the age-specific disease burden.

Results: Of the 15 counties analyzed, SF had the highest HBsAg prevalence (1.78%), followed by Santa Clara (1.63%) and Alameda (1.45%). The majority of CHB cases were estimated to be in LA County (83,770), followed by Santa Clara (31,273), and Alameda (23,764). Among the CHB cases, 12.7% is active HBeAg positive, 24.2% is active HBeAg negative, and 10.6% has cirrhosis.

Conclusion: This study confirms and quantifies the current burden of CHB in high endemic counties in the state of California using population-level estimates combined with clinical data including those from the community.

Keywords: HBV, Disease status, California, Burden of disease

Background

As a leading cause of liver disease, liver cancer, and liver transplantation, chronic hepatitis B (CHB) is an important public health problem globally [1]. In 2013, viral hepatitis took the lives of about 1.45 million people and was the seventh leading cause of death in the world, surpassing malaria and tuberculosis [1]. An estimated 850,000–2.2 million people in the United States (US) live with CHB and only 34.6% are aware of their infection [2]. The highest prevalence of CHB and CHB-related liver cancer in the U.S is in the state of California (CA), primarily in the San Francisco (SF) bay and Los Angeles (LA) areas [3]. However, only 34.6% are diagnosed [2], 33.3% of those diagnosed receive care [4], and 45% of those linked to care receive treatment if eligible according to treatment guidelines [5]. Without diagnosis, linkage to care and treatment, one in four people with CHB will die from cirrhosis, liver cancer, and/or liver failure [6]. In US regions with high proportion of immigrants, such as the SF Bay area, the vast majority of confirmed cases of CHB are Asian or Pacific Islander (API) [2]. A study from San Francisco found that of all hepatitis B virus (HBV) infection cases reported, 84% were API and of those 80% were foreign born [7]. In the U.S., the prevalence of CHB among foreign-born people is estimated to be 10 times higher than the national prevalence rate [8]. A

* Correspondence: mtoy@stanford.edu
[1]Asian Liver Center, Department of Surgery, Stanford University School of Medicine, 780 Welch Road, CJ130D, Palo Alto, CA 94304, USA
Full list of author information is available at the end of the article

seroprevalence survey study on Asian Americans in the SF Bay area concluded that 8.9% API were infected with CHB but 65.4% of the chronically infected adults were unaware of their infection [2]. One of the four overarching goals of the Department of Health and Human Services Action Plan for the Prevention, Care and Treatment of Viral Hepatitis is to increase the diagnosis rate of CHB from 33 to 66% by 2020 [9].

The National Health and Nutrition Examination Survey (NHANES) has been the primary data source for HBV [10] prevalence estimate in the US population. However, due to the small sample size in the survey, it is not an appropriate source for county- and state-specific prevalence estimates of CHB [11]. In addition, county-level and race/ethnicity-specific data are important for setting priorities in public health and resource allocation at the local level and since the distribution of CHB disease burden varies by race/ethnicity which itself varies by counties. Thus, to fill this gap, the aim of this study was to estimate the prevalence of HBsAg and quantify CHB active disease burden in the state of CA and certain specific counties by age, race/ethnicity, and disease activity status, using population-based data and clinical data from a large clinical and community consortium in the SF bay area.

Methods

As a first step, we obtained age-specific population for 12 counties in the SF Bay area and 3 large counties in the LA area (Los Angeles, San Bernardino and Orange counties) as well as county-specific race/ethnicity distributions in these populations from the US census [12]. We then categorized the population according to the following four major racial/ethnic groups: White, Hispanic, Black, and API. Nativity data for Black and API populations were also obtained from the US census bureau. Approximately, 10.3% of Blacks in the US are foreign born [13], of whom 36% were born in Africa, 35% in Jamaica and Dominican Republic, 15% in Haiti, and 9% in East and South America, and 5% elsewhere [14]. Within the API population, we further divided the groups into: South Asian (23.3%), Korean (8.6%), Japanese (6.7%) and other East Asian (61.4%) [15, 16]. Secondly, we calculated age-specific API foreign-born population distribution from the US census data [17] and used these age-specific distributions for the East Asia, Korea and South Asia group. For example, the Japanese foreign born distribution was reported to be 27% in the US [15]. Next, we collected race/ethnicity- and nativity-specific HBsAg prevalence data among White [11], Hispanic [11, 18], Black [11, 19–21] and APIs [2, 11, 19, 22–24] in the US from the literature. Jung et al. reported a 0% (353 people tested) of HBsAg prevalence among 70+ year old Hispanic population, which we decided not to take and assume the same prevalence for 60 + as the 60–69 age-group (0.38%). Table 1 shows the race/ethnicity- and nativity- as well as age-specific prevalence rates, where reported, in the studies that we used as prevalence data to calculate the overall prevalence for the SF Bay area, the LA area and for the entire state of California.

In all race/ethnicity groups of ages 0–19 years, except for the Black foreign-born Africa and Haiti groups as well as the API foreign-born East Asia, we used the NHANES 2015 data. NHANES reported a prevalence of 0.03% (0.01–0.08) among 6–19 year old group, which we used for 0–19 year olds in the White, Hispanic, Black US-born, API US-born Korea, Japan and South Asia groups, as well as the Japanese foreign-born group. We used the prevalence that was 10-fold greater than the general population explanation of the NHANES study and applied it to the Black foreign-born in Jamaica and Dominican Republic, API US-born East Asian and API foreign-born Korean groups for estimating the prevalence among 0–19 year olds.

In order to quantify the age-specific "active" disease burden in relation to CHB activity and cirrhosis, we analyzed clinical baseline data such as HBV DNA and alanine aminotransferase (ALT) levels of 2000 consecutive new treatment-naïve CHB patients who presented between 2009 and 2014 at several hepatology and community gastroenterology and primary care clinics as of the SF Bay Area Consortium (SFBAC). Following the American Association for the Study of Liver Disease (AASLD) guidelines [6], disease status was defined as "active" by the following criteria: presence of cirrhosis or an elevation of ALT > 2 times the upper limit of normal (ULN) or evidence of significant histological disease plus elevated HBV DNA above 2000 IU/mL for HBeAg-negative and above 20,000 IU/mL for HBeAg-positive non-cirrhotic cases.

Results

Estimates of HBsAg prevalence and burden

The age-specific foreign-born distribution for API for age groups 0–19, 20–29, 30–39, 40–49, 50–59, 60–69, and 70+ were 22, 64, 83, 87, 89, 87, 90%, respectively. Combining population distribution by county, race/ethnicity and nativity with race/ethnic specific HBsAg-prevalence, we estimated that overall, all race-combined, there are 104,734 (range 70,952–153,598) CHB cases or 1.18% (range 0.80–1.73%) in the SF Bay area. Table 2 shows the estimated overall age-specific HBsAg-prevalence (all race combined) and related number of CHB cases in the SF Bay area.

As shown, the highest prevalence was amongst ages 40–49 (2.08%) with a total of 25,627 (24.5% of all cases), followed by 1.86% for those between the ages of 30 and 39. In the LA area, with a population of 15.5 million, we estimated that the overall prevalence is 0.71% (range 0.46–1.12%), with a total of 109,442 (range 71,363–172,482) with CHB. For California as a state with

Table 1 Race/ethnicity- and nativity-specific HBsAg prevalence data from literature review

Race/Ethnicity	Ages 0–19 Prevalence (range)	Reference	Ages > 19 Prevalence (range)	Reference
White	0.03% (0.01–0.08)	Roberts et al. [11]	0.10% (0.05–0.20)	Roberts et al. [11]
Hispanic	0.03% (0.01–0.08)	Roberts et al. [11]	20–29 0.16% (0.05–0.47)	Jung et al. [18]
			30–39 0.14% (0.04–0.42)	
			40–49 0.49% (0.24–1.00)	
			50–59 0.39% (0.21–0.72)	
			60–69 0.38% (0.10–1.37)	
			70 + [a] 0.38% (0.10–1.37)	
Black US-Born	0.03% (0.01–0.08)	Roberts et al. [11]	0.10% (0.05–0.20)	Roberts et al. [11]
Black Foreign-Born				
Africa	7.30% (6.50–8.00)	Ugwu et al. [20]	20–29 10.45% (9.50–11.30)	Ugwu et al. [20]
			30–39 11.20% (9.70–12.70)	
			40–49 6.99% (5.60–8.30)	
			50–59 10.86% (9.70–12.00)	
			60+ 10.86% (9.70–12.00)	
Jamaica and Dominican Rep.	0.30% (0.10–0.80)	Roberts et al. [11]	2.10% (0.70–4.00)	Din et al. [19]
Haiti	2.50% (2.10–3.00)	Tohme et al. [21]	2.50% (2.10–3.00)	Tohme et al. [21]
South & Central America	0.30% (0.10–0.80)	Roberts et al. [11]	0.60% (0.2–2.00)	Din et al. [19]
API US Born				
East Asia	0.30% (0.10–0.80)	Roberts et al. [11]	1.40% (0.65–1.90)	Din et al. [19]
Korea	0.03% (0.01–0.08)	Roberts et al. [11]	1.40% (0.65–1.90)	Din et al. [19]
Japan	0.03% (0.01–0.08)	Roberts et al. [11]	0.10% (0.05–0.20)	Roberts et al. [11]
South Asia	0.03% (0.01–0.08)	Roberts et al. [11]	1.40% (0.65–1.90)	Din et al. [19]
API Foreign Born				
East Asia	1.10% (0.90–1.90)	Shuler et al. [23]	20–29 5.40% (3.10–8.50)	Lin et al. [2]
			30–39 11.50% (8.30–15.20)	
			40–49 12.20% (9.70–15.00)	
			50–59 8.80% (7.00–10.80)	
			60–69 8.00% (5.90–10.60)	
			70–79 6.70% (4.00–10.40)	
			80+ 3.70% (1.00–9.30)	
Korea	0.30% (0.10–0.80)	Roberts et al. [11]	20–29 1.18% (0.43–2.55)	Hyun et al. [22]
			30–39 2.53% (1.61–3.77)	
			40–49 2.76% (2.00–3.70)	
			50–59 2.90% (2.23–3.69)	
			60–69 2.06% (1.37–2.96)	
			70–79 1.37% (0.59–2.68)	
			80+ 2.17% (1.17–2.77)	
Japan	0.03% (0.01–0.08)	Roberts et al. [11]	1.02%[b] (1.01–1.02)	Tanaka et al. [24]
South Asia	0.30% (0.10–0.80)	Roberts et al. [11]	2.70% (1.60–4.00)	Din et al. [19]

Definitions of race and ethnicity according to the US Census Bureau: White- A person having origins in any of the original peoples of Europe, the Middle East, or North Africa. Black or African American- A person having origins in any of the Black racial groups of Africa. Asian- A person having origins in any of the original peoples of the Far East, South East Asia, or the Indian subcontinent including, for example, Cambodia, China, India, Japan, Korea, Malaysia, Pakistan, the Philippine Islands, Thailand and Vietnam. Native Hawaiian or other Pacific Islander- A person having origins in any of the original peoples of Hawaii, Guam, Samoa, or other Pacific Islands. Hispanic origin can be viewed as the heritage, nationality, lineage, or country of birth of the person or the person's parents or ancestors before arriving in the US

The foreign born population includes anyone who is not a U.S citizen at birth, including those who became U.S citizens through naturalization

API Asian Pacific Islander, *US* United States, *HBsAg* hepatitis B surface antigen

[a]We adapted from Jung et al. and assumed a 0.38% for 70+

[b]We took a weighted average of Tanaka et al.'s HBV screening cohort ages 40–74 which we calculated to be 1.02%

Table 2 Estimated HBsAg prevalence and estimated number of HBsAg-positive cases in the San Francisco Bay area

Age Group (Years)	Population[a] (2015)	HBsAg-positive cases (range)	HBsAg-prevalence (range)
0–19	2,202,500	2607 (1474–5577)	0.12% (0.07–0.25%)
20–29	1,254,437	11,106 (6113–18,053)	0.89% (0.49–1.44%)
30–39	1,311,988	24,436(16,842–33,961)	1.86% (1.28–2.59%)
40–49	1,230,512	25,627 (19,102–33,946)	2.08% (1.55–2.76%)
50–59	1,192,159	19,120 (14,218–25,231)	1.60% (1.19–2.12%)
60–69	898,217	12,940 (8709–19,866)	1.44% (0.97–2.21%)
70–79	473,888	6117 (3455–10,572)	1.29% (0.73–2.23%)
80+	310,260	2781 (1039–6393)	0.90% (0.34–2.06%)
Total	8,873,961	104,734 (70,952–153,598)	1.18% (0.80–1.73%)

[a]Total population year 2015, counties: San Francisco, Santa Clara, Alameda, San Mateo, Contra Costa, San Joaquin, Merced, Monterey, Stanislaus, Marin, Santa Cruz and San Benito
HBsAg hepatitis B surface antigen

a population of 39.1 million, the prevalence was estimated to be 0.78% (0.51–1.21%), with a total estimated case number as 305,419 (range 200,100–475,523).

County-, race/ethnicity-, and nativity-specific HBsAg prevalence and burden

Of the 15 counties analyzed, SF County had the highest HBsAg prevalence (1.78%), followed by Santa Clara (1.63%), Alameda (1.45%), San Mateo (1.40%) and Contra Costa (0.88%), as shown in Fig. 1. However, LA County (83,770), Santa Clara (31,273), Alameda (23,764) and Orange County (15,091) have high number of individuals with HBsAg due to its large population.

Figure 2 shows the population and HBsAg distribution in the SF Bay area (Fig. 2a), Santa Clara County (Fig. 2b), and San Benito County (Fig. 2c). As shown, the SF Bay area has a 24.5% API population, but accounts for 88.5% of all CHB cases. Santa Clara County has the highest API population (36%) and they account for 94% of the HBsAg-positive cases in the county. San Benito County has the highest Hispanic population (59%), and they account for 38% of the HBsAg-positive cases in the county. In contrast, although API constitutes only 4% of the population in San Benito, they account for 50% of the HBsAg cases in this county.

In the SF Bay area, the HBsAg prevalence in API is estimated to be 4.26%. Although API comprises of 24.5%

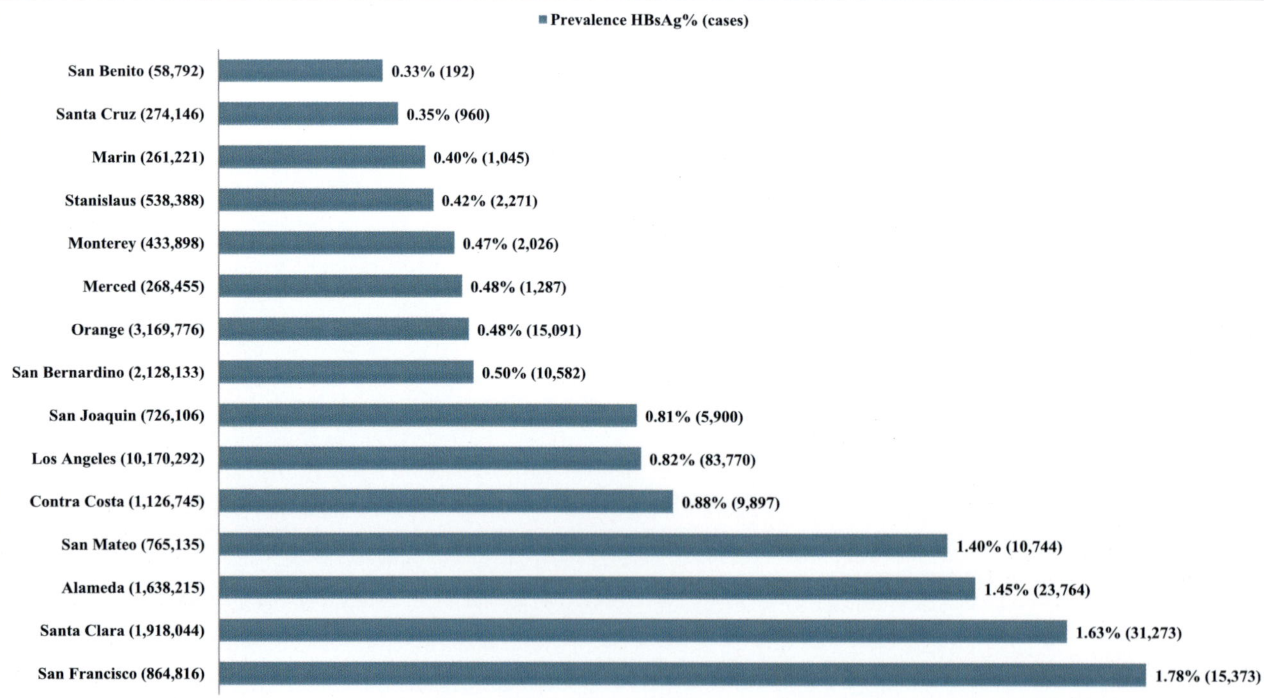

Fig. 1 HBsAg prevalence and number of chronic hepatitis B cases in 15 counties in the State of California

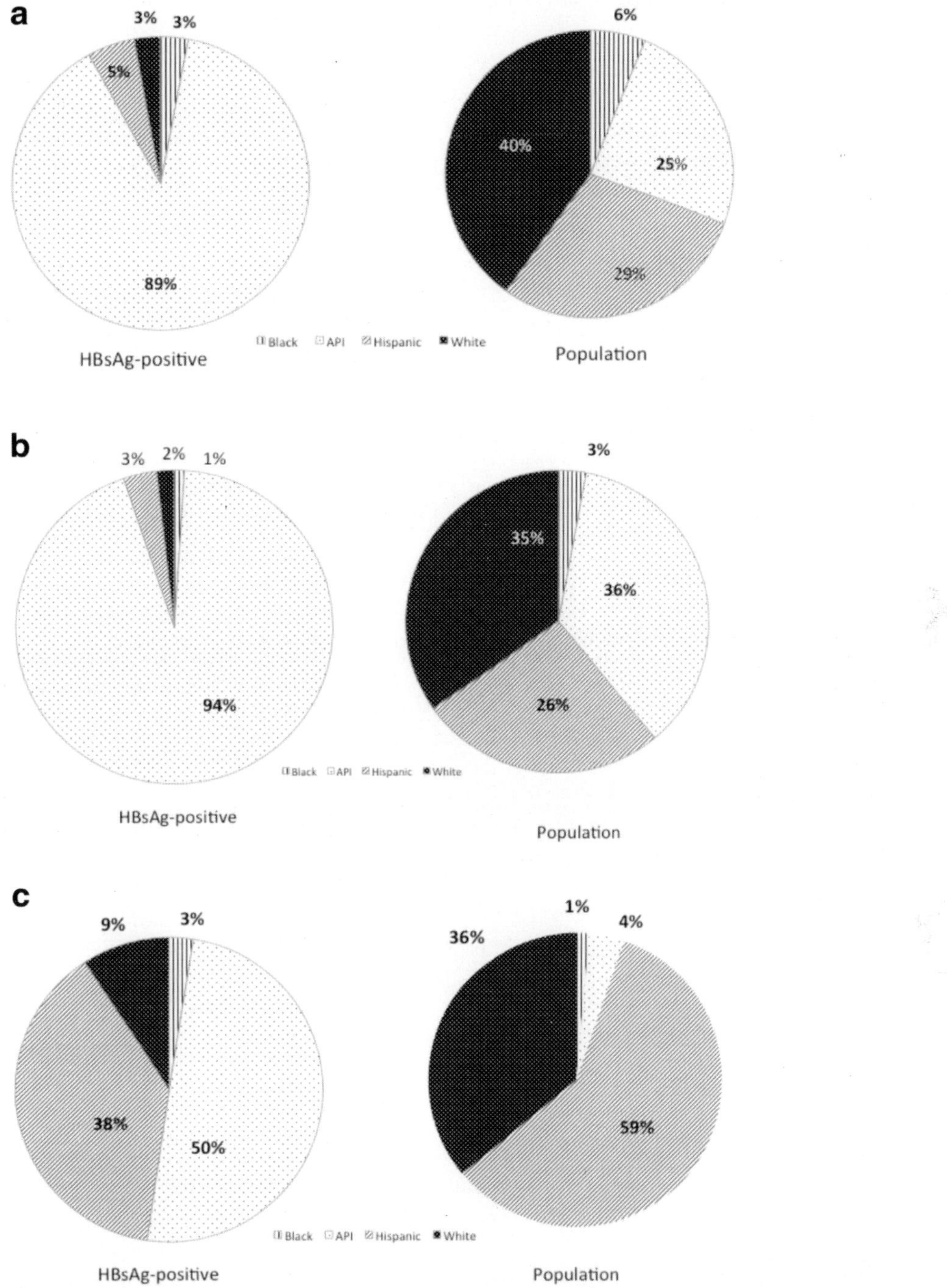

Fig. 2 Racial and ethnic distribution among HBsAg-positive and general population in the San Francisco Bay area (**a**), Santa Clara County (**b**), and San Benito County (**c**)

of the total population it accounts for 88.5% (92701) of the 104,734 HBsAg-positive cases. Of the HBsAg-positive cases among API cases, 4.93% were estimated to be US born and 84.0% foreign born (Table 3). Black cases (2886) made up 2.76% of total cases, with 0.39% being US born and 2.37% being foreign born.

Active disease burden

Table 4 shows the patient characteristics of the 2000 CHB patients in the Stanford and community clinic consortium from the SF Bay area (SFBAC). Of these, 55.8% were male, and the median age at diagnosis was 43. About 22% were positive for HBeAg, with 14% non-cirrhotic

Table 3 HBsAg-positive cases and its distribution by age, race/ethnicity and nativity within each age group in the total 104,734 estimated cases in the San Francisco Bay area

Age Group (Years)	API		Black		Hispanic	White	Total
	Foreign-Born	US-Born	Foreign-Born	US-Born			
0–19	889 (34.1%)	781 (30.0%)	435 (16.7%)	36 (1.38%)	204 (7.83%)	262 (10.0%)	2607
20–29	8059 (72.6%)	1497 (13.5%)	394 (3.55%)	69 (0.62%)	589 (5.30%)	498 (4.48%)	11,106
30–39	22,106 (90.5%)	777 (3.18%)	437 (1.79%)	73 (0.30%)	523 (2.14%)	520 (2.13%)	24,436
40–49	22,512 (87.8%)	540 (2.11%)	289 (1.13%)	68 (0.27%)	1724 (6.73%)	494 (1.93%)	25,627
50–59	16,399 (85.8%)	450 (2.35%)	386 (2.02%)	66 (0.35%)	1336 (6.99%)	483 (2.53%)	19,120
60–69	10,878 (84.1%)	377 (2.91%)	291 (2.25%)	50 (0.39%)	976 (7.54%)	368 (2.84%)	12,940
70–79	5077 (83.0%)	154 (2.52%)	151 (2.47%)	26 (0.43%)	515 (8.42%)	194 (3.17%)	6117
80+	2068 (74.4%)	137 (4.93%)	99 (3.56%)	17 (0.61%)	333 (12.0%)	127 (4.57%)	2781
Total	87,988 (84.0%)	4713 (4.50%)	2482 (2.37%)	405 (0.39%)	6200 (5.92%)	2946 (2.81%)	104,734 (100%)

active HBeAg-positive and 26% non-cirrhotic active HBeAg-negative. Approximately 9% of all cases had cirrhosis.

Applying clinical data from Table 4 to the SF Bay area CHB population, in Table 5, we show the estimated data on HBeAg, CHB activity, and cirrhosis. The number of active CHB cases, who are considered to be eligible for antiviral treatment by the AASLD guideline because they have significant viremia and evidence of on-going inflammation or hepatic fibrosis, included 14,3149 (12.6%) in the HBeAg-positive group, and 25,636 (24.5%) in the HBeAg-negative group, with 11,112 (10.6%) cirrhosis cases at baseline. In the LA area, a total of 51,952 people out of the 15.5 million population and 109,442 CHB cases are estimated to need antiviral treatment. When projected to the state of California as a whole, out of an estimated 305,419 CHB cases, 38,158 are active HBeAg-positive, 73,700 are active HBeAg-negative and 33,091 are cirrhotic. In total, an estimated 144,949 (47.5%) people with CHB in CA meet the AASLD criteria for treatment.

Table 4 Characteristics of the chronic hepatitis B patients from the hepatology and community gastroenterology and primary care clinics of the San Francisco Bay area consortium

Parameters	Results
Total number, N	2000
Male	1117 (55.8%)
Age	43 (18–88)
HBeAg-positive	444 (22.2%)
Active HBeAg-positive (non cirrhotic)*	272 (14%)
Active HBeAg-negative (non cirrhotic)*	510 (26%)
ALT (U/L)	39 (3–2809)
HBV DNA (log_{10} IU/mL)	4.0 (1.3–11.3)
Cirrhosis	185 (9%)

*Active is defined by an elevation of ALT > 2× upper limit of normal or evidence of significant histological disease plus elevated HBV DNA above 2000 IU/mL for HBeAg-negative, and above 20,000 IU/mL for HBeAg-positive [6]
HBeAg hepatitis B e antigen, *ALT* alanine aminotransferase

Discussion

This study confirms and quantifies the current burden of CHB in high endemic counties in the state of CA using population-level estimates combined with real-world clinical data including those from the community. We estimated the overall all race-combined HBsAg-prevalence of the SF Bay area, LA area, and the state of CA to be 1.18, 0.71 and 0.78%, respectively. The national US HBsAg prevalence estimated by NHANES is only 0.3% [11]. According to our estimates, SF Bay area prevalence surpasses the 0.3% by about 4-fold. The prevalence is highest in the SF (1.78%), Santa Clara (1.63%), and Alameda (1.45%) counties. However, the burden based number of patients is highest in the LA (83,770), Santa Clara (31,273) and Alameda (23,764) counties, due to the large population, especially APIs, in these counties. As expected, a significant portion of the burden is among the API population, with an estimated 4.26% HBsAg-prevalence. This rate is higher than the 3.1% reported by the NHANES 2015 study as the true prevalence of CHB infections for Asians [11], including both immigrants and naturalized citizens. Our estimate is comparable to the 3.8% prevalence reported by Levy et al. among men aged 18–35 years residing in low-income neighborhoods in Northern California [25]. Although the Centers for Disease Control and Prevention (CDC) estimates that Asians account for 50% of all CHB cases in the US [26], our study estimated that in CA, especially in the SF Bay area, APIs make up 88.5% of all the CHB cases. Particularly relevant is the high proportion of total CHB cases among the API foreign-born group that account for 84.0% of all the cases in the SF Bay area. It is estimated that the overall burden of CHB in the U.S. will continue to increase with ongoing immigration from countries with intermediate (2–8%) to high (> 8%) HBV prevalence [8]. For the foreign born population, we

Table 5 Prevalence of chronic hepatitis B in the San Francisco Bay area by age and disease status

Age Group (Years)	Population (2015)	Inactive[a] CHB	Active HBeAg positive	Active HBeAg negative	Cirrhosis
0–19	2,202,500	1805 (69.2%)	602 (23.1%)	201 (7.69%)	0
20–29	1,254,437	5360 (48.3%)	2744 (24.7%)	2701(24.3%)	300 (2.70%)
30–39	1,311,988	12,218 (50.0%)	4680 (19.2%)	6834 (28.0%)	704 (2.88%)
40–49	1,230,512	13,111 (51.2%)	2930 (11.4%)	7450 (29.1%)	2136 (8.33%)
50–59	1,192,159	9770 (51.1%)	1199 (6.27%)	5154 (27.0%)	2997 (15.7%)
60–69	898,217	7939 (61.4%)	438 (3.38%)	1813 (14.0%)	2751 (21.3%)
70–79	473,888	3186 (52.1%)	382 (6.25%)	1020 (16.7%)	1529 (25.0%)
80+	310,260	1448 (52.1%)	174 (6.25%)	463 (16.7%)	695 (25.0%)
Total	8,873,961	54,837 (52.4%)	13,149 (12.6%)	25,636 (24.5%)	11,112 (10.6%)

[a]Inactive CHB are those who are HBsAg positive with low HBV DNA or high HBV DNA but normal alanine aminotransferase or ALT levels
HBeAg hepatitis B e antigen

tried to use prevalence data from the US immigrant studies where available rather than the prevalence in their home country.

It is noteworthy that although currently both prevalence of HBV infection and incidence of hepatocellular carcinoma (HCC) due to HBV are high in the API population, data from SEER registries have shown a decline in HCC incidence among Asians, while rates in other racial/ethnic groups will continue to rise [27, 28]. In fact, in a national forecast study using SEER national data, by 2030, Hispanics will have the highest HCC in the country, while Asians will have the lowest HCC rates [28]. It is important to note that Hispanic is the largest racial/ethnic population in the state of California, accounting for 39% of the total CA population [29]. Relative to Asians, Hispanics tend to have lower CHB infection but higher HCV infection. Although our HBsAg-prevalence estimate of the Hispanic population in the SF Bay area is only 5% of the total, in counties that have large Hispanic populations such as San Benito and Merced, the Hispanic population makes up to 38% of all CHB cases. During the 2006–2010 period, among individuals aged 50–64 years, Hispanics experienced higher HCC incidence and mortality rates than Asians and Whites [30]. Few studies have investigated risk factors for HCC in Hispanics and the reasons for the rising trend in this ethnic group, although one study did show that HBV infection is one of the risk factors for HCC in Hispanic [30].

Although we analyzed 62% of the total population of California, it is unclear whether we can generalize the data from SF and LA reported here to the entire state of California, as SF and LA cover counties that are more densely populated and more diverse, and the remainder 43 counties in the state are quite different. However, our clinical data, including HBeAg status, among CHB patients from the university liver and community gastroenterology and primary care clinics were comparable to those reported by a North American multicenter study [31], suggesting some utility of generalizing our estimates to the state of CA. As there are many immigrants in California from the Middle East, which historically had a higher HBV prevalence than Western Europe or the European settlers of North America, the NHANES study we used to estimate the prevalence among whites does not differentiate among the white population which is likely a limitation in our study.

Given the high burden of CHB and HCC in the SF Bay area and California, targeted prevention and control efforts are needed to minimize the burden in these communities. A recent CDC-funded study showed that in cities with large populations of Asia- and Africa-born immigrants, community-based and refugee clinic-based HBV testing initiatives can identify substantial numbers of individuals with CHB [32], and stresses the fact that culturally and linguistically specific approaches were necessary in all phases of the initiatives. Our data and estimates can be used for resource allocation planning to target specific geographic areas and subpopulations, race/ethnicities for effective interventions, such as screening and linkage to care with appropriate therapies, to minimize the burden of CHB and its clinical consequences, such as liver cirrhosis, and liver cancer. These interventions are urgently needed as currently most of the CHB patients (70%) in the US are not aware of their HBV infection and there are also large gaps at various levels of the cascade of care for those with known CHB [5, 33–35]. Importantly, improved linkage to care can identify patients who may benefit from antiviral therapy which has been shown in both randomized control studies as well as large cohort studies in the US to substantially reduce HCC risk in CHB patients [36, 37].

Conclusion

In summary, our data suggest that there are approximately 305,000 persons living with CHB in the State of CA, and about half of these (47.5%, 150,000) have cirrhosis and/or meeting AASLD guideline criteria for antiviral therapy. We also found significant variation in the racial/ethnic make-up of the CHB population in different regions and counties of the State, highlighting the need for region/county-specific approach for public health efforts targeting CHB patients. Our methodology can be applied in other states or regions to estimate specific county, age, racial/ethnic prevalence and the overall and distribution active/advanced disease burden that would be crucial in the planning of local public health efforts in those areas.

Abbreviations
AASLD: American association for the study of liver disease; ALT: Alanine aminotransferase; API: Asian or pacific islander; CA: California; CDC: Centers for Disease Control and Prevention; CHB: Chronic hepatitis B; DNA: Deoxyribonucleic acid; HBsAg: Hepatitis B surface antigen; HCC: Hepatocellular carcinoma; LA: Los Angeles; NHANES: National Health and Nutrition Examination Survey; SF: San Francisco; SFBAC: San Francisco Bay Area Consortium; ULN: Upper limit of normal; US: United States

Funding
Funding for this study was provided by the Stanford Cancer Institute Award Program.

Authors' contributions
MT, MHN, SKS: Designed the study, analyzed the data, and wrote the manuscript. BW, TSV, AL, HT, JL, JZ, AWH: Gathered the data, analyzed the data, and wrote the manuscript. All authors read and approved the final manuscript.

Competing interests
Mehlika Toy, Bin Wei, Tejpal S Virdi, An Le, Jiayi Li, Jian Zhang, Ann W. Hsing, and Samuel K So have no disclosures.
Huy Trinh: Grant/research support: Gilead Sciences, Abbvie; Advisory board: Gilead Sciences; Speaker: Gilead Sciences.
Mindie H. Nguyen: Grant/research support: Bristol Myer Squibbs, Gilead Sciences, Janssen Pharmaceutical; Advisory board/consultant: Dynavax Laboratories, Gilead Sciences, Intercept Pharmaceutical, Anylam Pharmaceutical.

Author details
[1]Asian Liver Center, Department of Surgery, Stanford University School of Medicine, 780 Welch Road, CJ130D, Palo Alto, CA 94304, USA. [2]Division of Gastroenterology and Hepatology, Department of Medicine, Stanford University Medical Center, Palo Alto, CA, USA. [3]San Jose Gastroenterology, San Jose, CA, USA. [4]Palo Alto Medical Foundation, Mountain View, CA, USA. [5]Chinese Hospital, San Francisco, CA, USA. [6]Stanford Prevention Research Center, Department of Medicine and Stanford Cancer Institute, Stanford University School of Medicine, Palo Alto, CA, USA.

References
1. Stanaway JD, Flaxman AD, Naghavi M, Fitzmaurice C, Vos T, Abubakar I, Abu-Raddad LJ, Assadi R, Bhala N, Cowie B, et al. The global burden of viral hepatitis from 1990 to 2013: findings from the global burden of disease study 2013. Lancet. 2016;388(10049):1081–8.
2. Lin SY, Chang ET, So SK. Why we should routinely screen Asian American adults for hepatitis B: a cross-sectional study of Asians in California. Hepatology. 2007;46(4):1034–40.
3. Gish RG, Cooper SL. Hepatitis B in the greater San Francisco Bay Area: an integrated programme to respond to a diverse local epidemic. J Viral Hepat. 2011;18(4):e40–51.
4. Hu DJ, Xing J, Tohme RA, Liao Y, Pollack H, Ward JW, Holmberg SD. Hepatitis B testing and access to care among racial and ethnic minorities in selected communities across the United States, 2009-2010. Hepatology. 2013;58(3):856–62.
5. Kim LH, Nguyen VG, Trinh HN, Li J, Zhang JQ, Nguyen MH. Low treatment rates in patients meeting guideline criteria in diverse practice settings. Dig Dis Sci. 2014;59(9):2091–9.
6. Terrault NA, Bzowej NH, Chang KM, Hwang JP, Jonas MM, Murad MH, American Association for the Study of Liver D. AASLD guidelines for treatment of chronic hepatitis B. Hepatology. 2016;63(1):261–83.
7. CDC. Characteristics of persons with chronic hepatitis B: San Francisco, California, 2006. Morb Mortal Wkly Rep. 2007;56(18):446–8.
8. Kowdley KV, Wang CC, Welch S, Roberts H, Brosgart CL. Prevalence of chronic hepatitis B among foreign-born persons living in the United States by country of origin. Hepatology. 2012;56(2):422–33.
9. Services HaH. In: Services DoHaH, editor. Action plan for the prevention, care, & treatment of viral hepatitis. Washington, DC; 2017.
10. Chen CJ, Yang HI, Su J, Jen CL, You SL, Lu SN, Huang GT, Iloeje UH, Group R-HS. Risk of hepatocellular carcinoma across a biological gradient of serum hepatitis B virus DNA level. JAMA. 2006;295(1):65–73.
11. Roberts H, Kruszon-Moran D, Ly KN, Hughes E, Iqbal K, Jiles RB, Holmberg SD. Prevalence of chronic hepatitis B virus (HBV) infection in U.S. households: National Health and nutrition examination survey (NHANES), 1988-2012. Hepatology. 2016;63(2):388–97.
12. United States Census Bureau [http://www.census.gov/]. Accessed 15 Aug 2017.
13. Current Population Survey, Annual Social and Economic Supplement. 2013. https://www.census.gov/programs-surveys/saipe/guidance/model-input-data/cpsasec.html. Retrieved February 17, 2017.
14. Pewsocialtrends: A rising share of the US black population is foreign born [http://www.pewsocialtrends.org/2015/04/09/a-rising-share-of-the-u-s-black-population-is-foreign-born/]. Accessed 18 Aug 2017.
15. PewSocialTrends: The Rise of Asian Americans [http://www.pewsocialtrends.org/files/2013/04/Asian-Americans-new-full-report-04-2013.pdf]. Accessed 18 Aug 2017.
16. Total Asian alone or in any combination population 2015 American Community Survey 1-Year Estimates [https://factfinder.census.gov/faces/tableservices/jsf/pages/productview.xhtml?src=bkmk]. Accessed 21 Aug.
17. U.S. Census Bureau, P. D."Table 13. Projections of the Population by Nativity, Hispanic Origin, and Race for the United States: 2015 to 2060 (NP2014-T13)". 2014. Retrieved January 9, 2017. https://www.census.gov.
18. Jung M, Kuniholm MH, Ho GY, Cotler S, Strickler HD, Thyagarajan B, Youngblood M, Kaplan RC, Del Amo J. The distribution of hepatitis B virus exposure and infection in a population-based sample of U.S. Hispanic adults. Hepatology. 2016;63(2):445–52.
19. Din ES, Wasley A, Jacques-Carroll L, Sirotkin B, Wang S. Estimating the number of births to hepatitis B virus-infected women in 22 states, 2006. Pediatr Infect Dis J. 2011;30(7):575–9.
20. Ugwu C, Varkey P, Bagniewski S, Lesnick T. Sero-epidemiology of hepatitis B among new refugees to Minnesota. J Immigr Minor Health. 2008;10(5):469–74.
21. Tohme RA, Andre-Alboth J, Tejada-Strop A, Shi R, Boncy J, Francois J, Domercant JW, Griswold M, Hyppolite E, Adrien P, et al. Hepatitis B virus infection among pregnant women in Haiti: a cross-sectional serosurvey. J Clin Virol. 2016;76:66–71.
22. Hyun CS, Kim S, Kang SY, Jung S, Lee S. Chronic hepatitis B in Korean Americans: decreased prevalence and poor linkage to care. BMC Infect Dis. 2016;16(1):415.
23. Shuler CM, Fiore AE, Neeman R, Bell BP, Kuhnert W, Watkins S, Kilgour K, Arnold KE. Reduction in hepatitis B virus seroprevalence among U.S.-born children of foreign-born Asian parents – benefit of universal infant hepatitis B vaccination. Vaccine. 2009;27(43):5942–7.
24. Tanaka J, Koyama T, Mizui M, Uchida S, Katayama K, Matsuo J, Akita T, Nakashima A, Miyakawa Y, Yoshizawa H. Total numbers of undiagnosed carriers of hepatitis C and B viruses in Japan estimated by age- and area-specific prevalence on the national scale. Intervirology. 2011;54(4):185–95.

25. Levy V, Yuan J, Ruiz J, Morrow S, Reardon J, Facer M, Molitor F, Allen B, Ajufo BG, Bell-Sanford G, et al. Hepatitis B sero-prevalence and risk behaviors among immigrant men in a population-based household survey in low-income neighborhoods of northern California. J Immigr Minor Health. 2010;12(6):828–33.
26. Asian Americans and hepatitis B [https://www.cdc.gov/features/aapihepatitisb/]. Accessed 21 Aug
27. Ha J, Yan M, Aguilar M, Bhuket T, Tana MM, Liu B, Gish RG, Wong RJ. Race/ethnicity-specific disparities in cancer incidence, burden of disease, and overall survival among patients with hepatocellular carcinoma in the United States. Cancer. 2016;122(16):2512–23.
28. Petrick JL, Kelly SP, Altekruse SF, McGlynn KA, Rosenberg PS. Future of hepatocellular carcinoma incidence in the United States forecast through 2030. J Clin Oncol. 2016;34(15):1787–94.
29. In 2014, Latinos will surpass whites as racial/ethnic group in California [http://www.pewresearch.org/fact-tank/2014/01/24/in-2014-latinos-will-surpass-whites-as-largest-racialethnic-group-in-california/]. Accessed 21 Aug.
30. Setiawan VW, Wei PC, Hernandez BY, Lu SC, Monroe KR, Le Marchand L, Yuan JM. Disparity in liver cancer incidence and chronic liver disease mortality by nativity in Hispanics: the multiethnic cohort. Cancer. 2016; 122(9):1444–52.
31. Ghany MG, Perrillo R, Li R, Belle SH, Janssen HL, Terrault NA, Shuhart MC, Lau DT, Kim WR, Fried MW, et al. Characteristics of adults in the hepatitis B research network in North America reflect their country of origin and hepatitis B virus genotype. Clin Gastroenterol Hepatol. 2015;13(1):183–92.
32. Beckett GA, Ramirez G, Vanderhoff A, Nichols K, Chute SM, Wyles DL, Schoenbachler BT, Bedell DT, Cabral R, Ward JW, et al. Early identification and linkage to care of persons with chronic hepatitis B virus infection–three U.S. sites, 2012-2014. MMWR Morb Mortal Wkly Rep. 2014;63(18):399–401.
33. Liou IW, Nguyen MH. The cascade of care in chronic hepatits B. Curr Hepatol Rep. 2016;15:209–19.
34. McMahon BJ. Editorial commentary: sliding down the Cascade of Care for Chronic Hepatitis B Virus Infection. Clin Infect Dis. 2016;63(9):1209–11.
35. Spradling PR, Xing J, Rupp LB, Moorman AC, Gordon SC, Teshale ET, Lu M, Boscarino JA, Trinacty CM, Schmidt MA, et al. Infrequent clinical assessment of chronic hepatitis B patients in United States general healthcare settings. Clin Infect Dis. 2016;63(9):1205–8.
36. Liaw YF, Sung JJ, Chow WC, Farrell G, Lee CZ, Yuen H, Tanwandee T, Tao QM, Shue K, Keene ON, et al. Lamivudine for patients with chronic hepatitis B and advanced liver disease. N Engl J Med. 2004;351(15):1521–31.
37. Lin D, Yang HI, Nguyen N, Hoang J, Kim Y, Vu V, Le A, Chaung K, Nguyen V, Trinh H, et al. Reduction of chronic hepatitis B-related hepatocellular carcinoma with anti-viral therapy, including low risk patients. Aliment Pharmacol Ther. 2016;44(8):846–55.

25

Strategies for achieving viral hepatitis C micro-elimination

P. A. M. Kracht[1*], J. E. Arends[1], K. J. van Erpecum[2], A. Urbanus[3], J. A. Willemse[4], A. I. M. Hoepelman[1] and E. A. Croes[5]

Abstracts

The Netherlands is striving to achieve national elimination of the hepatitis C virus (HCV) as one of the first countries worldwide. The favorable HCV epidemiology with both low prevalence and incidence, together with access to care and treatment, present excellent conditions to further build on towards this objective. The Dutch national plan on viral hepatitis, introduced in 2016, defines targets in the HCV healthcare cascade and provides a structural framework for the development of elimination activities. Since many different stakeholders are involved in HCV care in the Netherlands, focus has been placed on micro-elimination initiatives as a pragmatic and efficient approach. These numerous micro-eliminations projects have brought the Netherlands closer to HCV elimination. In the near future, efforts specifically have to be made in order to optimize case-finding strategies and to successfully accomplish the nationwide implementation of the registration and monitoring system of viral hepatitis mono-infections, before this final goal can be reached. The upcoming years will then elucidate if the Dutch' hands on approach has resulted in sufficient progress against HCV and if the Netherlands will lead the way towards nationwide HCV elimination.

Keywords: Hepatitis C virus, Micro-elimination, Hep-CORE, HCV cascade of care

Background

Global elimination and eradication of the hepatitis C virus (HCV) has become the ultimate endeavor and final objective ever since the introduction of highly effective direct-acting antivirals (DAAs). The once fatal disease has thus been transformed into an infection that can effortlessly be cured, provided that one has access to care and therapy. Consequently, the World Health Organization (WHO) even envisioned universal elimination of the HCV to be accomplished by the year 2030 [1]. To this end, the WHO urged countries to develop and implement national policies on viral hepatitis. However, the European Liver Patients Association (ELPA) Hep-CORE study revealed that 14/27 countries still did not have a written national plan for the management of hepatitis C and / or hepatitis B (HBV) in 2016. The Netherlands therefore subsequently introduced a national plan on viral hepatitis in 2016 defining targets for each step in the Dutch HCV healthcare cascade: 1) awareness and prevention; 2) testing and diagnosis; 3) linkage to care; 4) access to medication and 5) monitoring and evaluation, in order to eventually achieve HCV elimination [2]. National coordination of HCV elimination however is complicated by (regional) differences in HCV patient subpopulations and the high number of stakeholders involved in HCV care. Considering these diversities, a uniform nationwide strategy targeting all HCV patients is unlikely to be the key solution to finally eliminate HCV. A more pragmatic approach would be to apply more focus and work towards 'micro-elimination' in different HCV subpopulations (e.g., individuals with HIV or hemophilia, (ever) injection drug users, migrants from high endemic countries, health care workers, prisoners). Micro-elimination, by way of targeting smaller and clearly delineated HCV risk groups, allows for faster and more efficient delivery of interventions. For this reason, micro-elimination as a 'bottom-up' approach may be a more feasible and efficient path to nationwide HCV elimination [3]. Various stakeholders involved in HCV

* Correspondence: p.a.m.kracht@umcutrecht.nl
[1]Department of Internal medicine and Infectious disease, Utrecht University, University Medical Center Utrecht, Utrecht, the Netherlands
Full list of author information is available at the end of the article

care have devoted their efforts to micro-elimination initiatives in the Netherlands, including: a) awareness campaigns directed at (ever) injection drug users and migrants but also health care workers; b) screening strategies in risk-groups to find undiagnosed persons with HCV, as recommended by the national Health Council [4]; c) regional and nationwide retrieval projects of lost to follow-up previously diagnosed patients; d) HCV healthcare pathways in addiction clinics and primary care to promote and guide linkage to care; e) registry and close monitoring of HCV subpopulations (registry of HIV/HCV coinfected managed by the Dutch HIV monitoring foundation and the hemophilia treatment center follows all HCV patients with hemophilia). However, the success of all (micro-) elimination efforts hinges on solid epidemiologic data on HCV prevalence and incidence in all HCV risk groups. Adequate registration and monitoring is an imperative element of HCV elimination and achieving this may be one of the most difficult obstacles to overcome in the elimination process.

This paper will describe (trends in) HCV epidemiology in the Netherlands, the micro-elimination progress in different HCV risk groups and also outline the strategies that have been employed by different stakeholders to improve uptake and retention in each step of the Dutch HCV healthcare cascade. Finally, we will elaborate on the Dutch progress towards nationwide HCV elimination and elucidate if the Netherlands may be among the first countries to achieve this final ambition in the near future.

Hepatitis C prevalence and incidence in the Netherlands

Although it is generally accepted that the Netherlands is a low prevalence region for HCV, only few studies have ever been performed to ascertain its prevalence in the general population. Two cross-sectional serosurveys in 1996 and 2007 calculated a national prevalence of 0.1% and 0.3%, respectively [5, 6]. Of note, groups from HCV endemic regions were considered underrepresented in the '96 survey and therefore a higher proportion (70%) of non-Dutch nationalities were included in the '07 survey. In 2012, Vriend et al. applied a different approach (i.e. the Workbook method) to estimate HCV prevalence in the Netherlands. The Workbook method incorporates lowest and highest available risk group based prevalence estimates which are subsequently multiplied by the different population sizes to generate an absolute number of HCV infected individuals per risk group. This study reported an estimated HCV seroprevalence of 0.22% which had been averaged from the lowest and highest total estimate of 0.07% and 0.37% respectively [7]. A recent update of this estimate, with more extensively defined prevalence estimates in different migrant populations, reported a 0.16% HCV seroprevalence in the Netherlands in 2017, which is still very similar to the older estimates from '96 and '07. This would correspond to 23,000 anti-HCV positive individuals in the Netherlands [8]. From a global perspective, it shows that the aforementioned HCV prevalence rate of 0.16% in the Netherlands is not only among the lowest in Western Europe but also one of the lowest worldwide [9–11]. Considering the HCV prevalence in distinct risk groups, the Dutch situation to some extent mimics the distribution in North America, Western Europe, and Australia, meaning that HCV infection is hyper endemic among people who (ever) inject(ed) drugs (PWID) (seroprevalence 39–74%) [12–16]. However, ongoing viral transmission of hepatitis C in the Dutch PWID group seems virtually non-existent: 44 cases of acute HCV were reported nationwide in 2016 of which < 5 were associated with intravenous drug use [17]. This is in line with the very low level of injecting among current drug users (estimated to be less than 1000 drug injectors in the whole country, with high access to clean injecting equipment). Nevertheless, underreporting due to an asymptomatic disease course cannot be ruled out. The low HCV incidence in PWID can also in part be explained by the decline in injection drug use (IDU) after the problematic 1960–1970's as a consequence of overall diminished popularity but also due to the availability of physician-prescribed methadone treatment, needle exchange and other harm reduction programs [18, 19]. In 2015, the national number of recent injecting drug users was historically low (±500 i.e. 6% of all opiate users in addiction care) [20]. In the Netherlands, the first generation migrants emerge quantitatively as the major contributor to the Dutch national HCV burden (41–70%) [6–8]. However, the number of new infections due to immigration is not considered to have great impact on the total pool of chronically infected since the annual Dutch population growth as a cause of immigration is < 0.5% at the time of writing [21]. Also, the HCV prevalence in migrant populations in different nations has been described to be lower in comparison to the country of origin prevalence estimates [22]. The Netherlands, next to having a low prevalence, is also characterized by a low incidence of HCV infections that are mainly observed in the subgroup of HIV-infected persons (49 acute HCV infections in HIV-infected in 2016, i.e. 5.5/1000 person years, 95% CI 4.1–7.2). It was recently reported that the Dutch incidence rate of acute HCV in this group has decreased considerably, which is illustrative of an effective "treatment as prevention" approach [23]. However, current re-infection rates in HIV-infected (34/1000 person years in 2016) are still high and predominantly related to the involvement of men who have sex with men (MSM) in high-risk sexual activities (including 'chemsex', i.e. sex under the influence of psychoactive drugs) [24].

Hepatitis C treatment effectiveness in different subpopulations

Various Dutch subpopulations with increased risk and/or prevalence of HCV can be identified as possible target groups for micro-elimination: the 'low risk population', migrants from high endemic countries, PWID, individuals with HIV, prisoners, MSM, patients with hemophilia, hemodialysis patients and health care workers (Table 1). As mentioned previously, to determine the success of HCV therapy uptake in subpopulations or otherwise assess the HCV micro-elimination progress, adequate patient monitoring systems are essential. In the Netherlands, several risk groups are closely monitored and (detailed) information on HCV therapy uptake is available in subpopulations such as HCV/HIV coinfected and HCV patients with an inherited bleeding disorder [24, 25]. With regard to the Dutch HIV population, annual screening for HCV infection is performed in those HIV positives in treatment with ongoing risk factors / behavior, irrespective of the presence of symptoms. Data from the Dutch HIV monitoring foundation (SHM), that includes 98% of all HIV-infected individuals who are retained in care, indicated that virtually all patients ($n = 1439$; 96.6%) had been screened at least once for HCV infection in 2017 [24]. Of note, the number of undiagnosed HIV/HCV coinfections is believed to be low (6% of the estimated 1750 undiagnosed Dutch HIV-infections) [24, 26]. Of those monitored HCV/HIV coinfected patients, 76% had been cured by February 2017 and from another 6% DAA therapy results were pending, totaling more than 80% clearance rate for this population [27]. Secondly, the van Creveldkliniek hemophilia treatment center (University Medical Center

Table 1 Hepatitis C micro-elimination progress in target populations in the Netherlands in 2017

	Population size (N)	HCV seroprevalence (%)	Total chronic HCV infections (HCV RNA (+)) (N)	HCV infections cured (N)/(%)	Source/Comments	Main actions/interventions to facilitate HCV elimination
HIV-infected	22,900	12%	1471 (R)	1124/76%	[24, 27]	• Behavioral counseling. • Once in a lifetime or frequent[c] screening (depending on risk behavior).
Hemophilia patients (born < 1992)	NA	NA	700 (R)	190/27.1%	[25] (Combined Dutch & UK cohort)	• Once in a lifetime screening. • Treatment scale-up.
High-risk MSM (HIV-negative)[b]	NA	4,8%	NA	NA/NA	[57]	• Behavioral counseling. • Frequent[c] screening • Early treatment in case of (re) infection.
Migrants from high endemic countries	1,527,032	NA	13,819 (E)	NA/NA	[58]	• Raise awareness of HCV through local/multimedia information campaigns. • Once in a lifetime screening for first-generation migrants with HCV prevalence ≥2% in country of origin.
PWID	14,000	39–74%	4040–7666 (C)	NA/NA	[7, 12–16, 59]	• Once in a lifetime or frequent[c] screening (depending on risk behavior). • Treatment scale up.
Prisoners	10,194/each day	7.4–13.9%	558–1049 (C)	NA/NA	[60–62]	• Educate prison doctors on HCV. • Once in a lifetime or frequent[c] screening (depending on risk behavior). • Include detainees in regular health insurance.
Hemodialysis patients	17,132	NA	NA	NA/NA	[63]	• Once in a lifetime screening.
Health care workers[d]	NA	NA	NA	NA/NA	–	• Once in a lifetime screening by employer.
General Dutch population	17,081,507[a]	0.1–0.4%	12,640–50,561 (C)	4427/8–35%	[7, 29]	• Raise awareness of HCV through multimedia information campaigns. • Educate general practitioners on HCV to increase compliance with viral hepatitis screening and referral guidelines. • Trace and treat HCV infected lost to follow-up.

PWID people who (have ever) inject(ed) drugs, *MSM* men who have sex with men, *NA* not available. (R) = reported numbers from publications of registries; (E) = estimated numbers reported in studies; (C) = calculated from seroprevalence estimates multiplied by .74 (assumed spontaneous clearance rate of 26%)

[a] https://opendata.cbs.nl/statline/#/CBS/nl, Dutch population numbers in 2017

[b] MSM with high-risk sexual activities

[c] One to four times per year

[d] Health care workers who perform hazardous tasks, putting them at risk for acquiring of transferring a hepatitis C infection (definition from the National Health Council) [4]

Utrecht, The Netherlands) reported that 27% of all 700 chronic HCV patients with an inherited bleeding disorder from a combined Dutch and UK cohort had been cured in April 2012 [25]. This proportion of cured patients, like in the HCV/HIV co-infected population, is expected to have increased dramatically since DAA-therapy became available.

Also, the transmission of HCV to hemophilia patients due contaminated blood products has been halted with the introduction of anti-HCV testing in blood donors and of recombinant clotting factors [28]. Finally, data obtained from the Drug Information System of the National Health Care Institute (GIP) illustrate that between the years 2009 until the availability of DAAs in 2015 an estimated 4427 persons with HCV have been cured in the Netherlands (i.e. 19% of the ±23,000 estimated HCV antibody positive individuals) [29]. With regard to the remaining HCV risk groups, exact data is lacking and no reliable estimate of DAA therapy uptake in these subpopulations could be made. A HCV prevalence estimate was available in a number of groups (Table 1).

Dutch hepatitis C healthcare cascade: Strategies towards micro-elimination

Awareness and prevention

A summary of the main Dutch strategies towards HCV elimination is depicted in Fig. 1. In the Netherlands, several institutions involved in public healthcare are dedicated to increasing awareness and knowledge of HCV in risk groups and as well as in the general population. To this end, a large nation-wide multimedia HCV awareness campaign was implemented in 2009/2010, targeting individuals attending methadone clinics and also risk groups in the general population. In participating methadone clinics HCV test uptake was 62% during the campaign. At the end of the project, 257 additional HCV-carriers had been identified in methadone clinic attendees and the intervention was judged to be cost-effective in this group. In contrast, the intervention was not cost-effective in the general population although the number of anti-HCV tests in 25 laboratories had increased by 12.9% in comparison with previous years [30]. At the annual Dutch National Hepatitis Day in November 2017, another compendious media campaign with both radio and television broadcasts was launched by the Dutch Liver Patient Association (NLV) to raise awareness among patients, physicians but also health policymakers for the increasing Dutch mortality rates as a cause of viral hepatitis [31]. This campaign has reached over ten million persons in the Netherlands (personal communication José Willemse, Executive director NLV).

Testing and diagnosis: Screening and retrieval projects

A key factor in achieving HCV elimination lies in augmenting the case finding rate. Case finding can be further classified as: i) the identification of undiagnosed HCV patients (i.e. screening) and ii) tracing of previously diagnosed patients who are no longer in clinical care (i.e. retrieval). Since migrants have been shown to account for the majority of HCV infections in the Netherlands, several large screening projects in migrant groups from high endemic countries (a.o. Afghanistan, China, Egypt, Iraq, Turkey, Poland) have been performed. The yield of these projects however was low, despite the use of peers in some projects, and only a handful of viremic HCV (1–10 persons per project, i.e. 0.1–4.8%) were identified of which also a small number was already aware of their disease [32–38]. These low results could be explained by a 'healthy volunteer' effect which indicates that the participants of screening projects are in fact healthier than the index population [39]. Further initiatives are therefore still needed to encourage more individuals with a migration background to get tested for HCV. This is also supported by the Dutch National Health Council (HC) who as of November 2016 recommends HCV screening in all first generation migrant populations with

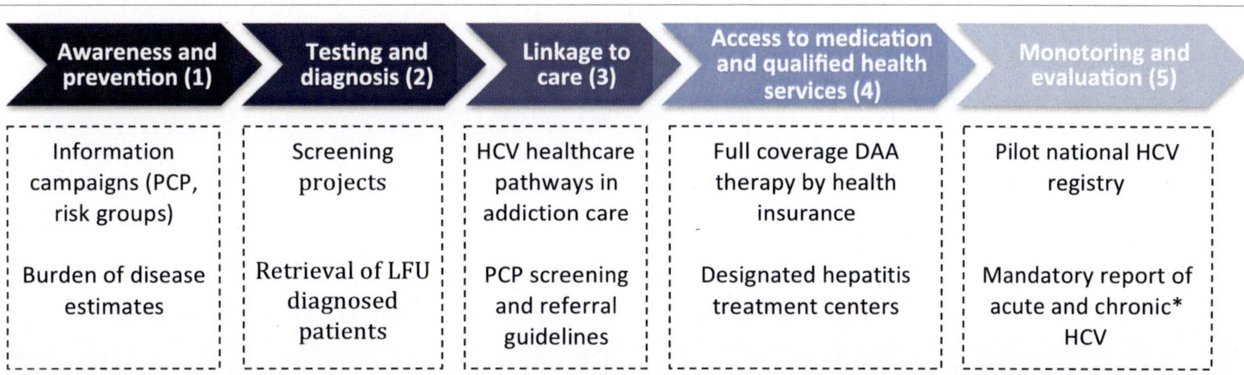

LFU, lost to follow-up; PCP, primary care physician. * implementation of mandatory report of chronic HCV is advised

Fig. 1 Dutch HCV care cascade

a known HCV prevalence in the country of origin of ≥2%. At the moment however, screening projects targeting migrant populations at locations other than primary care practices, require approval from the Ministry of Health, Welfare and Sport (VWS) [4]. This prerequisite poses a barrier for renewed screening efforts in migrant subgroups (last project dates from 2013) in the present DAA-era in which therapeutic options have improved immensely. Consequently, HCV screening in first generation migrants currently falls under the responsibility of Primary Care Physicians (PCPs) in the Netherlands who are guided by their evidence-based professional 'guideline on viral hepatitis' from the Dutch College of General Practitioners (NHG) [40]. The NHG guideline in addition promotes screening in individuals with an increased ALT (≥1.5 times the upper limit of normal) in the general population who may have been at risk for HCV infection. However, due to the small number of hepatitis patients in each PCP practice and the limited knowledge on hepatitis, screening of hepatitis in PCP practices is suboptimal. Another subgroup with high HCV prevalence (Table 1) deserving enhanced screening efforts is the detention population. Although the Dutch Custodial Institution Agency introduced updated guidelines on HCV screening in 2016, promoting HCV screening upon confinement for those who have been at risk, non-compliance with those guidelines occurs regularly and the frequent relocation of detainees further complicates treatment initiation and adherence. In addition, the Ministry of Justice finances the Dutch prison healthcare system and reimbursing DAA-therapy poses a heavy burden on its total health care budget. This constitutes another barrier for testing and treating HCV-infected detainees.

Next to screenings projects, several retrieval projects of diagnosed patients who have been lost to follow-up have been executed in various regions in the Netherlands. Projects were initiated by different physicians involved in care for hepatitis patients: hospital based specialists (Gastroenterology, Infectious Diseases and Microbiology), PCPs, but also Public Health physicians. The most commonly applied method in those retrieval projects was the reevaluation of positive HCV diagnostics from the past 10–15 years from microbiological laboratories in order to identify untreated patients. Patients with presumed persistent HCV would then be reevaluated by their PCP and, if appropriate, invited back into clinical care. The proportion of chronic HCV patients who were lost to follow-up was reported to be as high as 38% [41–43]. Results of the main (published) Dutch retrieval projects are summarized in Fig. 3. The largest retrieval effort in the center of the Netherlands (REACH-project) has been the most successful thus far with 28.3% of all lost to follow-up patients traced [44]. One of the success factors may be that, in contrast to other endeavors, in the REACH-project patients were invited directly at the outpatient clinic without interference of the general practitioner. The REACH-project served as a pilot and subsequent nationwide roll-out of HCV retrieval is scheduled to start in 2018 (CELINE). The CELINE initiative constitutes a collaboration between hepatologists and Infectious diseases physicians of all eight Dutch Academic Medical Centers (HepNED) and aims to realize case ascertainment in > 50% those who previously tested positive for HCV in the next 3 years and also to include 95% of retrieved patients in a national registry [45].

Linkage to care

The Dutch national plan on viral hepatitis underlined the importance of regional, multi-stakeholder, healthcare networks (i.e. hepatitis teams) in order to monitor and safeguard the local identification and linkage to care of HCV patients from all different risk group [2]. Such hepatitis teams have been installed successfully in various regions (Arnhem, Utrecht) and may serve as an example for other districts [32]. The "Breakthrough Project", initiated by the Netherlands Institute of Mental Health and Addiction (Trimbos Institute) is another example of a collaborative between various stakeholders. The Trimbos Institute aspired to structurally improve the detection and linkage to care of HCV in Dutch addiction care clinics and to develop sustainable HCV referral cascades. To this end, two implementation projects based on the Breakthrough methodology (Breakthrough Project) were initiated between 2013 and 2016. Multiple multidisciplinary teams, including Gastroenterology specialists from a (nearby) hepatitis treatment center and nurses, medical doctors and managers from the local addiction care center, created a local and sustainable HCV referral pathway to secure linkage to care. Final results of the project are pending.

Access to medication and qualified health services

In the Netherlands, virtually all patients have good access to healthcare and also, once diagnosed with HCV, to DAA therapy. As of November 2015, all available DAAs are reimbursed by basic health care insurance (which is obligatory in the Netherlands) irrespective of fibrosis stage, alcohol or drug use status. Basic healthcare insurance in the Netherlands however includes obligatory deductible excess, which added up to 385 euro per year in 2017 and 2018. This amount has to be paid by the policy holder before an insurance providers covers any expenses and may negatively affect one's willingness to get tested for HCV, especially in individuals with lower socio-economic status. On average, the obligatory deductible excess is fully spend by 50% of all insured individuals annually [46]. As described previously, the Ministry of Justice pays DAA therapy costs for individuals in detention. Asylum seekers can be considered for HCV treatment, but only when a residence permit is granted.

Although a wide variety of stakeholders is involved in the detection of and care for patients with a chronic HCV infection in the Netherlands (Fig. 2), until now treatment of HCV remains under the responsibility of hospital-based-physicians (specialists in hepatology or infectious diseases physicians working in designated hepatitis centers). There are 45 designated hepatitis centers in the Netherlands (Fig. 3) which can all be attended to on referral by the PCP. Physicians in all hepatitis treatment centers can consult the Dutch national "guidebook" on HCV treatment (www.HCVrichtsnoer.nl) that summarizes the recommendations of the main international guidelines on HCV treatment. The 'HCV richtsnoer' provides guidance for the appropriate DAA regimen selection with an update being published after each major international guideline revision [47].

Monitoring and evaluation

Adequate monitoring and registration of all patients in each step of the HCV healthcare cascade is essential to achieve HCV elimination. When drop out at any of the stages of the HCV healthcare cascade has been reduced to zero, elimination will have been achieved. By the Dutch public health act, in 1999 it became mandatory to report acute HCV infections to the local Public Health Services and hence incident infections are recorded since then. Until now, chronic HCV infections do not require notification but this is about to change in 2018. In addition, a pilot project was initiated in 2017 by the Dutch Association of Internal Medicine (NIV) and Gastroenterology and Hepatology (NVMDL) specialists with 8 participating hospitals aiming to create a registry for treatment uptake and outcome of all viral hepatitis B & C mono-infections. This project was able to benefit from the existing registration system of the HIV Monitoring Foundation (SHM) that has already been used to monitor both HIV-mono and HIV/hepatitis B or C co-infected patients for decades [48]. The previously mentioned national retrieval project CELINE aspires to further, both retrospectively and prospectively, complete this registry in the upcoming years.

The Dutch Central Bureau of Statistics (CBS) collects data on the primary cause of death in the general population and based on this information, the annual viral hepatitis C and B related mortality was estimated at +/–

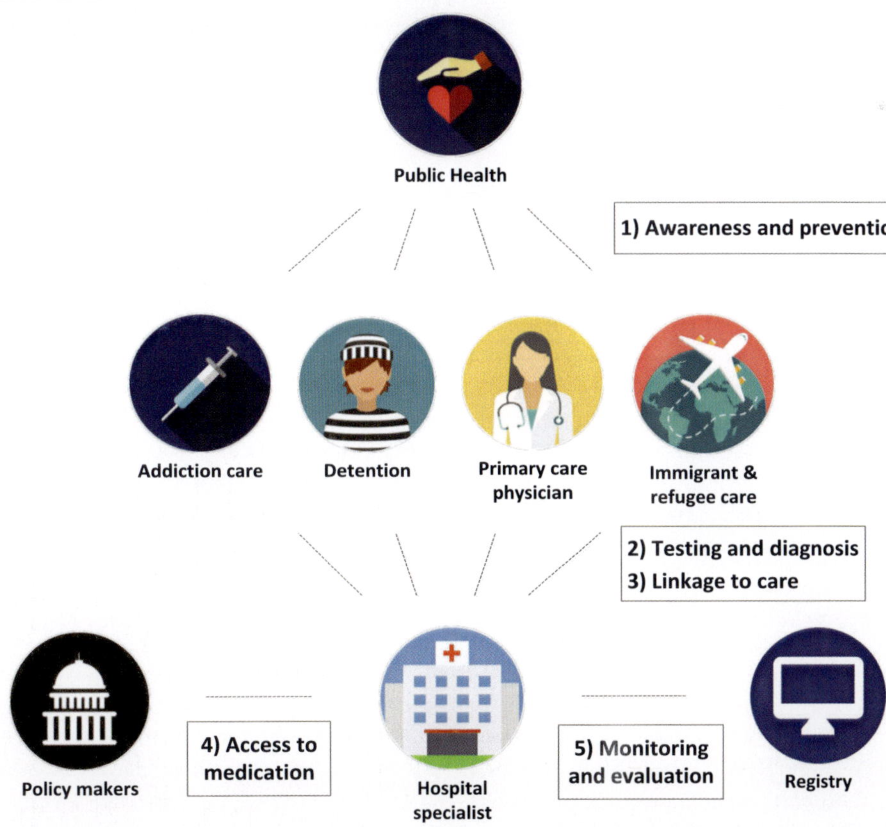

Fig. 2 Dutch HCV healthcare stakeholders

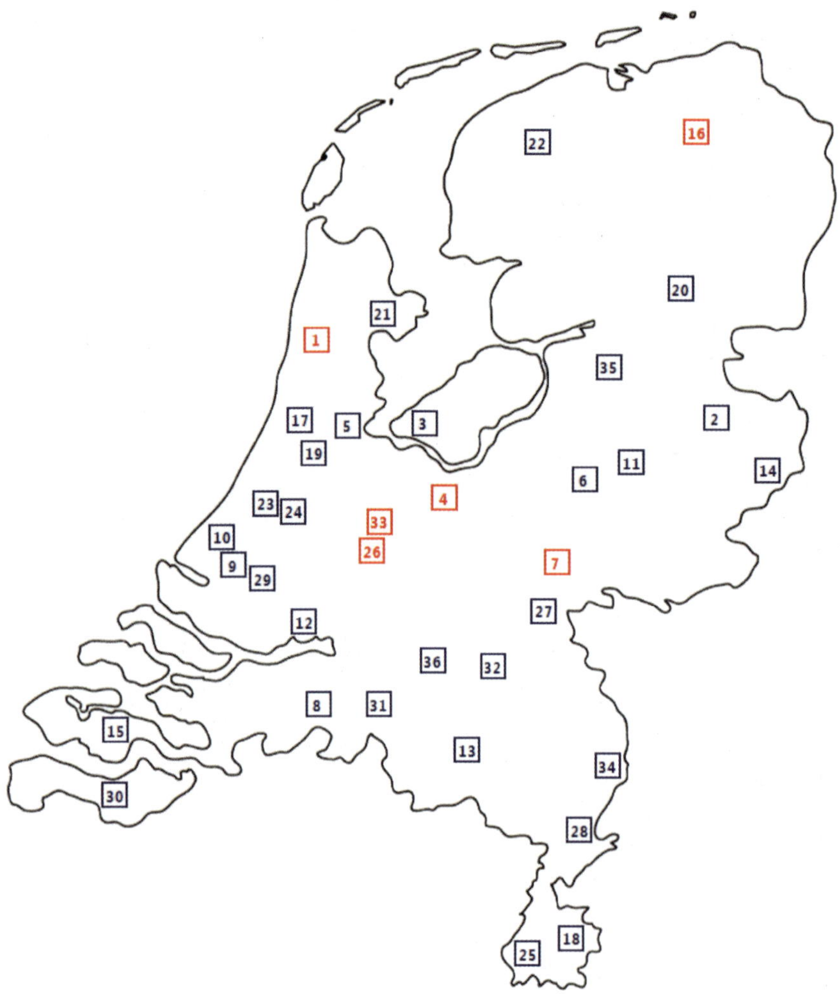

1. Alkmaar
2. Almelo
3. Almere
4. Amersfoort
5. Amsterdam (four hospitals)
6. Apeldoorn
7. Arnhem
8. Breda
9. Delft
10. Den Haag (two hospitals)
11. Deventer
12. Dordrecht
13. Eindhoven (two hospitals)
14. Enschede
15. Goes
16. Groningen
17. Haarlem
18. Heerlen
19. Hoofddorp
20. Hoogeveen
21. Hoorn
22. Leeuwarden
23. Leiden
24. Leiderdorp
25. Maastricht
26. Nieuwegein
27. Nijmegen (two hospitals)
28. Roermond
29. Rotterdam (three hospitals)
30. Terneuzen
31. Tilburg
32. Uden
33. Utrecht (two hospitals)
34. Venlo
35. Zwolle
36. 's-Hertogenbosch

Retrieval projects of previously diagnosed patients (in red)

	Region	**Years screened**	**Eligible for retrieval (N)**	**Evaluated (N)**
Beekmans et al. [41]	Alkmaar	15	20	4
Spruijt et al. [42]	Groningen	10	110	18
Wevers et al. [43]	Arnhem	15	1	0
Kracht et al. [44]	Utrecht / Nieuwegein / Amersfoort	15	269	47

Fig. 3 All 45 hepatitis treatment centers in the Netherlands [41–44]

500 deaths per year between 2002 and 2015 [31]. The viral hepatitis related mortality has not yet decreased as a consequence of the introduction of DAA-therapy. The van Creveldkliniek hemophilia treatment center reported a mortality rate of 28% in patients with hemophilia and chronic HCV of which 28% was liver-related (median follow-up of 31 years since HCV infection) [25]. These numbers however date from the pre-DAA era. The SHM registers the cause of death in HIV mono- and HIV/HCV coinfected however viral hepatitis related mortality in HIV/HCV coinfected individuals has not been explicitly described [24].

Future direction for hepatitis C (micro-) elimination in the Netherlands

The present Dutch situation with low HCV seroprevalence (0.1–0.4%) [7, 11] and a limited number of new infections [17, 23] is an excellent starting point for final HCV elimination. Some experts argue that the proportion of undiagnosed or 'hidden' HCV patients may actually be smaller than previously estimated as exemplified by a large high prevalence birth cohort screening project in the South of the Netherlands ($n = 3434$ patients) that did not identify any active HCV infections [49]. A study modelling the future HCV burden of disease in the Netherlands estimated an 85% reduction in chronic HCV infections by the year 2030, if treatment rate can be scaled up adequately [50]. In the past years, numerous Dutch micro-elimination projects have consequently put their efforts into enhancing the screening, linkage to care and finally the HCV treatment uptake in various risk group populations [27, 30, 32–35, 37, 38, 41–43]. Taking all endeavors into account, a drastic future reduction in the Dutch pool of chronic HCV-infected can be envisioned.

Important caveats however do remain in various stages of the Dutch HCV continuum of care which will have to be addressed before HCV micro-elimination can be achieved. First of all, the proportion of chronic HCV patients who has been lost to follow-up is substantial [41–43]. The nationwide roll out of the pilot project for retrieval but also registration of viral hepatitis C mono-infections (CELINE) therefore constitutes an important challenge to complete in the near future [45]. Secondly, as can be observed in the micro-elimination table, data on exact prevalence and therapy uptake is still unknown for many target groups (Table 1). The progress against HCV can thus not be tracked appropriately. When successfully executed, CELINE will substantially contribute to overcoming this issue by entering the data of > 95% of previously diagnosed HCV patients who have been retrieved in a central registry. Thirdly, despite the existence of various professional HCV screening guidelines, current screening strategies do not adequately target several high prevalence risk groups and a considerable group might still be unware of their disease. Specific improvements have to be made in the identification and linkage to care of HCV patients in addiction care centers, those originating from high endemic HCV countries immigrating to the Netherlands and also the general population as they constitute the major contributors to the Dutch HCV burden of disease (although overestimation of the HCV prevalence cannot be ruled out) [7]. Also, HIV-negative MSM who engage in high-risk sexual behavior (e.g. those receiving HIV Pre-Exposure Prophylaxis or PrEP) recently emerged as another subgroup with a relatively high HCV incidence (0.7–1.3 per 100 person-years) [51–53]. In the SHM HIV/HCV coinfected cohort, high DAA-therapy uptake of 76% has led to a decrease in HCV incident infections by half (from 11.2 to 5.5 per 1000 person-years) but a substantial (re-) infection rate remains [23]. Modeling studies describe that behavioral counseling in addition to treatment scale-up may be effective in further reducing the long-term HCV prevalence [54, 55].

With the current diminishing prevalence, the upcoming challenge will be to improve case finding strategies in order to accomplish higher treatment rates and to avoid a 'diagnostic burn-out' (i.e. the amount of treatments is reduced to zero because patients remain unware of their disease and therefore will not receive therapy) [56]. This diagnostic endeavor is preferably taken on by the PCPs as they encounter the majority of the Dutch population at risk for HCV in their practices. Since knowledge of HCV in Dutch PCPs is deemed insufficient, focus should shift towards educating PCPs about viral hepatitis C. With the current simplified DAA therapy regimens, treatment of patients with none to mild fibrosis may even be transferred to the PCPs in the future.

Conclusion

The current Dutch HCV epidemiology with both low prevalence and incidence in combination with universal access to DAA therapy, favors a future HCV elimination scenario. The micro-elimination method, that delivers targeted interventions at pre-defined HCV risk groups, is frequently applied to improve the Dutch HCV healthcare cascade and constitutes a pragmatic and efficient approach. To avoid an eventual diagnostic burn-out, efforts towards case-finding should be intensified. Although challenges remain, the Netherlands continues to be one of the global frontrunners in its efforts to national viral hepatitis C elimination. Whether this goal may actually be achieved by the year 2030, remains to be elucidated in the next couple of years.

Abbreviations

DAA: Direct-acting antiviral; ELPA: European liver patients association; GIP: Drug information system of the national health care institute; HCV: Hepatitis C virus; HIV: Human immunodeficiency virus; NHG: Dutch college of general practitioners; NIV: Dutch association of internal medicine; NVMDL: Dutch association of gastroenterology and hepatology; PCP: Primary care physicians; PWID: People who (ever) inject(ed) drugs; SHM: Dutch HIV monitoring foundation; WHO: World health organization

Funding

This research received no specific grant from any funding agency in the public, commercial or not-for-profit sectors.

Declarations

Publication charges for this article have been funded by MSD.

Authors' contributions

PK, JA and EC contributed to drafting the manuscript; KE, AU, JW and AH critically revised the manuscript for intellectual content. All authors read and approved the final to be submitted manuscript.

Competing interests

AH: advisory boards: Abbvie, BMS, Gilead, Janssen, MSD; consultancy: AbbVie; financial support for HCV retrieval project from Abbvie, BMS, Gilead and MSD; JA: advisory boards: Abbvie, BMS, Gilead, Janssen, MSD and ViiV; research grants: AbbVie, BMS; KvE: advisory boards: Abbvie, BMS, Gilead, Janssen-Cilag; Support for HCV patient care path from Abbvie, Gilead, Janssen-Cilag. The other authors declare that they have no competing interest.

Author details

[1]Department of Internal medicine and Infectious disease, Utrecht University, University Medical Center Utrecht, Utrecht, the Netherlands. [2]Department of Gastroenterology and Hepatology, Utrecht University, University Medical Center Utrecht, Utrecht, the Netherlands. [3]Centre for Infectious Disease Control, National Institute for Public Health and the Environment, Bilthoven, The Netherlands. [4]Dutch Liver Patient Association (NLV), Hoogland, the Netherlands. [5]Netherlands Institute of Mental Health and Addiction (Trimbos Institute), Utrecht, the Netherlands.

References

1. World Health Organization. Global health sector strategy on viral hepatitis 2016–2021. 2016. http://apps.who.int/iris/bitstream/handle/10665/246177/WHO-HIV-2016.06-eng.pdf;jsessionid=C9A6E8F12C8AFB281EAEDC0C2ABA6EE9?sequence=1. Accessed 2 Apr 2018.
2. Hogenbirk R, David S, van Steenbergen J, Urbanus A. Meer dan opsporen, Nationaal hepatitisplan: een strategie voor actie. 2016. http://www.rivm.nl/dsresource?objectid=119820d5-d1fe-440f-83cf-ffb7478f0282&type=pdf&disposition=inline. Accessed 2 Apr 2018.
3. Lazarus JV, Wiktor S, Colombo M, Thursz M. EASL international Liver Foundation. Micro-elimination – a path to global elimination of hepatitis C. J Hepatol. 2017;67(4):665–6.
4. Health Council of the Netherlands. Screening risk groups for hepatitis B and C. The Hague: Health Council of the Netherlands; 2016. https://www.gezondheidsraad.nl/documenten/adviezen/2016/11/01/screening-van-risicogroepen-op-hepatitis-b-en-c. Accessed 2 Apr 2018
5. Veldhuijzen IK, Conyn-van Spaendonck MAE, Dorigo-Zetsma JW. Seroprevalence of hepatitis B and C in the Dutch population. Infect Bull. 1999;10:182–4.
6. Vriend HJ, Op de Coul ELM, van de Laar TJW, Urbanus AT, van der Klis FRM, Boot HJ. Hepatitis C virus seroprevalence in the Netherlands. Eur J Pub Health. 2012;22(6):819–21.
7. Vriend HJ, Van Veen MG, Prins M, Urbanus AT, Boot HJ, Op De Coul ELM. Hepatitis C virus prevalence in the Netherlands: migrants account for most infections. Epidemiol Infect. 2013;141(6):1310–7.
8. Koopsen J, van Steenbergen J, Richardus JH, Prins M, Op De Coul ELM, Croes EA, et al. Chronic hepatitis B and C infections in the Netherlands: estimated prevalence in risk groups and the general population. J Hepatol. 2018;68:S156–7.
9. Blach S, Zeuzem S, Manns M, Altraif I, Duberg A-S, Muljono DH, et al. Global prevalence and genotype distribution of hepatitis C virus infection in 2015: a modelling study. Lancet Gastroenterol Hepatol. 2017;2(3):161–76.
10. Petruzziello A, Marigliano S, Loquercio G, Cacciapuoti C. Hepatitis C virus (HCV) genotypes distribution: an epidemiological up-date in Europe. Infect Agent Cancer. 2016;11(1):53.
11. European Union HCV Collaborators H, Robbins S, Zeuzem S, Negro F, Buti M, Duberg A-S, et al. Hepatitis C virus prevalence and level of intervention required to achieve the WHO targets for elimination in the European Union by 2030: a modelling study. Lancet Gastroenterol Hepatol. 2017;2(5):325–36.
12. Lindenburg CEA, Lambers FAE, Urbanus AT, Schinkel J, Jansen PLM, Krol A, et al. Hepatitis C testing and treatment among active drug users in Amsterdam: results from the DUTCH-C project. Eur J Gastroenterol Hepatol. 2011;23(1):23–31.
13. van den Hoek JA, van Haastrecht HJ, Goudsmit J, de Wolf F, Coutinho RA. Prevalence, incidence, and risk factors of hepatitis C virus infection among drug users in Amsterdam. J Infect Dis. 1990;162(4):823–6.
14. Rondy M, Wiessing L, Hutchinson SJ, Matheï C, Mathis F, Mravcik V, et al. Hepatitis C prevalence in injecting drug users in Europe, 1990–2007: impact of study recruitment setting. Epidemiol Infect. 2013;141(03):563–72.
15. van Santen DK, van der Helm JJ, Lindenburg K, van der Schim Loeff M, Prins M. HIV and hepatitis C treatment uptake among people who use drugs participating in the Amsterdam cohort studies, 1985–2015. Int J Drug Policy. 2017;47:95–101.
16. Schreuder I, van der Sande MA, de Wit M, Bongaerts M, Boucher CA, Croes EA, et al. Seroprevalence of HIV, hepatitis b, and hepatitis c among opioid drug users on methadone treatment in the Netherlands. Harm Reduct J. 2010;7(1):25.
17. Visser M, van Aar F, van Oeffelen A, van den Broek I, Op De Coul E, Hofstraat S, et al. Sexually transmitted infections including HIV, in the Netherlands in 2016. RIVM Rep 2017–0003. 2017. https://www.rivm.nl/dsresource?objectid=7b76e243-ca01-40d2-b50d-af67c2a0b83f&type=pdf&disposition=inline. Accessed 2 Apr 2018.
18. van de Laar TJW, Langendam MW, Bruisten SM, Welp EAE, Verhaest I, van Ameijden EJC, et al. Changes in risk behavior and dynamics of hepatitis C virus infections among young drug users in Amsterdam, the Netherlands. J Med Virol. 2005;77(4):509–18.
19. Van Den Berg C, Smit C, Van Brussel G, Coutinho R, Prins M, Amsterdam Cohort. Full participation in harm reduction programmes is associated with decreased risk for human immunodeficiency virus and hepatitis C virus: evidence from the Amsterdam cohort studies among drug users. Addiction. 2007;102(9):1454–62.
20. Wisselink DJ, Kuijpers WGT, Mol A. Kerncijfers Verslavingszorg 2015. Landelijk Alcohol en Drugs Informatie Systeem (LADIS). 2015. http://www.ggznederland.nl/uploads/assets/Werkdocument%20KC%202015%20.pdf KC 2015.pdf. Accessed 2018 Apr 2.
21. Central Bureau of Statistics Open data StatLine. Dutch population numbers in 2017. https://opendata.cbs.nl/statline/#/CBS/nl/dataset/37556/table?ts=1537815690008. Accessed 2 Apr 2018.
22. European Centre for Disease Prevention and Control. Epidemiological assessment of hepatitis B and C among migrants in the EU / EEA. 2016. https://ecdc.europa.eu/sites/portal/files/media/en/publications/Publications/epidemiological-assessment-hepatitis-B-and-C-among-migrants-EU-EEA.pdf. Accessed 2 Apr 2018.
23. Boerekamps A, Van den Berk GE, Fanny LN, Leyten EM, Van Kasteren ME, van Eeden A, et al. Declining HCV incidence in Dutch HIV positive men who have sex with men after unrestricted access to HCV therapy. Clin Infect Dis. 2018;66(9):1360–5.
24. van Sighem A, Boender S, Wit F, Smit C, Matser A, Reiss P. Monitoring report 2017. Human immunodeficiency virus (HIV) infection in the Netherlands. Stichting HIV Monitoring. 2017. https://www.hiv-monitoring.nl/files/1115/1117/7706/HIV_Monitoring_Report_2017.pdf. Accessed 2 Apr 2018.
25. van de Fransen Putte DE, Makris M, Fischer K, Yee TT, Kirk L, van Erpecum KJ, et al. Long-term follow-up of hepatitis C infection in a large cohort of patients with inherited bleeding disorders. J Hepatol. 2014;60(1):39–45.
26. van Sighem A, Nakagawa F, De Angelis D, Quinten C, Bezemer D, de Coul EO, et al. Estimating HIV incidence, time to diagnosis, and the undiagnosed HIV epidemic using routine surveillance data. Epidemiology. 2015;26(5):653–60.
27. Boerekamps A, Newsum AM, Smit C, Arends JE, Richter C, Reiss P, et al. High treatment uptake in HIV/HCV-coinfected patients after unrestricted access to direct-acting antivirals in the Netherlands. Clin Infect Dis. 2018;66(9):1352–9.
28. Mauser-Bunschoten EP, Bresters D, van Drimmelen AA, Roosendaal G, Cuypers HT, Reesink HW, et al. Hepatitis C infection and viremia in Dutch hemophilia patients. J Med Virol. 1995;45(3):241–6.
29. Hofman R, Schalm SW, Richardus J. How many hepatitis B and C patients have been treated in the Netherlands? [article in Dutch]. LEVER. 2017;2:11–2.
30. Helsper CW, Janssen MP, van Essen GA, Croes EA, van der Veen C, de Wit AG, et al. Effectiveness and cost-effectiveness of nationwide campaigns for awareness and case finding of hepatitis C targeted at people who inject

drugs and the general population in the Netherlands. Int J Drug Policy. 2017;47:117–25.

31. Hofman R, Nusselder WJ, Veldhuijzen IK, Richardus JH. Mortality due to chronic viral hepatitis B and C infections in the Netherlands. Ned Tijdschr Geneeskd. 2016;160(0):D511.
32. Richter C, Ter Beest G, Gisolf EH, Van Bentum P, Waegemaekers C, Swanink C, et al. Screening for chronic hepatitis B and C in migrants from Afghanistan, Iran, Iraq, the former soviet republics, and Vietnam in the Arnhem region, the Netherlands. Epidemiol Infect. 2014;142(10):2140–6.
33. Van Diemen AJ, Van Heerwaarden A, Schout C, Medisch U, Utrecht C. Onderzoek in het kort China onder de Dom Hepatitis B- en C-screening bij Chinese migranten in Utrecht. Infect Bull. 2011;1:19–21.
34. Grintjes K, MANP ASM, Dofferhoff F, Stelma RPM, Koene R, van Crevel M, Van den Muijsenbergh PPK. Hepatitis C-opsporing onder migranten in Nijmegen (HECOM). 2014;9(5):126–33.
35. Zuure FR, Bouman J, Martens M, Vanhommerig JW, Urbanus AT, Davidovich U, et al. Screening for hepatitis B and C in first-generation Egyptian migrants living in the Netherlands. Liver Int. 2013;33(5):727–38.
36. Urbanus AT, Steenbergen van JE. Hepatitis B-virus en hepatitis C-virus screeningsprojecten voor migranten in Nederland : stand van zaken 2014. Tijdschr voor Infect. 2015;10(2):31–6.
37. Hepatitis Info. http://www.hepatitisinfo.nl/projecten/screening/DU2558_Screening-en-bewustzijnsbevordering-hepatitis-B-en-hepatitis-C-bij-Chinezen-in-Nederland-2009-2013.aspx. Accessed 2 Apr 2018.
38. Richter C, Ter BG, Sancak I, Aydinly R, Bulbul K, Laetemia-Tomata F, et al. Hepatitis B prevalence in the Turkish population of Arnhem: implications for national screening policy? Epidemiol Infect. 2012;140(4):724–30.
39. Froom P, Melamed S, Kristal-Boneh E, Benbassat J, Ribak J. Healthy volunteer effect in industrial workers. J Clin Epidemiol. 1999;52(8):731–5.
40. Numans ME, Perquin MJ, van Putten AM, Richter C, Vrolijk JM, Bouma M. MS. Virushepatitis en andere leveraandoeningen, derde herziening. [Dutch College of General Practitioners Guideline "viral hepatitis and other liver conditions," third revision]. Huisarts Wet. 2016;3:108–19.
41. Beekmans N, Klemt-Kropp M. Re-evaluation of chronic hepatitis B and hepatitis C patients lost to follow-up: results of the northern Holland hepatitis retrieval project. Hepatol Med Policy. 2018;3(1):5.
42. Spruijt AG, Wilting KR, Mithoe GD, Niessen WJM. Tracing patients with chronic viral hepatitis. Ned Tijdschr Geneeskd. 2016;160(0):D414.
43. Wevers K, Puts G, Waegemaekers C, Hautvast J, Tostmann A. Detection and evaluation of chronic hepatitis B and C patients who were lost to medical follow up. Eur J Pub Health. 2017;27(Suppl 3):261.
44. Kracht PAM, Arends JE, van Erpecum KJ, Thijsen SFT, Vlaminckx BJM, Weersink AJL, et al. REtrieval and cure of chronic hepatitis C (REACH): results of micro-elimination in the Utrecht province. Liver Int. 2018. https://doi.org/10.1111/liv.13959.
45. Drenth JPH, et al. Nationale registratie van hepatitis B en C http://regist2.virology-education.com/Presentations/2017/NHD2017/11_Drenth.pdf. Accessed 2 Apr 2018.
46. Zorgthermometer: Verzekerden in beeld 2017 [report in Dutch]. Zeist; 2017. https://www.vektis.nl/uploads/Publicaties/Zorgthermometer/Verzekerden in beeld 2017.pdf. Accessed 2 Apr 2018.
47. HCV richtsnoer. http://www.hcvrichtsnoer.nl/. Accessed 2 Apr 2018.
48. van Sighem A, Smit C, Holman R, Gras L, Stolte I, Bezemer D, et al. Monitoring report 2012. Human immunodeficiency virus (HIV) infection in the Netherlands. Stichting HIV Monitoring. 2012; https://www.hiv-monitoring.nl/files/1013/5365/4371/HIV_MReport2012_web.pdf. Accessed 2 Apr 2018.
49. Heil J, Hoebe CJPA, Cals JWL, ter Waarbeek HLG, van Loo IHM, Dukers-Muijrers NHTM. Detecting hepatitis B and C by combined public health and primary care birth cohort testing. Ann Fam Med. 2018;16(1):21–7.
50. Willemse SB, Razavi-Shearer D, Zuure FR, Veldhuijzen IK, Croes EA, van der Meer AJ, et al. The estimated future disease burden of hepatitis C virus in the Netherlands with different treatment paradigms. Neth J Med. 2015;73(9):417–31.
51. Volk JE, Marcus JL, Phengrasamy T, Hare CB. Incident hepatitis C virus infections among users of HIV Preexposure prophylaxis in a clinical practice setting. Clin Infect Dis. 2015;60(11):1728–9.
52. Molina J-M, Capitant C, Spire B, Pialoux G, Cotte L, Charreau I, et al. On-demand preexposure prophylaxis in men at high risk for HIV-1 infection. N Engl J Med. 2015;373(23):2237–46.
53. McCormack S, Dunn DT, Desai M, Dolling DI, Gafos M, Gilson R, et al. Pre-exposure prophylaxis to prevent the acquisition of HIV-1 infection (PROUD): effectiveness results from the pilot phase of a pragmatic open-label randomised trial. Lancet (London, England). 2016;387(10013):53–60.
54. Salazar-Vizcaya L, Kouyos RD, Fehr J, Braun D, Estill J, Bernasconi E, et al. On the potential of a short-term intensive intervention to interrupt HCV transmission in HIV-positive men who have sex with men: a mathematical modelling study. J Viral Hepat. 2018;25(1):10–8.
55. Martin NK, Thornton A, Hickman M, Sabin C, Nelson M, Cooke GS, et al. Can hepatitis C virus (HCV) direct-acting antiviral treatment as prevention reverse the HCV epidemic among men who have sex with men in the United Kingdom? Epidemiological and modeling insights. Clin Infect Dis. 2016;62(9):1072–80.
56. Hill AM, Khan A, Nath S, Simmons B. "Diagnostic Burn-out" for Hepatitis C: when will countries run out of diagnosed people to treat with DAAs? Hepatology. 2017;66(Supplement 1):522A.
57. Hoornenborg E, Achterbergh RCA, Schim van der Loeff MF, Davidovich U, Hogewoning A, de Vries HJC, et al. MSM starting preexposure prophylaxis are at risk of hepatitis C virus infection. Clin Infect Dis. 2017;31(11):1603–10.
58. Koopsen J, van Steenbergen J, Richardus JH, Prins M, Op De Coul ELM, Croes EA, et al. Chronic hepatitis B and C in the Netherlands: prevalence in high-risk groups and the general population (submitted). 2018.
59. van de Laar MW, van Ooyen-Houben MMJ, Cruts AAN, Meijer RF, Croes EA, Ketelaars PM, van der P PM. Netherlands National Drug Monitor: NDM Annual Report 2016. Utrecht / Den Haag: Trimbos Instituut / Den Haag: WODC. 2016. https://assets.trimbos.nl/docs/3fdeab39-f34e-4aa0-97af-5dbf111c05a0.pdf. Accessed 2 April 2018.
60. Custodial Institutions Agency Ministry of Health. This is the Custodial Institutions Agency (DJI). 2017. https://www.dji.nl/binaries/LR_103353_ditisDJI_EN_tcm41-121757.pdf. Accessed 2 April 2018.
61. Leemrijse CJ, Bongers M, Nielen M, Devillé W. Hepatits C in penitentiary: a prevalence study [report in Dutch]. Nivel. 2010. https://www.nivel.nl/sites/default/files/bestanden/Rapport-hepatitis-C-penitentiaire-inrichtingen.pdf. Accessed 2 April 2018.
62. Schreuder I, Van der Sande M, Osterhaus A, Boucher C, Pinxt J, Hoebe C, et al. Prevalence of HIV, hepatitis B and C in institutionalized men in Sittard [report in Dutch]. 2010. RIVM Rapport 210502001. https://www.rivm.nl/dsresource?objectid=5aed8fcd-1b2b-44bf-b610-8d80b21c2e18&type=org&disposition=inline. Accessed 2 April 2018.
63. Nefrovisie. Renine (Dutch registry of dialysis treatments for kidney patients). 2016. https://www.nefrovisie.nl/wpcontent/uploads/2018/03/RENINE-year-report2016-web.pdf. Accessed 2 April 2018.

"B in IT" - a community-based model for the management of hepatitis B patients in primary care clinics using a novel web-based clinical tool

Debra A. O'Leary[1*], Eleanor Cropp[1], David Isaac[2,3], Paul V. Desmond[1], Sally Bell[1], Tin Nguyen[1], Darren Wong[1], Jessica Howell[1], Jacqui Richmond[4,5,6], Jenny O'Neill[7] and Alexander J. Thompson[1]

Abstract

Background: The current model of care for the treatment of chronic hepatitis B (CHB) in Australia is through specialist Hepatology or Infectious Diseases clinics, and limited accredited primary care practices. Capacity is limited, and less than 5% of Australians living with CHB currently access therapy. Increasing treatment uptake is an urgent area of clinical need. Nucleos(t)ide analogue therapy is safe and effective treatment for CHB that is suitable for community prescribing. We have evaluated the success of a community-based model for the management of CHB in primary care clinics using a novel web-based clinical tool.

Methods: Using guidelines set out by the Gastroenterological Society of Australia, we developed an interactive online clinical management tool for the shared care of patients with CHB in primary care clinics, with remote oversight from tertiary hospital-based hepatologists and a project officer. We call this model of care the "B in IT" program. Suitable patients were referred from the specialist liver clinic back to primary care for ongoing management. Compliance with recommended appointments, pathology tests and ultrasounds of patients enrolled in "B in IT" was assessed and compared to that of the same patients prior to community discharge, as well as a matched control group of CHB outpatients continuing to attend a specialist clinic.

Results: Thirty patients with CHB were enrolled in the "B in IT" program. Compliance with attending scheduled appointments within 1 month of the suggested date was 87% across all 115 visits scheduled. Compliance with completing recommended pathology within 1 month of the suggested date was 94% and compliance with completing recommended liver ultrasounds for cancer screening within 1 month of the suggested date was 89%. The compliance rates for visit attendance and ultrasound completion were significantly higher than the control patient group ($p < 0.0001$) and the "B in IT" patients prior to community discharge ($p = 0.002$ and $p = 0.039$, respectively).

Conclusions: The "B in IT" program's novel web-based clinical tool supports primary care physicians to treat and monitor patients with CHB. This program promotes community-based care and increases system capacity for the clinical care of people living with CHB.

Keywords: Chronic hepatitis B, Shared care, Hepatologists, Specialists, General practitioners, Primary care, B in IT, Compliance, Liver cancer, HCC screening

* Correspondence: oleary.debra@gmail.com
[1]Gastroenterology Department, St Vincent's Hospital Melbourne, 35 Victoria Parade, Fitzroy, VIC 3065, Australia
Full list of author information is available at the end of the article

Background

Approximately 1 % of Australians are living with chronic hepatitis B (CHB) [1]. If left untreated, hepatitis B-related cirrhosis, liver failure and hepatocellular carcinoma (HCC) result in mortality of up to 25% for people living with CHB [2–4]. In Australia, the second National Hepatitis B Strategy (2014-2017) set targets for diagnosis and care of people living with CHB, including increasing diagnosis rates of CHB to 80%, and increasing the proportion of patients receiving antiviral treatment to 15% (currently < 5%) [5]. The National Strategy highlights the need for primary care to play a central role in CHB monitoring and calls for the development of models of care to increase the involvement of general practitioners (GPs).

The recommended clinical management for the majority of people living with CHB is now protocol-based [6]. The introduction of safe and effective antiviral therapies for CHB, as well as simple clinical protocols for virological monitoring and HCC screening, makes shared care between specialist liver clinics and primary care physicians attractive, with community-based treatment possible for the majority of people with CHB. As of 1 July 2015 antiviral medications for CHB can be dispensed by community pharmacies in Australia, however there remain a limited number of GPs who are accredited prescribers. Shared care arrangements can help overcome this hurdle by promoting management in the primary care setting with clinical oversight and support provided by the specialist. This model will increase system capacity in both primary and tertiary care settings. Another potential advantage of community-based shared care of CHB is the convenience for patients in seeing their GP for review appointments, rather than needing to visit a hospital outpatient clinic. This may improve adherence of stable patients with six monthly blood tests ± liver ultrasounds for cancer screening recommended by the Gastroenterological Society of Australia (GESA) [6].

Published data describing the implementation of community-based shared care models for the treatment and monitoring of patients living with CHB in Australia are lacking. Here we describe the design and implementation of the "B in IT" program, a community-based model for the management of people living with CHB in primary care clinics using a novel web-based clinical tool overseen remotely by a project officer and specialists in tertiary hospitals.

Methods

"B in IT" program

The "B in IT" model of care is outlined in Fig. 1. For new patients, following a standard GP referral to a specialist liver clinic, the patient's CHB phase of disease is established over several consultations and the need for oral antiviral therapy ± HCC screening is determined. As outlined in the GESA algorithm for CHB management [6], there are four recognized phases of disease for CHB. Phases 1 and 3 are monitored by twice yearly serum alanine transaminase (ALT) testing and annual hepatitis B deoxyribonucleic acid (HBV DNA) testing, whereas patients with CHB phases 2 or 4 (characterized by elevated and/or fluctuating ALT and viral load) have these blood tests every 3 – 6 months while receiving antiviral therapy. Patients in any phase of disease who are at high risk of HCC (including Asian males > 40 years of age, Asian females > 50 years of age, those with cirrhosis or a family history of HCC) are also monitored via twice yearly liver ultrasound. Patients with cirrhosis or HCC, patients planned for interferon treatment, patients with a history of antiviral drug resistance, or people with complex medical co-morbidities, are not eligible for the "B in IT" program, and must remain in the care of the specialist liver clinic. All other patients with CHB attending the specialist liver clinic are eligible for the "B in IT" program and can elect to have ongoing care provided by their participating GP. Documented antiviral response is necessary prior to discharge of phase 2 and 4 patients.

EpiSoft cloud-based software was selected for the "B in IT" program because it enables GPs to monitor and treat CHB patients in the community, while still allowing for continued oversight by hepatologists and clinical nurse consultants, as part of a team care arrangement. The "B in IT" treatment protocol outlines when appointments, tests and prescriptions are due, with recall and reminder systems in the event of missed appointments. The system also includes "alarm bell" triggers for specialist review to inform GPs when a patient should be referred back to the specialist liver clinic. For patients being monitored in phase 1 or 3 of disease these triggers are an increase in ALT > 1.5 times the upper limit of normal, an increase in hepatitis B viral load > 2000 IU/ml (phase 3), an increase in fibroscan score > 2.5 kPa (or > 10 kPa score), or a new focal liver lesion detected via ultrasound. For patients being treated with oral nucleos(t)ide analogue therapy in phase 2 or 4 of disease the "alarm bell" triggers are an increase in hepatitis B viral load >10-fold (or from undetectable to detectable), an increase in serum creatinine or decrease in serum phosphate levels (in the case of tenofovir disoproxil fumarate therapy), a decrease in renal function, an increase in fibroscan score > 2.5 kPa (or > 10 kPa score), or a new focal liver lesion detected via ultrasound.

EpiSoft

Using guideline recommendations for the treatment and monitoring of CHB [6], custom "B in IT" treatment protocols of 12 month duration were developed within the

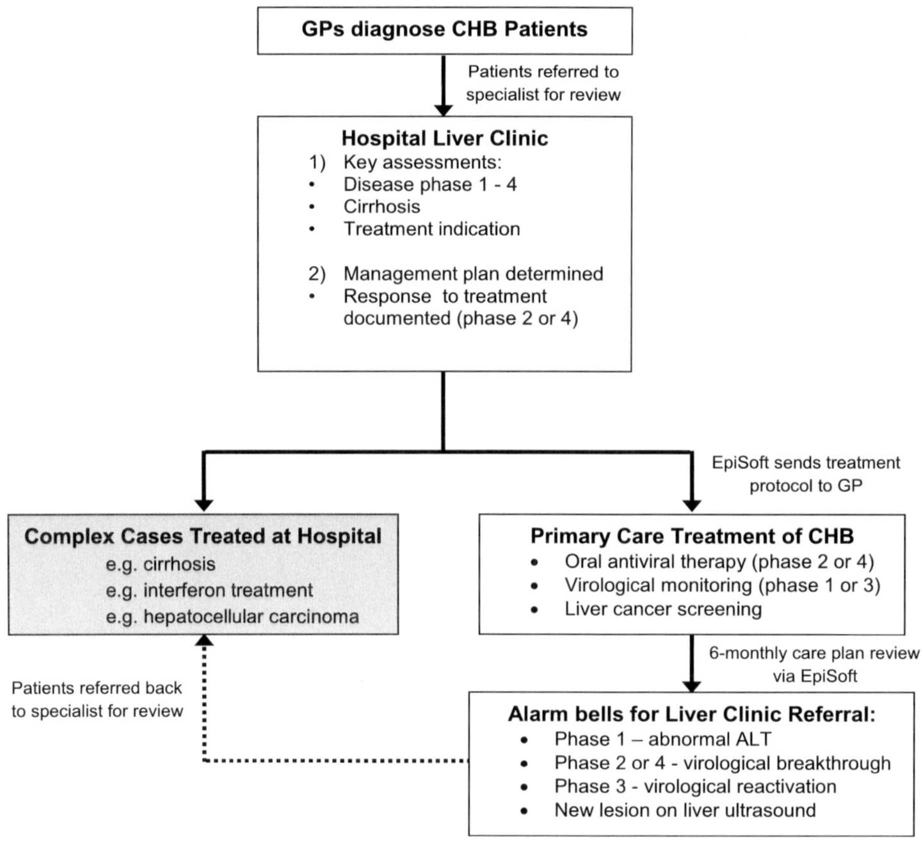

Fig. 1 The "B in IT" model of care. Following routine diagnosis at a community GP clinic and referral to the hospital liver clinic for assessment, patients with CHB suitable for discharge back to their GP were identified. For patients who chose to be monitored by their GP, compliance with recommended tests and review appointments was monitored remotely by hospital staff via the EpiSoft web-based clinical guide. Alarm bell messages built into each electronic treatment protocol were used to identify progression of disease and signal if and when a GP should refer the patient back to the hospital liver clinic

EpiSoft database framework to incorporate monitoring with or without twice yearly abdominal ultrasound for liver cancer screening, and with or without prescription of oral antiviral therapies. Fig. 2 outlines the algorithm for selection of the most appropriate "B in IT" shared care treatment protocol for a patient with CHB. EpiSoft was used to send treatment protocols into the relevant practice management software via secure HealthLink health level 7 (HL7) messaging in portable document format (PDF) that could be saved to the existing patient record at the primary care clinic. A hyperlink within the document allowed GPs to login to EpiSoft (via username and password or Medicare's National Authentication Service for Health (NASH) Public Key Infrastructure (PKI) token). Incorporation of goals and actions and electronic signatures of care team members enabled GPs to use this documentation to create Medicare billable GP chronic disease management plans and team care arrangements for patients participating in the "B in IT" program. Checkboxes allowed GPs to acknowledge when a patient had attended their appointment and latest ALT and (HBV DNA) test results (viral load) were manually entered within the patient's treatment protocol page. Checkboxes were used by GPs to indicate if any new focal liver lesions had been identified via ultrasound (where applicable). GPs could print pathology and radiology test request forms as PDF documents directly from EpiSoft, as well as prescriptions for antiviral medication (if required).

"B in IT" treatment protocols allowed secure electronic messaging between all care team members (e.g. when GPs wished to ask the liver specialist a question about a patient's test results), and email notification was used to alert clinicians of new messages in EpiSoft. Whenever new data was entered, the updated version of the treatment protocol was sent via HL7 messaging from EpiSoft into the GP's practice management software. Patients could be reminded of upcoming appointments by short message service (SMS) when mobile phone numbers were provided. Reminders were sent three weeks prior to the suggested appointment date, allowing enough time for completion of recommended tests prior to GP review. A

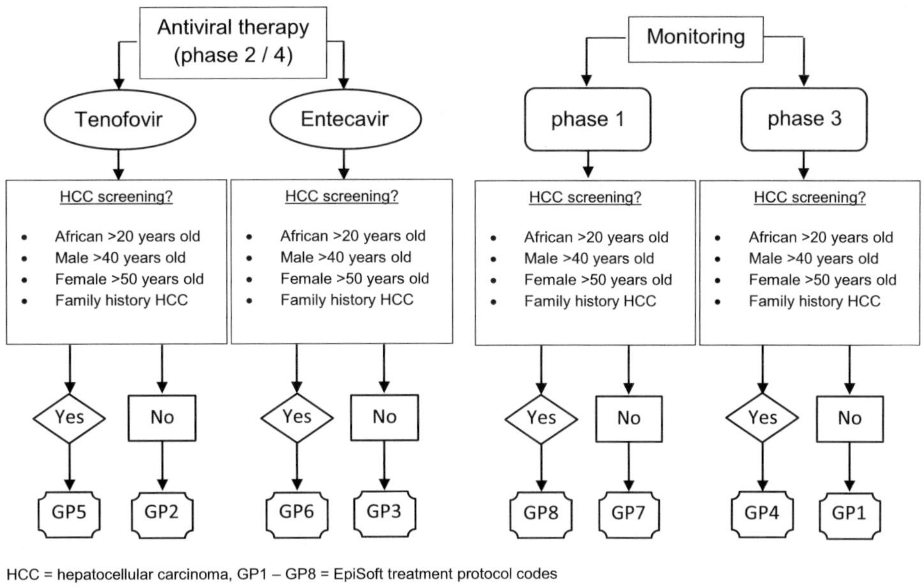

Fig. 2 Algorithm for selection of "B in IT" shared care treatment protocols. A hospital liver specialist would assess each patient with CHB to determine their phase of disease, and whether antiviral medication was required. Age, ethnicity and family history of HCC would determine whether twice yearly liver ultrasound was required for HCC screening. This allowed for selection of the most appropriate GP-managed treatment protocol (GP1 – GP8) for those patients who chose to be monitored by their community-based GP. EpiSoft was used to send electronic treatment protocols into the relevant practice management software via secure messaging

variety of user profile types were established within EpiSoft – program manager, hepatologist, clinical nurse consultant, GP and practice nurse. Access privileges varied between user types such that individual GPs and practice nurses could only see data from their own clinic's patients, whereas the program manager, hepatologists and clinical nurse consultants could access shared care records for all patients who had previously attended their hospital outpatient clinic (discharged to several different GP clinics).

Primary care site selection

Several GP clinics were identified as referring high numbers of patients with CHB by auditing the St Vincent's Hospital Melbourne (SVHM) outpatient liver clinic attendance records from June 2012 to July 2013 and cross-referencing against pathology testing for hepatitis B. Practice managers, practice nurses and GPs of four high referring clinics were invited to participate in shared care of their CHB patients. On-site group education sessions regarding diagnosis and management of CHB were conducted by specialists and one-on-one training in the use of the "B in IT" web-based tool was provided by the project officer.

Specialist engagement

Specialists working within the SVHM outpatient liver clinic with high CHB patient caseloads and who were already caring for patients referred by participating GP clinics were asked to participate in the "B in IT" program. No financial compensation was given to participating specialists, as the time required to review a shared care patient record took an average of less than 5 min every 6 months. This allowed specialists extra time to see CHB patients with more complex/advanced liver disease in a busy public hospital outpatient clinic.

"B in IT" patient enrolment

CHB patients identified as being referred to the SVHM outpatient liver clinic by participating GP clinics had their records physically flagged prior to their next appointment, and specialists were emailed by the project officer asking them to consider the patients' eligibility for shared care. Specialists noted in the electronic medical records which CHB patients were suitable and would prefer to see their GP for ongoing treatment/monitoring visits. Since the same level of care was to be continued with their GP (with specialist oversight), verbal consent from participants was adequate for enrolment.

Control patient identification

A database of all CHB patients attending SVHM outpatient liver clinic was used to identify a control patient cohort, matched in gender, ethnicity, age, treatment type. Two control patients (people continuing to attend the liver clinic) were selected for each "B in IT" patient. These control patients were selected randomly and could be referred from any GP clinic, so may never have been approached regarding participation in the shared care program.

Role of the project officer

A central project officer is necessary to manage the "B in IT" system. The project officer identified potential shared care patients attending participating GP clinics and SVHM specialist liver clinic by means of auditing appointment attendance from 2012 to 2013 and checking medical records of all new referrals to the liver clinic. The project officer created the custom CHB "B in IT" treatment protocols within EpiSoft, added all new patient records and linked them to the appropriate specialist, GP and treatment protocol based on clinician notes. Triggering of SMS reminders for each patient's appointments and auditing for compliance was also performed by the project officer using EpiSoft. The project officer reviewed all test results entered by shared care GPs and ensured that specialist and hepatitis nurse consultant care team members co-signed all care plans within EpiSoft following patient review with their GP. Reminder emails were sent from the project officer to GP clinics when "B in IT" patients were overdue for review, prompting their recall. The project officer also acted as a liaison between clinicians and the software provider regarding any software problems that could not be resolved independently.

Data collection and assessment of compliance

A reporting tool was built into EpiSoft, allowing for real-time monitoring of compliance with recommended dates for review appointments, pathology and ultrasound testing. Data was exported as a .csv file to enable custom sorting by variables such as treating GP, last appointment date or next appointment date, and test results were flagged as overdue if pending more than 6 months (ALT and ultrasound) or 12 months (HBV DNA level). Compliance of "B in IT" patients was assessed at two levels, the proportion of patients who attended a GP review visit and completed recommended tests within 1 month of the date suggested on their treatment protocol, and the proportion of patients who did so within 3 months of the suggested date. Patients were deemed lost to follow up at a GP clinic if they could not be contacted by phone or mail for 3 months after their suggested review date. Patients were deemed to be lost to follow up at a specialist liver clinic if they failed to attend three scheduled appointments. Due dates of recommended appointments and tests were included in compliance assessments when a patient was deemed lost. When comparing the compliance of "B in IT" patients before and during their participation in community-based care, patient data were excluded from the analysis if patients had only attended one specialist appointment. Any visit attended in the specialist liver clinic setting was deemed compliant (even if rescheduled several months later). Cancelled appointments were excluded from the analysis.

Outcomes

The primary endpoint assessed was compliance of "B in IT" patients with completion of pathology and ultrasound tests every 6 months, and attendance at their community GP clinics for shared care visits to review these results within 1 month of the recommended date. The secondary endpoint assessed was compliance of "B in IT" patients with test and visit completion within 3 months of the recommended date. Additional findings noted were enrollment rate, impact on outpatient liver clinic service and comparison of "B in IT" patient compliance with that of the same patient group prior to their enrolment in shared care. For further comparison of compliance, "B in IT" participants were compared to a control cohort of patients continuing to attend the hospital liver clinic - two control patients were selected for each "B in IT" patient, and groups were matched for gender, age, ethnicity and treatment type.

Statistical analysis

Parametric data is reported as mean ± standard deviation. Categorical data is reported as number (percentage). Exploratory, bivariate analyses of outcome variables were conducted using parametric or non-parametric tests as appropriate. Differences between characteristics of patient groups were assessed using two-tailed t-tests and two-tailed Fisher exact probability tests. Statistical differences between compliance of patient groups were assessed using the two-tailed Fisher exact probability test. For repeated measures testing in the B in IT group before and after enrolment in shared care, McNemar's test was used to determine statistical differences in compliance for visit attendance, pathology and ultrasound completion. A two-tailed significance threshold of $p < 0.05$ was used throughout. Analyses were performed using Stata version 12.1 (STATAcorp, Texas US).

Results

Two hundred patients with CHB attending SVHM outpatient liver clinics between August 2013 and June 2016 were referred by GPs from the four clinics participating in the "B in IT" program. As outlined in Fig. 3, 86 of the 167 potentially suitable patients with CHB still required further review at the time of this publication to determine phase of disease, leaving 81 patients with CHB eligible for enrolment in shared care. 45 (56%) patients provided consent to participate in the "B in IT" program. Of the 36 patients with CHB who declined to participate in shared care, only seven specified a reason. Six patients stated that the wait time from check-in until seeing a clinician was shorter at the hospital liver clinic than that at their community GP clinic (all six of these patients attend the same GP clinic), and one patient stated that the

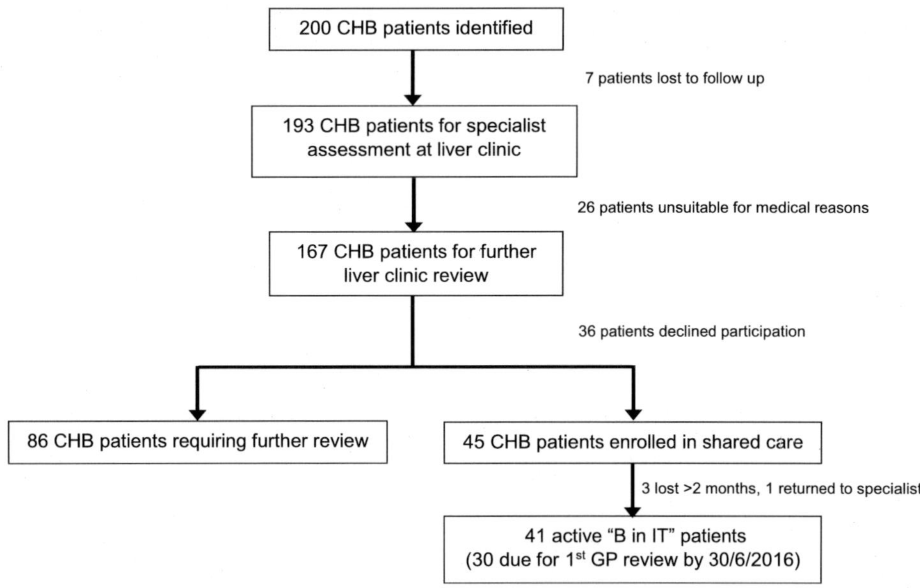

Fig. 3 Identification of CHB patients suitable for "B in IT" shared care. All patients with CHB referred to the hospital liver clinic by the four participating "B in IT" GP clinics between August 2013 and June 2016 were assessed for their suitability for shared care. Patients were deemed lost to follow up at the liver clinic if they failed to attend three scheduled appointments. Undetermined phase of disease, complex co-morbidities, history of HCC or cirrhosis were all reasons why patients were deemed unsuitable

hospital liver clinic was conveniently located on the way to their workplace.

Table 1 outlines the clinical features of the 30 patients enrolled in "B in IT" due for their first GP-led monitoring visit by the end of June 2016. Almost two thirds (63.3%) of the patients were female, the average patient age was 55.6 years. The majority of "B in IT" patients were Asian (80%), 40% of patients had previously attended more than ten liver clinic appointments and 80% of patients were in phase 1 or 3 of disease, requiring monitoring only. Eighty three percent of "B in IT" patients also required liver cancer surveillance, involving twice yearly ultrasound as per clinical guidelines [6]. Table 1 also describes the demographics of a group of 60 control CHB patients still attending the SVHM outpatient liver clinic, matched 2:1 to "B in IT" patients for age, gender, ethnicity and treatment type. One of the only statistically significant differences between the patient groups was that 78.3% of control patients had experienced a break in specialist care of more than 1 year compared to only 40% of "B in IT" patients ($p = 0.0005$ Fisher exact test). Also, fewer control patients had been seen in liver clinic for less than 1 year ($p = 0.005$ Fisher exact test).

Adherence to clinical monitoring and attendance of the 30 patients enrolled in "B in IT" is summarized in Table 2. Eighty three percent of patients attended their first shared care GP visit within 1 month of the suggested date and 87% of all shared care visits scheduled up until the end of 2016 (115 in total) were attended within 1 month of the suggested date. Adherence to the recommended pathology testing schedule within 1 month of the suggested date was 90% at the first shared care GP visit and 94% across all 115 review visits. Compliance of the 24 "B in IT" patients requiring twice yearly liver ultrasounds for cancer screening was 83% at the first visit and 89% across all visits. No significant improvement in adherence was noted if compliance was defined as completion up to 3 months after the suggested date.

The percentage of "B in IT" patients compliant with twice yearly visit attendance and completion of pathology tests and ultrasounds (as outlined in their shared care treatment protocols) was compared with that of the same patient group prior to their enrolment in shared care, as well as the control CHB group still attending SVHM liver clinic (see Table 3). Compliance when attending the specialist liver clinic was defined as completion of two liver function tests per year, two liver ultrasounds per year (if necessary), and attendance of all scheduled visits. Compliance of the "B in IT" patients with visit attendance was significantly improved following their enrolment in shared care, with only 50% of patients attending scheduled appointments at liver clinic compared to 86.7% attending twice yearly GP shared care appointments ($p = 0.002$). A higher percentage of "B in IT" patients also completed timely liver ultrasounds – 87.5% overall when enrolled in shared care versus only 26.3% of these patients completing two liver ultrasounds per year prior to community discharge ($p = 0.039$). A significant improvement was also seen in the percentage of "B in IT" patients completing

Table 1 Patient Demographics

Characteristic	"B in IT" patients	Control patients	*P* values
Total Number	30	60	
Female	19 (63.3%)	38 (63.3%)	1.000
Male	11 (36.7%)	22 (36.7%)	1.000
Age (years) mean ± SD	55.6 ± 12.6	55.3 ± 11.6	0.985
Female	53.8 ± 10.7	54.0 ± 10.4	0.867
Male	58.6 ± 15.4	57.6 ± 13.4	0.889
Ethnicity			
Asian	24 (80%)	48 (80%)	1.000
Sub-Saharan African	3 (10%)	6 (10%)	1.000
European	2 (6.7%)	4 (6.7%)	1.000
Pacific Islander	1 (3.3%)	2 (3.3%)	1.000
Preferred Language			
English	12 (40%)	30 (50%)	0.502
Vietnamese	6 (20%)	14 (23.3%)	0.794
Mandarin	4 (13.3%)	7 (11.7%)	1.000
Hakka Timorese	3 (10%)	1 (1.7%)	0.106
Cantonese	2 (6.7%)	4 (6.7%)	1.000
Other	3 (10%)	4 (6.7%)	0.682
Liver Clinic Visits			
< 5	10 (33.3%)	11 (18.3%)	0.185
5-10	8 (26.7%)	13 (21.7%)	0.791
> 10	12 (40%)	36 (60%)	0.116
Breaks in care (> 1 year)			
N/A (seen < 1 year)	9 (30%)	4 (6.7%)	0.005[a]
0	12 (40%)	47 (78.3%)	0.0005[a]
1	7 (23.3%)	6 (10%)	0.115
2	1 (3.3%)	3 (5%)	1.000
> 2	1 (3.3%)	0 (0%)	0.333
HBeAg Status			
Negative	29 (96.7%)	57 (95%)	1.000
Positive	1 (3.3%)	3 (5%)	1.000
Phase of disease			
1 – immune tolerance	0 (0%)	0 (0%)	1.000
2 – immune clearance	1 (3.3%)	3 (5%)	1.000
3 – immune control	23 (76.7%)	44 (73.3%)	0.802
4 – immune escape	5 (16.7%)	9 (15%)	1.000
Cleared (HBsAb positive)	1 (3.3%)	4 (6.7%)	0.661
Cirrhosis	0 (0%)	0 (0%)	1.000
Treatment type			
Monitoring	24 (80%) – 20 with HCC screening	48 (80%) – 40 with HCC screening	1.000
Antiviral therapy	6 (20%) – 5 with HCC screening	12 (20%) – 10 with HCC screening	1.000
Entecavir	5 (16.7%)	10 (16.7%)	1.000
Tenofovir	1 (3.3%)	2 (3.3%)	1.000

SD standard deviation, *N/A* not applicable, *HBeAg* hepatitis B e antigen, *HBsAb* hepatitis B surface antibody; [a]statistically significant

Table 2 "B in IT" patient compliance

	Attendance 1st visit	Attendance overall	Pathology 1st visit	Pathology overall	Ultrasound 1st visit	Ultrasound overall
Total scheduled	30	115	30	115	24	84
Completed +/− 1 month	25 (83.3%)	100 (87.0%)	27 (90.0%)	108 (93.9%)	20 (83.3%)	75 (89.3%)
Completed +/− 3 months	26 (86.7%)	109 (94.8%)	27 (90.0%)	111 (96.5%)	21 (87.5%)	79 (94.0%)

two pathology tests per year - 90.0% overall when enrolled in shared care versus 57.7% when attending the liver clinic ($p = 0.005$).

A similar pattern of compliance was observed for the control CHB patient group as the "B in IT" patients prior to their enrolment in shared care, with compliance decreasing after the first year of attendance. Only 63.3% of control patients completed twice yearly liver function tests compared to 90% of "B in IT" patients ($p = 0.011$) and only 40% of control CHB patients attended all visits scheduled, compared to 86.7% of "B in IT" patients ($p < 0.0001$). Again, the most dramatic effect of the "B in IT" program was seen when comparing HCC screening twice yearly liver ultrasounds – only 10% of control CHB patients were compliant overall compared to 87.5% of "B in IT" patients ($p < 0.0001$). This difference could also be seen during the first year of liver clinic attendance, with most control CHB patients (70.8%) only having one liver ultrasound per year, even though the GESA recommendation for CHB patients at high risk of HCC is twice yearly liver ultrasound [6].

Qualitative evaluation of participating GPs and specialists was performed using unstructured interview. Feedback from eight participating GPs was positive - GPs found the chronic disease management plan documentation and secure electronic messaging with specialists useful. Two GPs had a "B in IT" patient case load < 2 and reported some difficulty recalling how to use Episoft's web-based clinical tool, as each patient is only seen twice a year, so often had to contact the project officer and refer to their workflow user guide. The four GPs with "B in IT" patient caseloads > 5 soon became familiar with the web-based tool. All GPs reported feeling more confident in managing CHB since participating in the "B in IT" program, but still liked to have specialist oversight.

Feedback from participating specialists was similar – the more "B in IT" patients seen, the more familiar the clinicians are with use of the web-based tool. Specialists like the clinical summary view of latest pathology and imaging test results, which allows them to quickly review patient status and co-sign chronic disease management plans. Specialists were reliant on the project officer reminding them which patient records are due for review (which patients have recently seen their GP), and GPs were reliant on the project officer reminding them which patients are due for appointments.

At the time of this publication, 45 patients had been enrolled in the "B in IT" program (analysed compliance data is limited to those patients who completed their first shared care visit by end of June 2016), improving access to specialist care of an additional 45 patients with CHB who otherwise may have had their care delayed. This equates to two SVHM outpatient liver clinics per year – encompassing the time of four liver specialists per 3 h clinic. A project officer working 20 h per week has the capacity to oversee shared care of "B in IT" patients from approximately 10 GP clinics, assuming a maximum of 20 patients per GP clinic (up to a total of 200 patients). Expansion of the "B in IT" program greater than this would require an increase in the number of hours worked by one or several project officers.

Discussion

We have successfully piloted a shared care program for community-based management of people living with CHB using a novel web-based clinical platform – the "B in IT" program. Uptake of "B in IT" shared care to-date

Table 3 Comparison of compliance between patient groups

	Attendance compliance[a]		Pathology compliance[b]		Ultrasound compliance[c]	
	1st year	overall	1st year	overall	1st year	overall
"B in IT" patients	83.3%	86.7%	90.0%	90.0%	87.5%	87.5%
"B in IT" patients prior to discharge	63.3% $P = 0.083$	50.0%[d] $P = 0.002$	66.7%[d] $P = 0.020$	57.7%[d] $P = 0.005$	55.6%[d] $P = 0.031$	26.3%[d] $P = 0.039$
Control patients	68.3% $P = 0.205$	40.0%[d] $P < 0.0001$	80.0% $P = 0.369$	63.3%[d] $P = 0.011$	47.7%[d] $P = 0.002$	10.0%[d] $P < 0.0001$

[a]Attendance of all scheduled visits; [b]completion of two liver function tests per year; [c]completion of two liver ultrasounds per year; [d]statistically significant difference from "B in IT" patient group

has depended upon multiple factors - specialist recommendation to the patient, the existing relationship of the patient with their GP and specialist, convenience in location of the clinic, and languages spoken by the clinicians. For clinicians to find the "B in IT" program familiar and easy to use they need to have a high case load, as each patient is only seen once every 6 months. Compliance of community-based "B in IT" patients has met our expectation and been very good in comparison to patients with CHB attending hospital outpatient liver clinics, since people will generally have less travel time and shorter waiting times per visit when attending their local GP clinic. People also attend community clinics for a variety of other health reasons, so can be reminded of an upcoming CHB review when attending for a different reason. The improvement in compliance with regular ultrasound screening for liver cancer when patients were tracked through the "B in IT" program was drastic. Systematic measures to monitor compliance are required given that liver cancer incidence rates in the state of Victoria are increasing by more than 4% per year in both men and women, and CHB is a significant cause [7]. The "B in IT" program is such a mechanism and is currently being expanded to incorporate patients from additional GP clinics in Melbourne. Early detection of cirrhosis and prevention of liver cancer is difficult to quantify, but every case prevented saves the government hundreds of thousands of dollars in medical costs, with the annual cost of care being > $18,000 for each case of CHB-related HCC and a liver transplant costing > $150,000 [8].

Conservatively at least 25% of CHB patients seen at SVHM could be monitored in the community by their local GP (those in phase 3 of disease) if this program was expanded to include all GPs referring to the SVHM liver clinic. This proportion would be 40% (estimated from an audit of SVHM clinic lists performed during this study) if we include GPs prescribing antiviral medication in the community for treatment of stable phase 2 and 4 patients. There are currently 700 CHB patients seen at the SVHM outpatient liver clinic, which equates to 175-280 potential "B in IT" patients. Based on our observed enrolment rate, even if only 56% of eligible patients consented to participate in the "B in IT" program (98-156 people), this would still significantly increase involvement of GP clinics in CHB treatment and monitoring in Victoria, as called for in the second National Hepatitis B Strategy.

Another benefit of the "B in IT" program is the ability for GPs to send electronic messages to the other care team members, querying unexpected test results, if/when to refer back to liver clinic, or informing the project officer that a patient is overdue due to overseas travel. To-date more than 30 messages have been sent from participating GPs and responses from the care team are obtained within a week. This easy method of communication helps prevent unnecessary referrals back to liver clinic, while allowing specialists to maintain clinical oversight of "B in IT" patients and building capabilities in the primary care workforce for the treatment and monitoring of CHB. Confounders for B in IT attendance were not rigorously assessed in this study, however the trends appear positive for the program having impact.

A limitation of the "B in IT" program to-date is the small number of GP clinics engaged. Larger numbers of patients and clinicians will be needed to more accurately assess the success of this shared care model. As noted in the results, there were also fewer patients seen for less than a year in SVHM liver clinic in the control group compared to the "B in IT" group, so observation of the "B in IT" patients for several years will be necessary to see if their compliance remains high over time. The project officer role is required for this model of care, to ensure that clinician time is focused on the management of patients, not the day-to-day administrative tasks. So if patient and clinician numbers grow for the "B in IT" program the workload of the project officer will grow.

We will continue to monitor the success of the "B in IT" program via compliance of patients with recommended visits, pathology and imaging tests. Satisfaction of GPs and patients will also be determined via a survey. If employed as a long-term model of care, the "B in IT" program could dramatically increase the capacity for treatment of patients with complex cases of CHB at hospital liver clinics. Simplified treatment protocols have also been created within EpiSoft for use within specialist liver clinics to track compliance of all patients with CHB who require twice yearly HCC screening, and this is currently being trialed at SVHM. Monthly audit reports are being generated and any CHB patient overdue for HCC screening (>7 months since last liver ultrasound), and who does not already have a liver clinic appointment booked, is recalled via mailing test request forms with an appointment letter. Over the past 12 months 70% of overdue CHB patients have re-engaged with the liver clinic after first recall. Observation over the coming 6 months is required to determine if additional patients re-engage with the hospital's liver clinic after second recall.

Conclusions

The "B in IT" program for shared care of patients with CHB has been established, enabling GPs to treat and monitor patients with CHB in the community, with oversight from a project officer, hepatologists and nurse consultants in tertiary hospitals using EpiSoft. A centralized, secure cloud-based database allows for remote auditing of patient compliance against recommended appointment dates and pathology and ultrasound tests.

Compliance of "B in IT" patients has been > 85% to-date, proving this model of care can be successful. With government support and wide-reaching organisations such as primary health networks, the "B in IT" program would be amenable to broad use across the state of Victoria (and throughout Australia) for the treatment of patients with CHB. The "B in IT" program contributes towards the aims of the second National Hepatitis B Strategy to increase treatment uptake to 15% and is also aligned with the government's objectives to implement eHealth processes in the primary care setting and promote innovation and workforce development within the healthcare sector.

Abbreviations

ALT: Alanine transaminase; CHB: Chronic hepatitis B; DNA: Deoxyribonucleic acid; GESA: Gastroenterological society of Australia; GPs: General practitioners; HBV: Hepatitis B virus; HCC: Hepatocellular carcinoma; HL7: Health level 7; NASH: National Authentication Service for Health; PDF: Portable document format; PKI: Public key infrastructure; SMS: Short message service; SVHM: St Vincent's Hospital Melbourne

Acknowledgements

The authors would like to acknowledge the patients and GP clinic staff who have participated in the "B in IT" program, as well as Hepatitis Clinical Nurse Consultants at St Vincent's Hospital Melbourne Ms. Lucy McDonald, Ms. Chloe Layton, Ms. Lisa Stothers and Ms. Susanne Glasgow.

Funding

DAO and AJT were in part supported by a Cancer Australia Priority-driven Collaborative Cancer Research Scheme grant (No: 1,086,997). Additional funding was provided by North Western Melbourne Primary Health Network, Gilead Sciences Pty Ltd. and Bristol-Myers Squibb. None of these funding bodies were involved in the study design, collection, analysis or interpretation of the data included in this manuscript.

Authors' contributions

DAO managed the "B in IT" program, helped in the development of EpiSoft treatment protocols, collected and analysed compliance data and drafted the manuscript. EC managed the "B in IT" program for a period of 6 months. DI helped in the development of EpiSoft treatment protocols, participated as a GP seeing "B in IT" patients and provided advice as part of the project steering committee. PVD, SB, TN, DW and JH participated as care team members in the enrollment of "B in IT" patients and provided advice as part of the project steering committee. JH also assisted with statistical analyses. JR provided advice as part of the project steering committee, aided in patient survey design and patient enrolment through a nurse-led community clinic. JO designed the EpiSoft database and helped in the development of EpiSoft treatment protocols. AJT conceived of the study, provided content for EpiSoft treatment protocols, participated as a care team member in the enrollment of "B in IT" patients and oversaw the project steering committee. All authors read and approved the final manuscript.

Competing interests

Ms. Jenny O'Neill is a founder of Episoft Pty Ltd. Other author's declare that they have no competing interests.

Author details

[1]Gastroenterology Department, St Vincent's Hospital Melbourne, 35 Victoria Parade, Fitzroy, VIC 3065, Australia. [2]GP Liaison Department, St Vincent's Hospital Melbourne, 35 Victoria Parade, Fitzroy, VIC 3065, Australia. [3]North Richmond Community Health, 23 Lennox Street, Richmond, VIC 3121, Australia. [4]Victorian Infectious Diseases Service, The Royal Melbourne Hospital, 300 Gratten Street, Parkville, Melbourne, VIC 3000, Australia. [5]La Trobe University, The Australian Research Centre in Sex, Health and Society, 215 Franklin Street, Melbourne, VIC 3000, Australia. [6]Department of General Practice, The University of Melbourne, 200 Berkeley Street, Parkville, Melbourne, VIC 3000, Australia. [7]EpiSoft Pty Ltd, Suite 216, 20 Dale Street, Brookvale, NSW 2100, Australia.

References

1. MacLachlan JH, et al. The burden of chronic hepatitis B virus infection in Australia, 2011. Aust N Z J Public Health. 2013;37(5):416–22.
2. Hsieh CC, et al. Age at first establishment of chronic hepatitis B virus infection and hepatocellular carcinoma risk. A birth order study. Am J Epidemiol. 1992;136(9):1115–21.
3. Lavanchy D. Hepatitis B virus epidemiology, disease burden, treatment, and current and emerging prevention and control measures. J Viral Hepat. 2004; 11(2):97–107.
4. Mahoney FJ. Update on diagnosis, management, and prevention of hepatitis B virus infection. Clin Microbiol Rev. 1999;12(2):351–66.
5. Second National Hepatitis B Strategy 2014 - 2017, Australian Government Department of Health, 2014.
6. *Clinical update - Australian and New Zealand chronic hepatitis B (CHB) recommendations*, Gastroenterological Society of Australia, 2009.
7. Cancer Council Victoria. Cancer in Victoria - Statistics & Trends. V. Thursfield, et al., Editors. Carlton: Cancer Council Victoria; 2013.
8. Butler JR, et al. The direct cost of managing patients with chronic hepatitis B infection in Australia. J Clin Gastroenterol. 2004;38(10 Suppl 3):S187–92.

Permissions

All chapters in this book were first published in HMP, by BioMed Central; hereby published with permission under the Creative Commons Attribution License or equivalent. Every chapter published in this book has been scrutinized by our experts. Their significance has been extensively debated. The topics covered herein carry significant findings which will fuel the growth of the discipline. They may even be implemented as practical applications or may be referred to as a beginning point for another development.

The contributors of this book come from diverse backgrounds, making this book a truly international effort. This book will bring forth new frontiers with its revolutionizing research information and detailed analysis of the nascent developments around the world.

We would like to thank all the contributing authors for lending their expertise to make the book truly unique. They have played a crucial role in the development of this book. Without their invaluable contributions this book wouldn't have been possible. They have made vital efforts to compile up to date information on the varied aspects of this subject to make this book a valuable addition to the collection of many professionals and students.

This book was conceptualized with the vision of imparting up-to-date information and advanced data in this field. To ensure the same, a matchless editorial board was set up. Every individual on the board went through rigorous rounds of assessment to prove their worth. After which they invested a large part of their time researching and compiling the most relevant data for our readers.

The editorial board has been involved in producing this book since its inception. They have spent rigorous hours researching and exploring the diverse topics which have resulted in the successful publishing of this book. They have passed on their knowledge of decades through this book. To expedite this challenging task, the publisher supported the team at every step. A small team of assistant editors was also appointed to further simplify the editing procedure and attain best results for the readers.

Apart from the editorial board, the designing team has also invested a significant amount of their time in understanding the subject and creating the most relevant covers. They scrutinized every image to scout for the most suitable representation of the subject and create an appropriate cover for the book.

The publishing team has been an ardent support to the editorial, designing and production team. Their endless efforts to recruit the best for this project, has resulted in the accomplishment of this book. They are a veteran in the field of academics and their pool of knowledge is as vast as their experience in printing. Their expertise and guidance has proved useful at every step. Their uncompromising quality standards have made this book an exceptional effort. Their encouragement from time to time has been an inspiration for everyone.

The publisher and the editorial board hope that this book will prove to be a valuable piece of knowledge for researchers, students, practitioners and scholars across the globe.

List of Contributors

Stephen T. Barclay
Walton Liver Clinic, Glasgow Royal Infirmary, Glasgow, UK

Graham S. Cooke
Division of Infectious diseases, Imperial College London, London, UK

Elizabeth Holtham
NIHR Nottingham Digestive Diseases Biomedical Research Unit, University of Nottingham, Nottingham, UK

William L. Irving
NIHR Nottingham Digestive Diseases Biomedical Research Unit, University of Nottingham, Nottingham, UK
Microbiology, Queen's Medical Centre, Nottingham NG7 2UH, UK

Aline Gauthier, Jeremie Schwarzbard and Petar Atanasov
Amaris Ltd, London, UK

Martyna Gassowski, Benjamin Wenz, Viviane Bremer, Ulrich Marcus and Ruth Zimmermann
Department for Infectious Disease Epidemiology, Division for HIV/AIDS, STI and Blood-borne Infections, Robert Koch Institute, Berlin, Germany

Stine Nielsen
Department for Infectious Disease Epidemiology, Division for HIV/AIDS, STI and Blood-borne Infections, Robert Koch Institute, Berlin, Germany
Charité University Medicine, Berlin, Germany

Norbert Bannert and Claudia Kücherer
Department for Infectious Diseases, Division for HIV and other Retroviruses, Robert Koch Institute, Berlin, Germany

Claus-Thomas Bock
Department for Infectious Diseases, Division for Viral Gastroenteritis and Hepatitis Pathogens and Enteroviruses, Robert Koch Institute, Berlin, Germany

R. Stefan Ross
5Institute of Virology, National Reference Centre for Hepatitis C, University Hospital Essen, University of Duisburg-Essen, Essen, Germany

Hai-yang Zhou, Carol Duan and Zhao Wang
Wu Jieping Medical Foundation, Beijing, China

Shuang Liu, Su-jun Zheng, Yu Chen and Zhong-ping Duan
Beijing Youan Hospital, Capital Medical University, Beijing, China

Qing-fen Zheng
Beijing Youan Hospital, Capital Medical University, Beijing, China
Department of Gastroenterology, The First Affiliated Hospital of Zhengzhou University, Zhengzhou, China

Xiao-xia Peng
Department of Epidemiology and Biostatistics, School of Public Health and Family Medicine, Capital Medical University, Beijing, China

John F. Dillon
Division of Molecular and Clinical Medicine, School of Medicine, University of Dundee, Ninewells Hospital, Dundee, UK

Jeffrey V. Lazarus
Centre for Health and Infectious Disease Research (CHIP) and WHO Collaborating Centre on HIV and Viral Hepatitis, Rigshospitalet, University of Copenhagen, Copenhagen, Denmark

Homie A. Razavi
Center for Disease Analysis, Louisville, Colorado, USA

Partha Sarathi Mukherjee, Eliza Dutta, Dipesh Kr. Das, Shatabdi Ghosh, Suvadip Neogi and Arka Sarkar
Liver Foundation, West Bengal, 12, Kyd Street, Kolkata 7000016, India

Chari Cohen, Joan M. Block and Gang Chen
Hepatitis B Foundation, Doylestown, PA, USA

Alison A. Evans
Hepatitis B Foundation, Doylestown, PA, USA
Drexel University School of Public Health, Philadelphia, PA, USA

W. Thomas London
Hepatitis B Foundation, Doylestown, PA, USA
Fox Chase Cancer Center, Philadelphia, PA, USA

Peixin Huang
Haimen City Center for Disease Control and Prevention, Haimen City, China

Anastasios Fotiou, Eleftheria Kanavou, Argyro Antaraki and Manina Terzidou
Epidemiology Unit, Greek Reitox Focal Point of the EMCDDA, University Mental Health Research Institute, 2 Soranou tou Efesiou St., Athens 11527, Greece

Clive Richardson
Panteion University of Social and Political Sciences, 136, Leoforos A. Siggrou, Kallithea, Athens 17671, Greece

Anna Kokkevi
University Mental Health Research Institute, 2 Soranou tou Efesiou St., Athens 11527, Greece

Francisco Hevia-Urrutia, Ileana Alvarado-Echeverría, Alfredo Sanabria-Castro, Marta Sánchez-Molina, Luis Meza-Sierra, Alexander Parajeles-Vindas, Oscar Méndez-Blanca, Marcela Barguil-Gallardo, Iliana Chavarría-Quirós and Cecilia Monge-Bonilla
Hospital San Juan de Dios, Caja Costarricense del Seguro Social, 4917-1000 San José, Costa Rica

Álvaro Sánchez-Siles
Hospital México, Caja Costarricense del Seguro Social, San José, Costa Rica

Manuel Saborío-Rocafort
Hospital Nacional de Niños, Caja Costarricense del Seguro Social, San José, Costa Rica

Judith I. Tsui
Department of Medicine, Section of General Internal Medicine, University of Washington School of Medicine and Harborview Hospital, 325 9th Ave, Box 359780, Seattle, WA 98104, USA

Stephen C. Ko
Department of Global Health, Boston University School of Public Health, 801 Massachusetts Avenue, 3nd Floor, Boston, MA 02118, USA

Evgeny Krupitsky
St. Petersburg Bekhterev Research Psychoneurological Institute, Bekhtereva St., 3, St. Petersburg 192019, Russian Federation
First St. Petersburg Pavlov State Medical University, Lev Tolstoy St. 6/8, St. Petersburg 197022, Russian Federation

Dmitry Lioznov
First St. Petersburg Pavlov State Medical University, Lev Tolstoy St. 6/8, St. Petersburg 197022, Russian Federation
Pasteur Research Institute of Epidemiology and Microbiology, St. Petersburg, Russian Federation, Mira St. 14, St. Petersburg 197101, Russian Federation

Christine E. Chaisson
Data Coordinating Center, Boston University School of Public Health, 85 East Newton Street, 9th Floor, Boston, MA 02118, USA

Natalia Gnatienko
Department of Medicine, Section of General Internal Medicine, Clinical Addiction Research and Education Unit, Boston Medical Center, 801 Massachusetts Avenue, 2nd Floor, Boston, MA 02118, USA

Jeffrey H. Samet
Department of Medicine, Section of General Internal Medicine, Clinical Addiction Research and Education Unit, Boston University School of Medicine/Boston Medical Center, 801 Massachusetts Avenue, 2nd Floor, Boston, MA 02118, USA
Department of Community Health Sciences, Boston University School of Public Health, 801 Massachusetts Avenue, 2nd Floor, Boston, MA 02118, USA

Jeffrey V. Lazarus and Kelly Safreed-Harmon
CHIP, Centre for Health and Infectious Disease Research and WHO Collaborating Centre on HIV and Viral Hepatitis, Rigshospitalet, University of Copenhagen, Copenhagen, Denmark

Antons Mozalevskis and Irina Eramova
World Health Organization (WHO) Regional Office for Europe, Copenhagen, Denmark

Silvano Barbosa de Oliveira, Ana Roberta Pati Pascom, Juliana Machado Gisiviez and Fábio Mesquita
Department of STI, AIDS, and Viral Hepatitis, Brazil Ministry of Health, Brasília, DF, Brazil

Adele Schwartz Benzaken
Department of STI, AIDS, and Viral Hepatitis, Brazil Ministry of Health, Brasília, DF, Brazil
Fundação de Medicina Tropical Doutor Heitor Vieira Dourado (FMT-HVD), Avenida Pedro Teixeira 25, CEP: 69040-000 Manaus, AM, Brazil

Meritxell Sabidó
Fundação de Medicina Tropical Doutor Heitor Vieira Dourado (FMT-HVD), Avenida Pedro Teixeira 25, CEP: 69040-000 Manaus, AM, Brazil

Anne Marie Carew, Jean Long and Suzi Lyons
Health Research Board, Grattan House, 67-72 Lower Mount Street, Dublin 2, Ireland

Niamh Murphy, Kate Hunter and Lelia Thornton
HSE Health Protection Surveillance Centre, 25-27 Middle Gardiner Street, Dublin 1, Ireland

Cathal Walsh
Department of Statistics, Trinity College Dublin, Dublin, Ireland
Health Research Institute (HRI) and MACSI, University of Limerick, Limerick, Ireland

Ruchi Sogarwal, Varada Madge, Pratyush Bishi, Apam Woleng and Rishi Garg
MAMTA Health Institute for Mother and Child, New Delhi, India

Chul S. Hyun
Holy Name Medical Center, Teaneck, NJ, USA
Center for Viral Hepatitis, 35 Van Nostrand Avenue, Englewood, NJ 07631, USA

Seulgi Lee
Center for Viral Hepatitis, 35 Van Nostrand Avenue, Englewood, NJ 07631, USA

William R. Ventura
St. Joseph's Regional Medical Center, Patterson, NJ, USA

Soon S. Kim and Soyoung Yoon
Korean Community Services, Queens, NY, USA

Alexis Llewellyn, Mark Simmonds and Amanda J Sowden
Centre for Reviews and Dissemination, University of York, York, UK

Ginny Brunton
UCL Institute of Education, University of London, London, UK

Will L Irving
Faculty of Medicine and Health Sciences, University of Nottingham, Nottingham, UK

Swati Jha, Divyesh Devaliya and Shripad Desai
AmeriCares india Foundation, Mumbai, India

Susan Bergson
AmeriCares, Stamford, CT, USA

Ludmila Maistat and Natalija Kravchenko
Alliance for Public Health, Kiev, Ukraine

Amulya Reddy
London, UK

Rachel Thorpe
Australian Research Centre in Sex, Health and Society, La Trobe University, Bundoora, Victoria, Australia

Jack Wallace
Australian Research Centre in Sex, Health and Society, La Trobe University, Bundoora, Victoria, Australia
Disease Elimination, The Burnet Institute, Prahran, Victoria, Australia

Jacqueline A. Richmond
Australian Research Centre in Sex, Health and Society, La Trobe University, Bundoora, Victoria, Australia
Disease Elimination, The Burnet Institute, Prahran, Victoria, Australia
Department of General Practice, The University of Melbourne, Parkville, Victoria, Australia

Peter Higgs
Disease Elimination, The Burnet Institute, Prahran, Victoria, Australia
Department of Public Health, La Trobe University, Bundoora, Victoria, Australia

Margaret Hellard
Disease Elimination, The Burnet Institute, Prahran, Victoria, Australia
Department of Epidemiology and Preventive Medicine, Monash University, Melbourne, Australia
Department of Infectious Diseases, Alfred Health, Melbourne, Australia

Jeanne Ellard
Kirby Institute, University of New South Wales, Kensington, New South Wales, Australia

Alexander Thompson
Department of Medicine, University of Melbourne, Melbourne, Australia
Department of Gastroenterology, St Vincent's Hospital, Melbourne, VIC, Australia

Musomba Rachel, Castelnuovo Barbara, Charlene Komujuni, Patience Nyakato, Ponsiano Ocama and Mohammed Lamorde
Infectious Diseases Institute, Makerere University, Mulago Hospital, Kampala, Uganda

Claire Murphy
Centre for Communicable Diseases, Queen Elizabeth University Hospital, Glasgow, Scotland

Philippa Easterbrook
World Health Organizations, Geneva, Switzerland

Rosalind Parkes Ratanshi
Cambridge Institute of Public Health, Cambridge, UK

N. Beekmans and M. Klemt-Kropp
Department of Gastroenterology and Hepatology, Northwest Clinics, Alkmaar, The Netherlands

Vendula Belackova and Allison M. Salmon
Uniting Sydney Medically Supervised Injecting Centre (MSIC), Sydney, Australia

Marianne Jauncey
Uniting Sydney Medically Supervised Injecting Centre (MSIC), Sydney, Australia
School of Public Health and Community Medicine, University of New South Wales, Sydney, NSW, Australia

Eberhard Schatz
Correlation network, Foundation De Regenboog Groep, Amsterdam, The Netherlands

Aleksander Krag
Department of Gastroenterology and Hepatology, Odense University Hospital, University of Southern Denmark, Odense, Denmark

Marcus Schuchmann
Department of Internal Medicine, Constance Medical Centre, Constance, Germany

Hanna Sodatonou and Jeff Pilot
Norgine Ltd Clinical Development and Medical Affairs, Harefield, UK

James Whitehouse
Norgine Global Health Outcomes, Norgine Ltd, Uxbridge, UK

Simone I. Strasser
AW Morrow Gastroenterology and Liver Centre, Royal Prince Alfred Hospital and University of Sydney, Sydney, Australia

Mark Hudson
Liver Unit, Freeman Hospital, Newcastle upon Tyne Hospitals NHS Trust and Institute of Cellular Medicine, Newcastle University, Newcastle upon Tyne, UK

Marcelo Contardo Moscoso Naveira, Komal Badal, Jagadish Dhakal, Neichu Angami Mayer, Bina Pokharel and Ruben Frank Del Prado
UNAIDS Nepal, UN House, Pulchowk, Lalitpur GPO 107, Nepal

Mehlika Toy, Bin Wei, Tejpal S. Virdi and Samuel K. So
Asian Liver Center, Department of Surgery, Stanford University School of Medicine, 780 Welch Road, CJ130D, Palo Alto, CA 94304, USA

An Le and Mindie H. Nguyen
Division of Gastroenterology and Hepatology, Department of Medicine, Stanford University Medical Center, Palo Alto, CA, USA

Huy Trinh
San Jose Gastroenterology, San Jose, CA, USA

Jiayi Li
Palo Alto Medical Foundation, Mountain View, CA, USA

Jian Zhang
Chinese Hospital, San Francisco, CA, USA

Ann W. Hsing
Stanford Prevention Research Center, Department of Medicine and Stanford Cancer Institute, Stanford University School of Medicine, Palo Alto, CA, USA

P. A. M. Kracht, J. E. Arends and A. I. M. Hoepelman
Department of Internal medicine and Infectious disease, Utrecht University, University Medical Center Utrecht, Utrecht, the Netherlands

K. J. van Erpecum
Department of Gastroenterology and Hepatology, Utrecht University, University Medical Center Utrecht, Utrecht, the Netherlands

A. Urbanus
Centre for Infectious Disease Control, National Institute for Public Health and the Environment, Bilthoven, The Netherlands

J. A. Willemse
Dutch Liver Patient Association (NLV), Hoogland, the Netherlands

E. A. Croes
Netherlands Institute of Mental Health and Addiction (Trimbos Institute), Utrecht, the Netherlands

Debra A. O'Leary, Eleanor Cropp, Paul V. Desmond, Sally Bell, Tin Nguyen, Darren Wong, Jessica Howell and Alexander J. Thompson
Gastroenterology Department, St Vincent's Hospital Melbourne, 35 Victoria Parade, Fitzroy, VIC 3065, Australia

David Isaac
GP Liaison Department, St Vincent's Hospital Melbourne, 35 Victoria Parade, Fitzroy, VIC 3065, Australia
North Richmond Community Health, 23 Lennox Street, Richmond, VIC 3121, Australia

Jacqui Richmond
Victorian Infectious Diseases Service, The Royal Melbourne Hospital, 300 Gratten Street, Parkville, Melbourne, VIC 3000, Australia
La Trobe University, The Australian Research Centre in Sex, Health and Society, 215 Franklin Street, Melbourne, VIC 3000, Australia
Department of General Practice, The University of Melbourne, 200 Berkeley Street, Parkville, Melbourne, VIC 3000, Australia

Jenny O'Neill
EpiSoft Pty Ltd, Suite 216, 20 Dale Street, Brookvale, NSW 2100, Australia

Index